Too Good T[o]
Nutrients Quiet th[e]

A Four Generation Bipolar Odyssey

David Moyer
LCSW, BCD
Lt Col, USAF, Ret

Introduction by Robert Bransfield, M.D.

2003

Nu-Tune Press
P.O. Box 691
Penn Valley Ca 95946

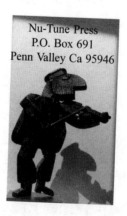

Nu-Tune Press
P.O. Box 691
Penn Valley Ca 95946

Printed in the United States of America
First Edition: January 2003

ISBN #0-9717990-0-8

When water gets caught in habitual whirlpools,
dig a way out through the bottom to the ocean.
There is a secret medicine
Given only to those who hurt so hard
They can't hope.

Rumi 13th century

This book is dedicated to Jeanette, Katherine, Tim, Raina, Dan, and Chris. May you all find the secret medicine you need.

A dream

I finally slept. I dreamed I was at the edge of a long, narrow frozen pond in the midst of a snow-covered forest. The ice was thick near the edge, thinner toward the middle. I saw people lying face-down on the ice near the center. I couldn't tell how many. My focus was only on the ones nearest to me. They were still; I thought they were dead at first. But then I noticed indentations in the ice from the warmth of their bodies, and I knew they were alive. Alive, but terrified that if they moved so much as a muscle, they would fall through. I couldn't get out to help them without breaking the ice myself, so I turned and trudged as fast as I could through the thigh-deep snow until I found a long branch poking out of a snowdrift. Slowly, breathlessly, I dragged it back to the pond. Someone else had come along while I was gone. He stood on the opposite side, gazing at me helplessly. I carefully pushed the branch across the ice to him. When both of us had a firm grip, we slid it toward some of the people and yelled for them to reach out and grab hold. They hadn't stirred while all this was going on, and even in the brief time I'd been away, the heat of their bodies had melted more of the ice. Yet for a long time, or what seemed like a long time, no one moved. Then, without lifting his half-frozen face from the ice, a man raised his right arm and carefully, blindly, swept it back and forth through the air, searching for the branch we were shouting for him to grab onto. Just as his hand touched the branch, I woke up.

Table of Contents

Any notes or footnotes follow each chapter.

Acknowledgments

First I want to thank an Internet poster whose name I never knew nor likely would have remembered, having visited so many chat rooms and Web sites in my search. The person could have lived right next door or thousands of miles away, but it felt like we were in the same room. Before I followed his or her links I had followed the threads left by hundreds of others, all of them, like me, looking for ways to cope, or to help others cope, with a world of brilliant lights and terrifying darkness, of grandiose fantasies and debilitating fears. They weren't having much success, though, and until that moment, neither was I. Thanks, anonymous poster, wherever you are, for referring me to Tony Stephan. Without your help, this book would have been written very differently. It would have sensitized readers to the pathos of bipolar disorder, encouraged patients to take their medicine, and offered them, at most, a way to manage their mental disorder between hospitalizations. Because of your input, my son can expect more, much more. He does not have to remain the giant of his dreams or the dwarf of his fears. He can look forward to more in his future than his past would suggest.

I am grateful to Barb and Tony Stephan, as well as David Hardy, for their courageous commitment to making a difference. Their search for effective solutions was born out of the same despair and helplessness my family experienced. Their pioneering work adds to an already existing and yet still relatively unknown body of knowledge addressing the usefulness of nutrients to promote proper brain functioning and to restore what I call the broken brains of those suffering from a number of central nervous system (CNS) disorders. These disorders have heretofore been conceptualized in our culture as mental disorders.

I want to thank Dr. Robert Bransfield for his consultation, encouragement, and for writing the introduction. As I sorted through increasingly technical material, he invited me to join an Internet discussion group he had developed for health care providers, scientists, and knowledgeable advocates for change. He started this group after he and some colleagues in the American Psychiatric Association noted that patients were being cured of mental illness by the use of antibiotics for underlying complex infectious diseases. In the belief that mainstream psychiatry was being unfairly dismissive of these results and their implications, he and his colleagues resolved to use the discussion group as a forum where others could explore their experiences and share research findings. Since the purpose of the group was to explore issues around microbes and mental illness, it was called MMI. Dr. Bransfield maintains a Web site at mentalhealthandillness.com.

My sincere thanks goes to Dr. William Burgdorfer, Dr. Robert Cade, Dr. Bruce Charlton, Mr. George Eby, Dr. Hugh Fudenberg, Dr. Bonnie Kaplan,

Dr. John Martin, Dr. Puneet Pakeet, Dr. Richie Shoemaker, Dr. Robert Yolken and Dr. Joh-Kar Zubieta for permission to share highlights of their leading-edge research, as well as for their invaluable feedback. They have helped this backyard mechanic keep his flights of fancy to a minimum. I also want to thank Dr. Richard Poel, my previous commander and mentor at Beale Air Force Base. Dr. Poel would remind our medical facility professional staff that we could do whatever we wanted with our clients as long we followed Poel's rule: Know what you know and know what you don't know. I want to thank my sister, Judith R. Shamp, for the pen and ink drawing, "The Fragility of Nature," a symbolic representation of the hemispheres of the brain in the photo section. Judy is an award-winning professional artist in Houston whose creations include church banners, hospital art, wearable art, bug purses, and now, pen and ink drawings in support of this project.

Thanks to editor Paul Witcover from New York for his uncanny knack in opening new doors for me to explore with my family and for his ability to condense my verbose verbiage into short, simple, highly focused statements that even I can understand. And for final proofing I owe a debt of gratitude to Kit Bailey from Second Look in Nevada City. Thanks to artist Michael Lierly from Little Rock Arkansas for the neuron illustrations, and graphic artist Teri Paulus-Bershaw from Design Works for her assistance on the cover. She is also from Nevada City.

To Chris, who has been to the mountains and the valleys, thank you for your self portrait, both in picture and words. Thanks for being willing to share your experiences in the hope that others can learn from them. To my father — your life work has been a series of valiant yet futile efforts to undo the consequences of a crippling set of illnesses we call bipolar disorder. Thanks for sharing your experiences in this book in the hope that others won't have to repeat them. What happened in your past does not have to be the prologue for what happens in their future. Most of all I want to thank you Gayle, for putting up with my monomania to understand something of these crippling and complex brain disorders and for your practical advice and editorial assistance.

Foreword

Some might call it a quiet revolution, others an evolution, still others a new renaissance. Whatever it is, it has already started, and it is transforming lives every day. Nutrients are restoring broken brains. Thousands of psychiatric patients who have spent years if not lifetimes plagued by weight gain, excessive tiredness, and structural changes in their brains, as well as by such esoteric-sounding afflictions as tardive dyskinesia, severe ketoacidosis, serotonin syndrome, status epilepticus and discontinuation syndrome, are experiencing hope for a normal life. Quietly, without a lot of fanfare and media hype, ordinary people are using nutritional solutions to restore brain functioning. They are talking about it on the Internet. From a province in Canada to Harvard University, innovative physicians and other professionals are investigating nutritional solutions to CNS disorders, recommending them to their patients, and researching and reporting the amazing results. This is the story of one family's odyssey in searching for and finding drug-free solutions to bipolar disorder.

But the story is not just about my family, which has lived under the shadow of bipolar disorder for four generations. It is about the many families suffering from the full array of CNS disorders and about the professionals in the justice, educational, and health care systems who deal with them. While there is no single "cure-all" for CNS patients, extensive research supports the premise that proper nutrients can assist many patients to recover from their illness, frequently without any drugs, or with significantly reduced amounts.

In addition, substantial evidence exists that bipolar disorder and other biologically based disorders have been prematurely conceptualized and labeled as Diagnostic and Statistical Manual (DSM-IV) disorders; that is, as "mental" disorders. Given that brain cells have both stimulating and inhibiting properties, and that highly complex processes keep those opposing functions balanced, it is only reasonable to assume that a multitude of causes disrupt that balance to produce the common behavioral manifestations of what we currently label "bipolar disorder."

Too Good To Be True? is about a journey, not a destination. Except for the book's bold and unambiguous central premise — that nutrients do in fact quiet the unquiet brain — the reader looking for a "one-size-fits-all" solution will not find it here. My intent is not to provide organized, complete, "shrink-wrapped" solutions. It is to ask questions. It is to describe our odyssey, a trip filled with both peril and promise. The odyssey involves visiting what I have come to call the American Gulag, exploring the parallel universe of alternative health care, and seeking refuge in the hoped-for safety of mainstream medicine. It involves plunging into the dark and dangerous world of bipolar madness, from the depths of hell to the equally terrifying heights of heaven. Like the illness, this odyssey includes stunning vistas and valleys of disappointment and despair. Each step of the odyssey points toward new questions, new paradigms, and ultimately new solutions.

While this book is based on a true story, I have changed the names and detailed circumstances of some ancillary persons. I have taken artistic license in writing fiction-like narrative, including details and dialogue based on actual events, in order to provide continuity and character development and to fill in portions of the story in which I was not a direct participant.

Some of the chapters deal with research into the causes and treatment of bipolar disorder. I claim no specialized expertise in this area, apart from having the persistence to track down leads by reading books, researching in local and university libraries, traveling through the vast universe of the Internet with my mouse, and talking with pioneers who are making inroads into our understanding of CNS disorders. Einstein once said, "Most fundamental ideas of science are essentially very simple and may be expressed in a language comprehensible to everyone." I have attempted to make these topics as easy to understand as possible while at the same time trying to avoid oversimplification. Any conclusions expressed herein regarding the etiology, assessment, or treatment of bipolar disorder are based on my best-faith efforts to apply the facts as I understand them and may not be definitive statements of scientific fact. I am a licensed clinical social worker, a grandnephew, a grandson, a son, and a father of individuals who have exhibited bipolar symptoms. I am not a scientist.

My search was based on the assumption that there are no inappropriate questions, only unrefined ones. In retrospect, some of my questions were naive to the point of being ridiculous. Some were more sophisticated than I knew, touching on topics already being pursued by leading-edge researchers. In the process of finding new questions to replace old ones, I learned there are few simple questions, fewer still simple answers.

In my research, I explored a number of methods for assessing and treating the symptoms of bipolar and other CNS disorders. I tried to be open to all points of view. This made for an interesting journey, especially when the perspectives were mutually exclusive. These viewpoints are shared to stimulate thinking "outside of the box," not necessarily to recommend a particular assessment or treatment plan. Given that things are not always as they seem, readers are advised to complete the entire book before exploring, with their health care provider, a particular assessment tool or treatment for themselves, a patient, or a family member or friend.

While I researched this book, various professionals told me certain alleged facts that had a profound influence on our family's journey. Some of those "facts" were incorrect or in conflict with other "facts" I was told. Some, to be frank, are still, as they say, up in the air. Areas of conflict not addressed in the narrative are listed in Appendix 3. They are listed at the end to pre-serve the integrity of the story and to illustrate the risks and benefits involved in leaving no stone unturned.

I invite readers to share any feedback on the ideas in this book at the email address provided below. If you know an answer or a resource for any of the unanswered questions you find herein, I would love to hear from you. Too Good To Be True? Volume II will incorporate this feedback as well as late-breaking developments. The odyssey continues.

Finally, some words of caution and a disclaimer are in order. First, while my intent is to introduce the reader to novel ways of thinking about CNS disorders and their treatment, this book is not intended to substitute for medical care or to provide specific solutions to those suffering from CNS disorders. Second, if you are suffering from a psychiatric illness and experience troubling thoughts while reading this book, please discuss these thoughts as soon as possible with a trusted support person or a professional. While such a warning may seem overly cautious, perhaps even demeaning to the average reader, one lesson I learned from our odyssey is that long-held and cherished assumptions about self-responsibility and self-control become irrelevant myths when a person's brain is broken. Lastly, my family and I have no financial or business relationship with Tony and Barb Stephan or David Hardy, except that we purchase nutritional supplements from Synergy Group, a non-profit company established by them to promote the research and utilization of nutritional supplementation for CNS disorders. The text mentions stocks I own or have owned in companies not involved in the assessment or treatment of CNS disorders, and which play a minor role in the story. I have written this book as objectively as possible and I have no financial or business relationship with companies or professionals who provide diagnostic assessment services or products discussed herein.

David Moyer, October 15, 2002
dave@bipolarodyssey.com

Introduction

Too Good to Be True? Nutrients Quiet the Unquiet Brain reads like a 21st century mystery novel. It is the story of four generations touched by bipolar disorder and the efforts of David Moyer, a mental health professional, to weave his way through the sometimes baffling justice and mental health systems. There are two particularly important points we learn from his journey. Be proactive and consider everything, while accepting nothing as an absolute.

The most challenging frontier is the human brain. Once considered too complex to understand, we can now use our minds to unlock the secrets of our brain. The 1990s were the "Decade of the Brain." The research of the last decade has launched us into a century and a millennium of increasing potential to understand the world within us. Already it is apparent that human consciousness and mental functioning are constantly impacted by a multitude of interactive systems within us and around us.

David Moyer's journey is energized by a very powerful motivation. His father and his adult son are ill and in need of assistance. He is unwilling to accept the status quo. So too, we all have the responsibility, freedom, and empowerment to pursue opportunities for the best possible health care for our family and ourselves. We live in a free country, with freedom of information and freedom of opportunity to pursue the health care provider and methods of our choice. The Internet offers unlimited opportunities to access uncensored, worldwide sources of medical information for researchers, health care professionals and patients. Unlike medical ethics, medical information evolves on a daily basis. To use this new information effectively, we need to retain humility and flexibility, as some of the dogmatic views of the present quickly become the rejected and outmoded ideas of the future.

David Moyer's father and son suffered from a condition we currently call "bipolar illness." Patients with this condition display an excessive intensity of mood, cyclic mood swings, and moods that do not always appropriately reflect their current life situation. The moods of these patients are not adequately regulated. Although the symptoms of this condition are readily described in the Diagnostic and Statistical Manual of the American Psychiatric Association, the actual cause or causes remain a mystery. There are theories, hypotheses, and speculation, but no one knows for sure.

Even without knowing the causes of this illness, we have treatments that are sometimes very effective, though not curative for everyone. Advances in medicine are discovered by a combination of determination, ingenuity, and luck. The most important discoveries in medicine are yet to be made. A treatment that is dramatically effective for one person may be a failure for someone else. No two people are the same, not even identical twins. Bipolar illness is a syndrome of a cluster of related symptoms that appear to have a number of different causes. But what are these causes? Knowing this will give us more insight into more effective treatment options. We must start by reviewing some basic biology.

All biological systems are in a dynamic balance with their environment. An adequately balanced ratio of different resources is needed to maintain health. An insufficient amount of any resource can result in a deficiency, while an excess of any resource or substance can cause toxicity. Either a deficiency or toxicity can cause an impairment of our functioning and regulatory processes. In addition, there is increasing evidence that low-grade trauma to the brain and body is caused by chronic low-grade infections. Some of this trauma is a direct effect from microbes such as viruses and bacteria, while some is caused by our own immune system as it is provoked into action by the presence of these microbes. Chronic stress can further compromise our recuperative abilities. The interactive effects of deficiencies, toxicity, infections, dysregulated immune effects, chronic stress and other possible causes result in a very slow and microscopic trauma to our brains. Injury to different neural pathways can result in a decline in our functional capacities, which may contribute to causing psychiatric illness and even criminal behavior in some cases.

These insights provide new treatment options. Lithium and herbs are ancient treatments. Research with infectious diseases has demonstrated that anti-microbial treatments cure some cases of mental illness. The distinction between a psychoactive medication and a nutrient is not always clear, and there is increasing evidence that nutritional approaches have their role in the treatment of mental illness. David Moyer's findings reflect some of my clinical experience, as I have seen patients demonstrate a significant improvement of their mental symptoms from nutritional approaches. This book raises some interesting and highly relevant questions for providers as well as recipients of mental health care. It has given me some new ideas, but it has also left me with a major question. How do we combine the best of traditional psychiatric treatments with the best of innovative approaches?

I have made some very broad statements. To look at these issues in more detail, read the book and discover how one family's journey transformed their understanding and their treatment of bipolar illness. I think you will find their journey to be most intriguing and thought-provoking. I certainly did.

Robert C. Bransfield, M.D.
Private Practice of Psychiatry
Red Bank, N.J.

Prologue - Intimations from the Past

James Mangram had scarcely moved since starting his trip early on the morning of July 26, 1932. Between his departure from Los Angeles and his arrival in Oakland in the late afternoon, he mostly sat slumped in the rail car holding his head in his hands, his elbows resting on his knees. Passengers embarked and disembarked, but he did not look up, and no one intruded upon his evident preoccupation. Only when the train pulled out of the Oakland station on the final leg of his long journey did his grief-weary eyes glance up to take in the sight of the early evening fog rolling in, half-shrouding the San Francisco skyline and covering the bay with an eerie blanket of gray. Each clack of the metal wheels took him one rail-length closer to his Napa destination. As the clatter increased, the train picking up speed, James put his head into his hands again. His thoughts were fixed on the car behind him. It held the remains of what had just two days earlier been his 36-year-old wife, Harriet, and their 7-year-old son, Lloyd. The bodies shared a casket.

Paying for two caskets would not have been a problem. James's career with the Associated Oil Company in Oakland and, later, Los Angeles, had flourished. Since he and Harriet had married in 1921, they had purchased and rented out three houses, all of which assured extra monthly income. Financially, in spite of the Depression, life had been good to them ... that is, until now. No, paying for two caskets was not the issue. The issue was the possibility of someone seeing him with two caskets, offering condolences and then, as if that gave them the right, asking unwanted, unanswerable questions. Besides, despite what had happened, he wouldn't have felt right separating mother and son.

As he had done repeatedly since their deaths, James retraced his actions prior to and during the day of July 24th. Had he said something unkind? Had he been too busy with his work? Had there been an unresolved argument? He couldn't identify anything out of the ordinary. Lloyd was a friendly, cooperative child. James could think of nothing that Lloyd might have done to provoke his mother's rage. James had never known Harriet to lose her temper, either at him or at Lloyd. He had noticed that Harriet had been quiet and not sleeping well, but she had experienced this problem before and it had always seemed to pass.

He replayed the unwanted scene over and over again in the back of his mind. He recalled how the shots had awakened him in the early morning, felt again the initial shock, the confusion, how his mind had almost immediately begun to search for explanations — engine backfires, an explosion, a lightning strike, anything but the murder-suicide of his son and wife. But when he'd stumbled into his son's bedroom, as much as he wanted to deny the evidence of his eyes, he could not. Even now, he could not escape the image of his mortally wounded wife lying over the lifeless body of their only child. He doubted he ever would.

The train made a special stop, as James requested, in Crockett near the Carquinez Straits a few miles south of Vallejo. As he stepped down the stairs of his railcar at 9:15 that night, the porters were placing the casket onto a gurney and transferring possession to the undertaker from Treadway Funeral Home. His in-laws, Ira L. Jones (known as I.L.), and Josephine, Ira's wife, had come to meet the train along with two of their daughters, Clara and Pearl. They greeted him awkwardly. Condolences were exchanged.

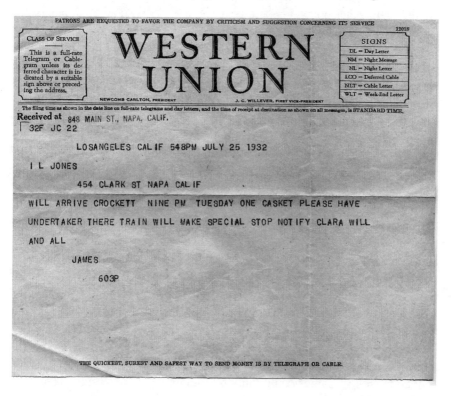

Leaving the casket with the undertaker, James rode with his in-laws up Highway 29 from Vallejo to Napa. They talked of how unusually hot and dry the season had been that year, how small the prune and apple crops were going to be. They spoke of their hope that the next year would see more rainfall so that the farmers could recoup their losses. They spoke of everything but what they had left behind at the train station. After they arrived at his father-in-law's home at 11:30, James went straight to bed.

The funeral the next day was small. Death by cancer or a car accident would have been a more acceptable route to the cemetery. The grief of the few immediate family members who were invited, and who came, was palpable, expressed in quiet sighs and, in a few cases, uncontrollable tears. Yet despite the outpouring of raw emotion, the funeral proceedings themselves, from the hymn, "Going Home," to Psalm 23, the Shepard's Psalm, to the homily by the reverend from the Methodist church, took on a brittle, restrained quality. The words to articulate the grief – or the blame – were held in check. The reverend would have had a tough time giving a eulogy. He didn't even try.

On the surface, his inlaws were cordial and supportive to him. Yet James, in the most private places in his heart, wondered if they had lingering questions about him. Maybe they wondered about his fitness as a husband just as he wondered about their fitness as parents. As he furtively stole glances toward them at the cemetery, he interrupted his own self reproach and speculated as to their possible culpability, perhaps some secret childhood trauma that had planted the seeds of despair in their daughter. The prospect of sharing the blame temporarily lightened the oppressive weight on his shoulders that he was destined to carry for the rest of his life.

Throughout the interminable day of funeral, wake, and burial, James felt as if he wasn't really present. What was happening was somehow a dream, even when the single casket was lowered with aching slowness into the ground at Mt. Veeder Cemetery, that little patch of land that Wilbur and Emma Taylor Moyer had deeded to the county in 1871.

The next day, Ira and Josephine drove James back to Crockett. On the way, the unasked questions remained unasked as conversation turned again to the manageable and the mundane, mostly weather and crops. When he arrived at the station, James bid his in-laws farewell and boarded the train that would take him back to Los Angeles. As the clacking of the wheels increased its tempo, James put his head in his hands and, as he would for the rest of his life, remembered.

Part I - Must the Past be Prologue?

I know the past and thence will essay to glean a warning for the future so that man may profit by his errors, and derive experience from his folly.

Shelly

1 - Family Trees, Roots, and Skeletons

A visit to Mt. Veeder

October 12, 2000 was one of those fall days of clear blue skies that makes it all but impossible to stay indoors. That morning, together with my 84-year-old father, Ray, and my 24-year-old son, Chris, I had driven 3 hours from Penn Valley to the Veterans Home in Yountville near Napa, where my father had a 10 AM meeting scheduled with the admissions committee. Ray was an overweight diabetic with a pacemaker. Because his health was slowly declining, he wanted to be in a place like the Veterans Home where he could transition from a retirement home setting to nursing care when he could no longer care for himself. The committee had turned him down once before, but this time the meeting went better than I had expected. The staff promised that they would favorably consider Ray's request for admission once he provided them with a physician's report on his current health. I was still skeptical that they would agree to admit him once they saw that report but said nothing to dampen my father's hopeful mood. Knowing how poorly Ray had fared in another retirement home two years previously, my wife Gayle and I did not expect that he would succeed in this latest effort, even if he were admitted. We had already agreed between ourselves that he would continue to live with us until he required more care and attention than we could provide for him. But he had asked to go, so I had taken him.

After the meeting, we had lunch at the cafeteria of the Veterans Home. Ray started to reminisce about the years he had spent in the Napa area as a boy and young man. On impulse, I suggested we visit some of his old haunts since we were in the neighborhood. And so we headed toward Mt. Veeder, a few miles northwest of Napa. Mt. Veeder is a mountainous area of oaks and coastal redwood forest with small farms and vineyards. With the exception of an occasional walled estate, it looks much as it did when Ray spent his formative years there from 1916 until 1936.

Soon we were driving on the old Mt. Veeder Road heading toward the cemetery that my great grandparents Wilbur and Emma Taylor Moyer had deeded to the county 129 years before. Wilbur and Emma had also deeded an equal portion of the remaining 640 acres of their property to each of their children: four boys, Rollin, Earnest, Frank, and Willard, and two girls, Ethel and Ruth.

We passed by the entrance to the Mt. Veeder Winery, its driveway blocked by a large and ornate wrought-iron gate. Once this had been the driveway of Ray's Uncle Frank. It had been more than 30 years since I had last paid a visit to the house my great-uncle had built by himself in 1961 when he was in his 60s. There would be no visit today. The gate was closed and locked. If Emma Taylor Moyer had been with us, she would not have been pleased.

Not that she would have objected to the gate being locked. No, what would have bothered her was that her son's 100-acre ranch had been converted since his death in 1985 into a vineyard and winery. And as if that weren't bad enough, the house he had built with his own two hands had been transformed into a place for tasting the wine from said vineyard.

Emma, a community activist, had been a member of the Woman's Christian Temperance Union. She had waged a successful battle in 1904 to keep a saloon near her Methodist Church from being built.[1] Now her efforts were forgotten by all but us. Maybe some other time, when the gate was open, we would drive up the expansive asphalt driveway that had replaced the narrow gravel road I still vividly remembered from childhood visits to see my great uncle and aunt. Maybe then we would raise a glass of the forbidden wine and drink a toast to the memory of my great-grandmother.

For now, though, we continued up Mt. Veeder Road for another mile before turning left down a dirt road that

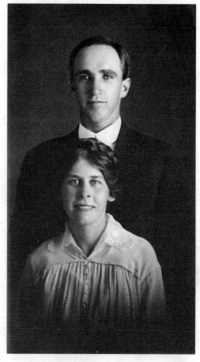

Rollin and Rose Moyer

led toward another 100-acre ranch, the one where Ray had spent his childhood. His mother, Rose, had sold that ranch in 1936, when my father was 19 years old, in spite of his arguments to the contrary. While Ray had recognized the inherent value of 100 acres of farm property, Rose had listened to a higher authority.

My grandmother, Rose, married my grandfather, Rollin Moyer, on May 24, 1914. The wedding was initially scheduled for sometime in June, but Rose's mother, Josephine, known in the family for her "second sight," asked the couple to move the date to May because she predicted she would die before June. She died the day after Rose and Rollin were married. Rose, who also claimed special "gifts" gave birth to her only child, Ray, in 1916 and raised him single-handedly following Rollin's premature death in 1928.

Rose was an eccentric Four Square Pentecostal. She obsessed about religious issues, receiving direction from the Lord Himself on matters great and small, from the salvation of Clara, her optimistic-minded younger sister,

4

who worshipped a more forgiving and less demanding God, to such issues as when and where to move her place of residence. Clara, a member of the Unity Church, was a warm, positive-minded person with a perpetual smile and a kind word for others, always ready to listen. But God was the only one Rose listened to. With everyone else, she did the talking.

When Rose spoke, what she said would be unrelated to what the other person had said. Even the infirmities of old age failed to counteract what seemed to be a congenital predisposition to dominate conversation. Though her mind was sharp, she never mastered the art of verbal give and take. The size of her handwriting ranged from normal to so small it couldn't be read without a magnifying glass. Some of her writing contained intense religious material, such as dire warnings to Clara regarding the perilous state of her immortal but unbelieving soul. While Rose was never formally diagnosed with any condition, those who knew her considered her to be eccentric.

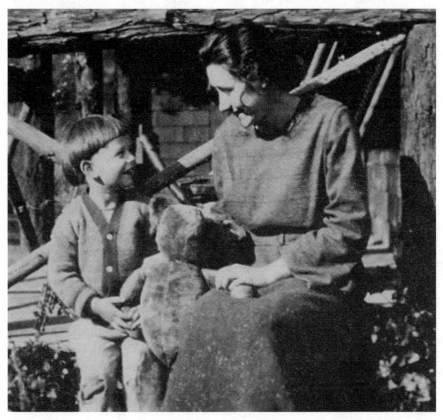

Ray and Aunt Clara, circa 1920

The sights and smells of his Mt. Veeder home evoked a stream of memories in my father's mind. The stories spilled out in rapid succession as we drove.

"See that rock?" He pointed to a large flat boulder near his childhood home. "That's where Aunt Clara used to tell me stories. I used to go play there when my mother would get a 'burden.'"

"A burden?" I asked.

"She would feel the Lord putting a burden on her heart to pray about something. She would pray and cry out loud. It scared me, so I would go out to the rock to play.... Look at that slope over there by the barn." Our eyes followed his finger to a huge barn to the left of the house. We could see a steep slope from the barn down to the pasture. "That's where the cow slipped and slid all the way down the hill one rainy day. When my father saw this he quoted a passage from the Bible, 'Israel slideth back as a backsliding Heifer.' I used to enjoy getting out of the house by going to the barn with my dad and feeding the chickens and milking the cows. Our kittens would come up and I would squirt the milk right into their mouths."

I turned the car around and headed back to the main road. Ray turned to the back seat where Chris was sitting. He interrupted the silence with a comment. "After my father died, I secretly wished that my mother had died instead of him."

Chris didn't say anything.

"How did your father die?" I asked, hoping to stimulate Chris's curiosity about our family history, since this was his first visit to the Mt. Veeder area.

"He and my grandfather both died of typhoid fever. My grandfather died of it directly. My father lived through the typhoid, but then later died from the flu when I was 12. We always thought that it was the typhoid that weakened his heart. He wasn't the same after that."

Ray started talking about our family tree as we drove back to Mt. Veeder Road. "During the War, when I was in Hawaii, I got some information about our family history from an old family Bible that belonged to Aunt Ethel. It traced the Moyer family all the way back to John Philip Meyer. He fought in the Revolutionary War. He was known for his wrestling ability. His descendants settled in Pennsylvania. After his first wife died, he married Anne Margaret Morr. They changed their name to Moyer. You know there were no divorces in eight generations until the day Ruthie divorced me in 1970." We had heard it before, but he enjoyed telling the story. As my father had grown older, his conversation had become difficult to follow at times, seeming to jump from topic to topic, but I had learned to recognize his inner logic — and the frequent endpoint of his mental wanderings, his divorce from Ruthie.

Family secrets

Back on the main road and headed down the hill, Ray pointed to what looked like a residential driveway that I had not noticed when we first drove up the road. I turned left, drove past a ranch-style house with toys in the front yard, and continued on for about 50 yards to a sign that read: "Keep Out, No Trespassing."

We had arrived at Mt. Veeder Cemetery. Chains blocked further passage with the car. "What kind of welcome is this?" I wondered aloud as I parked, only partly joking. "My great grandfather donates the land for a cemetery, our ancestors are buried here, and now, if we want to visit, we are trespassers?"

"Maybe they had a problem with vandals," Ray opined.

We got out of the car, stepped around the chains, and proceeded to trespass into the cemetery. The leaves of the oak and dogwood trees were in full color, drifting to the ground at the slightest touch of a breeze.

The last time I had been there was in 1978, for Rose's burial. Back then, the cemetery had been well maintained, filled with clear, uncluttered paths near interesting tombstones dating back into the late 1800s. There were no "keep out" signs then. Now many of the elegant old tombstones were gone, replaced by faded, plastic-covered cards on which the names of the deceased were all but illegible. The paths and many of what gravestones remained were covered with trees and bushes. Between the actions of vandals and the neglect of the groundskeepers, the cemetery was a "ghost" of what it had been.

Concerned about my 84-year-old, 200-pound father walking over the uneven ground without assistance, I asked him if he needed help. He said he didn't. Since his wide-legged gait was always interminably slow, Chris and I strolled ahead, down what used to be the main path, to find the Jones family plot. Save for the distant sound of a cowbell and a dog barking, the cemetery was quiet and still. We were the only living beings present. Amidst a stand of young trees, some of which were growing right out of the graves, we found Ira and Josephine Jones buried next to their son and five of their daughters. The grave site of the sixth daughter, Rose, was elsewhere in the cemetery.

The Jones family had originally come to Napa from eastern Nebraska in 1904. They had worked hard to make a life, laboring in the orchards and factories, and washing, ironing, and sewing for hire. The father, Ira Jones, taught himself to be a carpenter and a realtor. He bought some land from their combined earnings and built a house; then, with the rent money from that house, bought more land and built another until he had built a total of ten houses, renting them out for anywhere from eight to twelve dollars a month. Ira was able to support his growing family comfortably from the rental income and eventually put enough aside to purchase an eleven-room home in the Bragg Hill section of Napa. In 1917, he moved there with his wife, Josephine, and their six daughters and one son.

While the rest of the Jones girls remained in Napa, Harriet wandered far from the family's rural orb. She married at a young age and moved with her husband, James Mangram, to Oakland and, later, Los Angeles. The union between Mangram, a successful businessman, and Harriet Jones, a daughter of one of the wealthier men in the Valley had seemed full of promise. She married a successful businessman. He married one of the Jones girls. As the wedding announcement in the Napa Valley Register stated, "His bride is the daughter of Mr. and Mrs. I. L. Jones of Napa. Her father is one of the most prominent business men of that section, where as a realty dealer he amassed the fortune which has enabled him to retire from active business life."

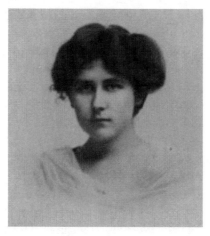

Harriet Jones

Yet that promise had been cruelly and inexplicably broken. Standing at the family plot, I looked down at Harriet's grave. On her tombstone were the words, "Harriet Mangram - Lloyd Mangram Died July 24, 1932." She had been buried with her young son.

In the nearly 70 years since, the graves had sprouted fir and pine trees that reached as high as 15 feet. Now, as I stood in their shadow, I thought that time and the elements would soon finish their tasks, and no sign would be left outside our memories that these people had ever lived or died.

Chris and I walked a few more feet down the hill to the Moyer family plot.

"Here's the Moyer side of the family," I told Chris. "Look, here's Wilbur Moyer's grave."

Wilbur and Emma were buried next to each other, underneath a huge oak tree and surrounded by all their children. I noticed that they occupied the best real estate in the cemetery, as was befitting since they had donated the land. Through the moss on Wilbur's white stone marker I could make out the words, "Born April 24, 1849, Dayton Ohio. Died Nov 24, 1899, Napa California." Another stone said that Emma Taylor Moyer, born in 1853, had died in 1932. I thought I had remembered that Rose's grave was here, with her husband, Rollin, but there was no marker. Yet even though her resting place seemed to have disappeared, it looked like both the Jones and Moyer families had been spared the indignity of having plastic index cards put on their graves to replace the headstones and tombstones stolen by vandals.

Chris looked at the graves.

I broke the silence around us. "Wilbur and Emma owned 640 acres, including the land in this cemetery. Imagine where we would be today if this land hadn't been sold."

He didn't say anything, just wandered around looking at the Moyer graves. Seemed like he really wasn't interested in learning about his family history. I didn't say anything, but I was disappointed he seemed so nonchalant.

I pointed to the grave of my grandfather, Rollin. "Here is Grampa Ray's father, Rollin." Chris looked at the weatherbeaten gravestone. "How many families do you know that have their own cemetery?" I asked.

Again, he didn't say anything. I looked back to see how my father was doing. He was teetering.

"Are you sure you're okay?" I yelled.

"I'm fine," he called back.

He didn't look it. Maintaining his balance was tough enough when the ground was flat. I hurried back up the hill to help him while Chris lingered at the graves. "Hold on a sec, Dad. I'll be right there." I walked faster, but not fast enough. I broke into a run as I saw him fall on a slightly raised, grass-covered grave, his head narrowly missing a tombstone.

"Chris! Grandpa Ray fell down!" I called, frightened now.

My father was trying to pick himself up when I got there. He seemed more embarrassed than hurt. "You could have hit your head, and we would have had to plant you here," I scolded.

"Got my feet tangled in the weeds. If I had hit one of those gravestones it would have been serious, but I didn't."

I tried to help him get up, but he was too heavy and weak, even with my help. "Okay, wait till Chris gets here; we'll pull you up."

Chris was slowly walking up the hill with his recently acquired methodical, almost mechanical, gait, a waxen facial expression obscuring any concern he might have had. I bit back my impatience and waited for him to reach us. "He didn't hurt anything. Can you help me get him up?"

Together we each grabbed an arm and took hold of Ray's blue overalls at the waist. We pulled him to his feet. Then we escorted him to a weathered chair and table under a similarly weathered old roof beside a shiny new headstone. The red and yellow flowers on the grave site were fresh.

"Here's a recent grave of some woman," I said. "The stone says she was a 'longtime friend' of a guy named Brandlin. Seems like a strange thing to put on a tombstone!"

"Yes, I knew Chester," said Ray. "Lived on the other side of the road; we used to go to school together. Must have been his girlfriend. He died a long time ago."

"Grampa Ray," I said. "We found all the great aunts and uncles from the Moyer and Jones families, but we couldn't find Grandma Moyer's gravestone."

Ray shrugged. "Maybe someone stole it for the marble."

"Oh well," I said. "Rose always was the black sheep of the family. Guess she still is. Speaking of black sheep, Harriet is buried with her son. The stone reads, 'Harriet Mangram-Lloyd Mangram Died July 24, 1932.' I didn't know they were buried together."

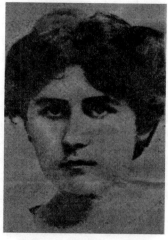

Wedding Announcement

Ray reminisced about his Aunt Harriet and his cousin Lloyd.

"I was about 13 or 14 at the time," he said. "When we found out what happened, the whole family was shocked. Folks wouldn't talk about it."

"Were you close to Harriet or Lloyd?" I asked.

"Not very. They were in LA. I remember a few visits with Aunt Harriet. Lloyd was a lot younger than me. I think he was about 7 when he died."

"So what did folks make of it? How did they explain what happened?"

"When I first heard about it, my mother told me there had been a terrible accident. I was suspicious though, because whenever other family members had died, people always talked about what had happened. No one talked about Harriet and Lloyd's death. Even at the funeral, whenever I came around, folks started talking in whispers. I figured that whatever had happened, I wasn't supposed to know about it. One day a while later I overheard Uncle Frank say she had shot herself and Lloyd. He said he couldn't understand, because Aunt Harriet was 'so gentle she wouldn't hurt a flea.' And that's how I learned the truth."

"Sounds like the family wasn't very open about it," I commented. I understood all too well what had kept the mourners from speaking openly, why they had shared their secrets in hushed tones beyond young Ray's hearing and understanding. Even though in those private conversations, at some level, they had talked about what Harriet had done and speculated as to why she did it, publicly, they had guarded the family secrets then, just as they would continue to do in the future. Aunt Clara was later to omit Aunt Harriet from a family scrapbook, and, likewise, Aunt Pearl, another of Harriet's

Family Trees, Roots, and Skeletons

sisters, was to leave her out of an extensive and detailed family history she had written for posterity. [2]

The Moyer-Jones clan was a hard-working, non-drinking, churchgoing group of farmers, carpenters and seamstresses. They were stable, productive contributors to their community, without any known history that could account for the inexplicable actions of Ray's Aunt Harriet, or, for that matter, for the unrestrained religiosity of her sister, Rose, Ray's mother. Harriet's actions were, all too literally, both un-speakable and unfathomable to these rural farm folk. No one knew the cause of this tragedy.

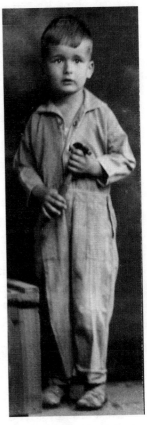

But perhaps we, their descendants, could understand more. Some of us had wrestled with the demons that had overwhelmed Harriet. Some of us were still wrestling with them. The family skeletons lay buried in the old cemetery, but the family secrets would remain hidden no longer. We had been given an opportunity to learn from them, regardless how painful the lessons might be. We would learn from them. We had no other choice.

The shadows were lengthening. We still had many miles to travel. Chris and I helped Ray to his feet and escorted him over the mounds of dirt to the car. We headed back to our home in the Sierra foothills, leaving the Mt. Veeder Cemetery empty and silent again, except for the slight rus-tling of branches in the breeze and the falling of the brown and yellow leaves over the final resting

Lloyd Mangram

places, marked and unmarked, of the dead. Ahead, though I did not yet know it, lay an odyssey that would span four generations, from Harriet and Rose to Ray and, finally, to my son, Chris.

Speaking of Chris, he didn't say much that day. Although he had cut his psychotropic medications by a third, they still caused him to be tired and uncommunicative.

11

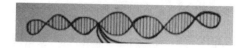

Notes

1. When Emma Taylor, a member of the Woman's Christian Temperance Union (WCTU), fought to keep a saloon from being built near the First Methodist Church of Napa, she and her fellow prohibitionists threatened a "Carrie Nation." Carry A. Nation and her followers had a smashing career storming into saloons. They used rocks and hatchets to demonstrate their displeasure at those who contributed to the nation's moral decline by serving liquor. The threat of local "hatchitation" caused the would-be saloon owner to blink. The WCTU chapter won. No "demon" rum would be served in that neighborhood.

Ray tells us how, when he was a teenager, he happened to be riding with his Aunt Pearl and Uncle Will through the neighborhoods of both the Methodist and Catholic churches. His uncle claimed that the lack of bars or brothels near the Methodist church was the direct result of the efforts of none other than Emma Taylor Moyer. For proof, he pointed to the bars and brothels that were flourishing near the Catholic church, where a saloon had been established without any community opposition. Ray remembered that Aunt Pearl blushed, and that he was confused. He didn't know what a brothel was.

2. In the years that followed the death of Harriet and her son, her sisters appeared to prune her branch from the family tree. Late in her life, Pearl, Harriet's oldest sister, wrote a five-page history of the Jones family, detailing their move from Nebraska, their early efforts to establish themselves in the Napa area, and the early deaths of sisters Margaret and Jenelle from TB. Her history makes no reference to Harriet. Clara, the baby of the family, produced a scrapbook of family notes and news clippings. These included such newspaper headlines as "Actress Hurt in Car Crash," "Banker Ends Life Over Insanity Fear," "Robber Shoots Ticket Agent," and one entitled "Shoots self through the Heart," about a businessman who ended his life after business reversals. Clara included family, marriage, and obituary notices, and a Personal Mention column announcing that "Miss Clara Jones from Walla Walla, Washington has arrived in Napa to spend time with her father, I.L. Jones." Nothing about Harriet was preserved. Her scrapbook was put together as if Harriet had never existed. Perhaps the clippings were her way to universalize similar tragedies of others in order to come to grips with the untimely deaths of her sister and nephew.

2 - A Shaky Start

I don't personally recollect what happened on January 19, 1946. However, the events of that night were indelibly imprinted into my mother's memory, so much so that when she told me about it, I felt like I had been there. Actually, I was. I was two and a half weeks old, blissfully sleeping in a crib in front of my mother and father's bed, satiated with my mother's milk and, thankfully, unable to comprehend the storm that was about to break.

The noise of traffic on the road in front of their two-bedroom rental home on Orange Avenue in Fresno was keeping my father awake. Every few minutes he would hear the sound of car tires hitting a flattened can. He kept tossing and turning, worried that he would wake up Ruth, his wife. The noise from the tires hitting the can was the least of his worries.

Vicarious memories

Ever since he was honorably discharged from the Army after World War II, Ray's readjustment to civilian life had been tenuous. D.T. Jamison, Ray's father-in-law, had gotten him a job selling life insurance, but he hadn't been able to sell any policies. Then Ray had taken a job pruning vineyards, but he worked so slowly that he couldn't make any money at it. He was disgusted with himself for his lackluster performance. He was confused, had no energy, and wasn't sleeping well. Negative thoughts circled around in his head on a pivot of fear. Could he provide for his family? Could he be a father to his children? Could he ever get out of this slump?

As a 16-year-old, Ray had single-handedly run the 100-acre, self-sustaining family farm after the death of his father, Rollin, from complications of typhoid fever. He had taken care of the animals; raised, killed, and prepared the chickens; pruned the pear and cherry orchards; planted, maintained, and fertilized the vegetable garden with chicken and cow manure; provided oversight for the fall harvest of the orchards. But now he couldn't even prune a few grapevines.

Having been raised in the Pentecostal tradition, Ray viewed depression as a spiritual malady. Lately he had confided in Ruth that he thought he had committed a sin that could not be pardoned. She hadn't been able to figure out what he was talking about.

During the war, my father had served with the Army Air Transport Command (ATC) at Hickam Field, where he was involved in processing secret communications regarding the planned bombing of Hiroshima and Nagasaki. Like most who fought in the war, he accepted the necessity of the bombings, believing they had saved the lives of countless U.S. Soldiers. His work was important, and Ray had performed well in the headquarters of the ATC, rising to the rank of Staff Sergeant. If he had any guilt over his role in communicating top secret messages that led to the slaughter of thousands of civilians, he wasn't aware of it. Yet here he was now, 30 years old, an unemployed veteran with a wife, a three-year-old daughter and a 2-week-old son, unable to provide for his family and obsessing over some unpardonable sin he felt he had committed.

Ruth's family had tried to help in other ways besides the insurance job. D.T. and Ethel, his wife, who were already helping with the rent, felt that Ray wasn't getting enough good-quality vegetables, fruits, and protein. If only Ray would eat the right foods, they intuitively thought, perhaps he would feel better. So they bought food they believed was fresh and wholesome from the stores in Fresno and gave it to the struggling young family. When that didn't seem to help, their focus turned from feeding Ray's body to feeding his soul. A month before I was born, D.T., Ethel, and my mother took Ray to a faith healer. The healer prayed as only Pentecostals can for God to intervene and release the evil forces that were holding him in bondage. After the family gave a small offering to the healer, Ray went home feeling more depressed than ever. Even the prayers of a healer to God Almighty, the creator of the universe, could not help him. He was convinced that God had truly given up on him. He had indeed committed the unpardonable sin, even though he couldn't think of what it was that he had done.

The tires continued to pound the flattened can on Orange Avenue. Ray got up and walked into the garage. He closed the door, opened the car door, leaned in, and started the engine. He lay down on the cold dirt garage floor. Now he would sleep — forever.

Minutes later Ruth woke up. She could hear the muffled sound of the car's engine running in the garage. She noticed that Ray wasn't in bed. She called for him. There was no answer. She called again, louder. Still no answer. Afraid, she ran in her pajamas through the house, out the back porch, and across the lawn into the garage. One sniff of the fumes, and her throat involuntarily tightened. Then she saw Ray lying motionless on the garage floor. The first thing she did was open the garage door and turn off the engine. Then she called his name. No response. She shook him and called again, louder. Still no response. Not knowing if he was alive or dead, she ran back into the house and frantically called an ambulance. When she returned to him, she pressed fingers to his throat, feeling for a pulse in the carotid artery. He was alive, but still unconscious. The ambulance took him to a local hospital, then ultimately to the Veterans Administration hospital in Palo Alto, where he was to stay for two months.

When Ray, an only child, had met Ruth, the eldest of four children, he had been attracted to her confident, take-charge style. Little could he have known that her ability to efficiently and quickly respond to a crisis would one day save his life. As strong as she was, her body protested in response to this grievous upset. Her milk stopped flowing, so from then on I was bottle-fed.

In the hospital, Ray received a series of shock treatments. In those days, the grand mal seizure precipitated by the electrical charge through the brain caused considerable muscle tension, so much so that physical injuries, from strained muscles to broken bones, were not uncommon. Ray's back was never the same after his first treatment. The shock therapy seemed to help, but at what cost, neither Ray nor his doctors could tell.

The VA medical board reviewed Ray's illness and determined it was service-connected. That decision ensured that my father would have access to a VA "safety net" for those times in the future when he needed hospitalization or would be unable to take care of himself.

During a long rehabilitation period, Ray used his occupational therapy time to create a game called Strategy. In it, players amassed land, air, and sea forces, and, when they had accumulated enough forces, launched an atomic bomb to wipe out the opposing forces. He was later to get a patent on the game. It was during this period of hospitalization that my father decided to utilize the GI bill and pursue a career in teaching. Five years later, he obtained his BA from Fresno State College with a 3.8 GPA.

A different kind of upbringing

Even though my childhood was not typical, there was a period of relative stability during my elementary school years. My father taught high school and worked as a California State Park ranger in the summers. He served in leadership positions in the Westminster Presbyterian Church in Fresno. He was also a team leader for 4-H classes in forestry.

I have fond memories of this period of relative normalcy with my father. I remember the thrill of spending days with him at Millerton Lake in the Sierra foothills northeast of Fresno, where he worked as a park ranger; the fun of riding with him on the tractor as he plowed our family orchard west of Fresno. I remember the summer when he organized our 4-H club to transplant trees after a forest fire near Sequoia Lake west of Fresno, and the "kick the can" games he organized on family camping trips.

But this period of stability and happiness was over by the time I entered eighth grade in 1957. It was then that Ray had the first of what would be a long series of hospitalizations for depression, each one lasting anywhere from two to four weeks. The shock therapy resumed and was continued, with increasing memory loss. Sometimes he couldn't talk at all. Then he would be sad and thin, almost a stranger. He would catatonically shuffle up and down the hall in the VA hospital in Fresno like a zoo animal pacing the perimeter of its cage. Sometimes he was so catatonic that he didn't move at all. During those times, he was oblivious to the world around him. But there were different times as well, times when he talked fast and didn't listen. He was very happy and fat then, yet also a stranger. Which of these men was my real father, I used to wonder. The man who was sad and thin or the one was irrationally happy and fat? Over the years, in the course of visiting him in the hospital when he was depressed and in jail when he was manic, I came to realize that my father was both of these men, as well as the teacher, farmer, forest ranger, Sunday school teacher, and church elder.

But even back then, when I was just a boy, I knew in the back of my mind that my father was different and that life with him was like walking along the edge of a precipice. When I was in the eighth grade, our family took a vacation trip to San Francisco. My father and I walked out onto the Golden Gate Bridge. I felt a kind of low-key, irrational fear as we walked. I glanced over the railing and looked down at the same silhouette of a body I had looked up at two hours earlier when we had taken the tour of Fort Point, a virtual replica of Fort Sumpter located under the San Francisco side of the Golden Gate Bridge. Our tour guide had informed the group with a kind of macabre relish that a suicidal person had crashed through the wooden roof of the fort. Whether I was looking up or down at the silhouette, I could still make out the pattern of arms, head, and legs where the person had crashed through the wooden roof. According to our guide, the man had jumped at night and missed the water but had succeeded nonetheless. As I thought of all the others who had successfully jumped through that seductive "Golden Gate," their destination the same regardless of whether they splashed into the cold, foreboding waters of San Francisco Bay or not, the realization struck me that I could be walking back alone. The subtle, haunting, persistent fear that crystallized inside me at that moment never left me for long; in fact, I realized as well that I had been feeling it for some time already, only without being able to put it into words. It was a kind of "precipice-dread" that would visit me on and off throughout my life. Even when things seemed stable, I knew they really weren't.

During my high school years, from 1960 to 1964, I succeeded in keeping my school and church life in tight compartments separated from my family life. At school, I was the viola player, the choir singer, a guy who hobnobbed with the college-bound students. At church, I was the choir and youth group member. At home, I was the son of a man whose increasingly poor judgment was threatening his employment at Tranquility Union High School, about 30 miles west of Fresno. Ray had taught there for 10 years. As I was finishing high school, preparing to begin life as a college student at Westmont College in Santa Barbara, my father's life was unraveling, thread by thread.

Starting in 1963, Ray began seeing bright lights that he interpreted as divine in origin. These powerful visions brought on profound oceanic feelings of connection with God. From what I now know, these experiences, and their perceived religious significance, were most likely manifestations of a kind of temporal lobe epilepsy, which is similar to both psychomotor epilepsy and complex partial seizures.

Epidemiological studies of epilepsy have found that psychotic symptoms occur about ten times more with these kinds of seizures compared to generalized epilepsy.[1] One researcher found that six of 12 consecutive bipolar patients had temporal lobe symptoms with symptoms of hallucinations with aura-like qualities. These included "olfactory hallucinations, visual misperception, déjà vu or mystical experiences, spontaneous anxiety, fear or rage, ideational viscosity (grandiose or self-deprecatory repetitive thoughts), driven speech, forced thoughts, memory blanks and depersonalization."[2] Another researcher found that 10 percent of patients from a clinic devoted to the treatment of affective disorders such as bipolar illness had what he called subictal affective disorder, one criterion of which he described as "brief euphorias, often with beatific religious colorations."[3]

To Ray, these transcendental experiences were a message from God. It was a message to change the world . . . starting with the educational system of California. That same year, 1963, he "founded" an "organization" he called California Teacher Association-13, or CTA-13. The purpose of this organization was to restore Christian values to the California schools. But CTA-13 remained an organization of one. It existed only in Ray's brain.

Ray's attempts to bring his message to the world coupled with his inability to perceive himself accurately in a social context, led, in 1964, to what was essentially a forced resignation from his teaching job during my senior year in high school. Like the prophets of old, Ray was becoming a suffering saint. His resignation did not dissuade him from further efforts to accomplish his "mission." If anything, it propelled him forward. He selected aspects of his religious faith that seemed to encourage his role as the "suffering saint," a term he, interestingly enough, used to address his children and our pets. "Are you a suffering saint?" he would ask, blissfully unaware of what we in the trade call "projective identification"; that is, projecting internal thoughts and qualities onto others. He became depressed.

At that time, psychiatrists treated depression with tricyclic antidepressants such as Elavil and Tofranil, a class of drugs now known to increase the cycling of moods for bipolar patients. Their attempts to treat Ray's depression probably increased his frequency of cycling between manic and depressive states. His several series of shock therapy treatments, while they didn't do much for his memory, did seem to help him to recover from his depression ... until the onset of the next cycle.

In 1966, while a sophomore at Westmont College, I read an article in *Life* Magazine about how Jack Dreyfus, a bipolar patient and the founder of the brokerage firm that bears his name, had discovered that Dilantin, an anti-seizure medication, helped him stabilize his moods. The drug was believed to reduce excessive reactivity of nerve cells, or neuronal excitotoxicity. I shared the article with the VA psychiatrist who was caring for my father during one of his hospitalizations, and he agreed to give it a try. It helped my father to get over his depression. I hoped that the Dilantin would help him get better control over his unstable behavior. Eventually, the Dilantin would be replaced with lithium, then Tegretol, none of which materially affected his gradual, relentless downhill slide.

My sister Judy and I, like so many children from families affected by mental illness, gravitated toward the helping professions. However, she stopped her occupational therapy training abruptly after being stalked by a patient for four terrifying months. She decided to become an art major instead. As for me, after finishing my undergraduate degree in psychology, I completed the training for the Peace Corps, only to decide that I wasn't ready to organize the barrios of Colombia after all, and took a job at the Seattle Mental Health Institute in Seattle, Washington. I began attending graduate school at the University of Washington School of Social Work in September, 1969.

While I was attending graduate school, Ray was teaching in the remote town of Herlong, California, not far from Susanville in the northeast corner of the state. Like most small towns, Herlong was a community in which unusual behavior stood out, providing grist for rumor mills that have voracious appetites. So it was that Ray's idiosyncratic views and behaviors became a cause for concern and gossip. I never heard all the specifics of the allegations, except through my father. I didn't really want to hear them; I was trying to establish my own identity as far removed from his as possible. Overt misbehavior was never the issue. The issue was the effect of his psychiatric illness on his ability to function as an effective teacher. After teaching there for two years, Ray's contract was not renewed. His conflicts with school administration officials and parents, his religious preoccupations and his repeated hospitalizations eventually led to the loss of not only his job but also his teaching credential.

After my sister and I left home and established ourselves, my mother told us she was going to divorce my father. She needed a life away from the precipice. She had the choice of staying with a sinking ship or finding a lifeboat for herself while there was still time to get some pleasure out of life. My mother chose the lifeboat. She had once saved Ray's life. Now she needed to save her own. She divorced him in 1969. It was crystal clear to me that in spite of the different medications, my father's prognosis was not improving as I had hoped it would. During the Christmas break of 1970, I stopped to visit him in Susanville on my way to visit my mom and her new boyfriend,

Dick Harrison, a bee keeper and farmer, as well as, coincidentally enough, an educator who had served as a school superintendent in Southern California. They would be married in July of 1971.

I drove through Northern California in the pelting rain in my little red Opal Kadett and arrived in Susanville at about 9 in the evening, where, in spite of the rain, I finally found my father's apartment. I suspected something was wrong when it took several minutes for him to come to the door and open it. While I was waiting, my suspicions were confirmed: In the faint porch light, I saw a poignant, hand-painted cardboard sign propped on a window sill. The sign read, "Counseling: Will pay one dollar." My father was in such dire straits that he was willing to pay anyone a dollar in order to counsel the person. The best I can figure it, he was sick, but if he could be well for someone else, then he would feel well. It was as if he had a bad cough and offered to pay a dollar for the privilege of treating another with the cough medicine. He projected illness onto others whom he would then counsel, as a way to assure himself he was well. By now, Ray had lost his teaching job in Herlong and was barely able to function. The next day, I drove him through the pouring rain to the VA hospital in Palo Alto, where he was again admitted.

In March of 1971, I obtained a Master of Social Work degree from the University of Washington. I found a job with the municipal probation department of Seattle and waited to see if I would get drafted into the Army or be able to obtain a commission in the Air Force. It was either one or the other. Meanwhile, I had resigned myself to the fact that my father's prognosis was poor. He could not keep a job. He would require intermittent hospitalizations for the foreseeable future, perhaps even for the rest of his life.

While the focus of this book is on the bipolar odyssey, I did have another life apart from the one revolving around my father and precipice-dread. I met Gayle Peterson at Whitworth College in April of 1970 on my first — and last — blind date.

In July of 1971, I received a commission into the Air Force as a First Lieutenant and received my first assignment to Travis Air Force Base in California, where I worked as a clinical social worker in the mental health department. How ironic that I should begin my Air Force career at the same base from which my father had been discharged in 1946, the year I was born. Seven months later, Gayle and I were married, and thus began an adventure that would take us almost around the world.

Since my mother was out of Ray's life, it fell upon me to watch over him. I already knew that his life would be sandwiched between periods of incapacitating depression and ill-fated jousting at windmills in the style of the fictional character Don Quixote.

And I, like a faithful Sancho Panza, would walk beside him along the precipice, trying to pull him back without falling over the edge myself.

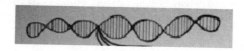

Notes

1. Gibbs, F.A., Dibbs, E.L., *Atlas of Electroencephalography*, Vol. 2, <u>Epilepsy</u>, Addison Press, Cambridge, Mass., 1952.

2. Lewis, D., Feldman,O., Greene, M., Martinez-Mustardo, Y., "Psychomotor epileptic symptoms in six patients with bipolar mood disorders," *American Journal of Psychiatry*, 141:1583-1586, 1984.

3. Himmelhoch, J.M., "Major Mood Disorders Related to Epileptic Changes," In: D. Blumer, (ed.), <u>Psychiatric Aspects of Epilepsy</u>, American Psychiatric Press, Washington, D.C., 271-294, 1984.

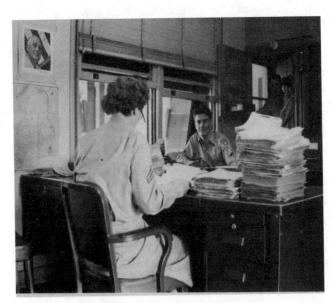

SSgt Ray Moyer - 1944 at Pearl Harbor

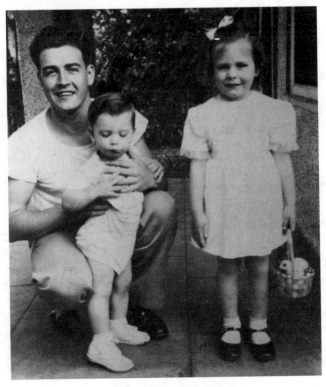

Ray, Author, Sister (Judy) at
Orange Avenue home - 1947

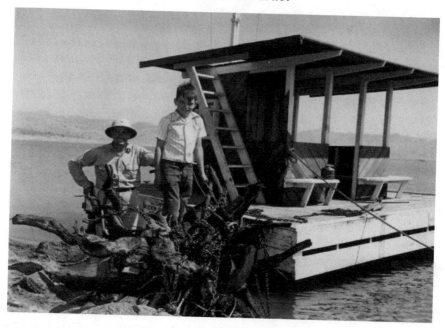

Father and Son - Millerton Lake 1954

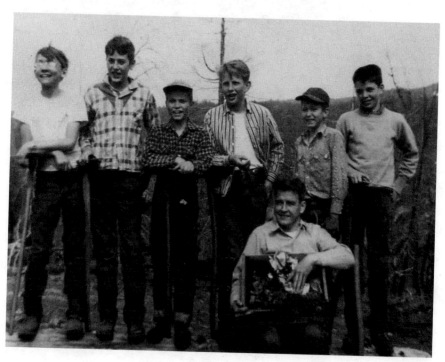

4-H Reforestation Project - 1957

3 - The Trip

It was four in the morning on June 25, 1984, when the Greyhound bus drove into Shasta, California. Among its passengers was a jovial, portly, overly friendly 67-year-old man wearing dirty, faded-blue overalls and old, scarred, leather shoes. He was a man on a mission.

Old friends meet

After sitting for ten hours on a bus that smelled of vinyl, smoke, and human sweat, Ray was last in line to step off the bus. He had a pack on his back, a suitcase in his right hand, and a large paper bag in his left. The pack held important papers, the suitcase contained clothes, and the paper bag bulged with assorted amenities ranging from horehound drops to underwear, as well as $85 worth of books he had bought in Seattle just a few days earlier. He had been visiting our family while we vacationed with family and friends there. Gayle and I had tried to get him to take his lithium, but he had refused.

As the last of the diesel fumes from the departing bus drifted away, Ray inhaled the cool, early morning mountain air. He felt that "good to be alive feeling" he had felt so many other times in his life. He walked toward the brick bus station, but the door was locked, and the lights were off. After circling the station and still finding it closed, he walked down the main street of town. Mt. Shasta looked gray and colorless in the early dawn, a dark silhouette against the lightening sky. The stars were starting to flicker out. Ray looked unsuccessfully for a telephone booth along the empty street. While walking toward the main business section of town, half-whistling to himself, he found a bench near a gurgling stream in a city park. He lay down on the bench and closed his eyes. This was the first time he had closed his eyes since he had started his trip thirteen hours earlier in Seattle. With all those people on the bus to talk to, he'd given no thought to sleep. He didn't need much sleep anyway, not when life was so good to him.

The rising sun over Mt. Shasta cast long shadows over the landscape. Ray heard the soft sounds of sneakers as a jogger ran nearby. He sat up and rocked forward several times to get momentum, then pushed his hefty body off the bench. He looked to his left and saw a beam of light breaking out of the clouds to touch the top of Mt. Shasta. The reflection on the snow-capped mountain seemed to sparkle. "The light shines in the darkness, and the darkness has not overcome it," he muttered to himself. The rest of the mountain was still gray. He walked in search of a pay phone with his own unique gait, leaning to one side, legs spread apart as if to balance his bulky frame to the asymmetry caused by a radical mastectomy some years before. He found a phone booth at a Chevron gas station a block from the park. He got out his address book and dialed. The phone rang for a long time.

"Hello?" said a sleepy-sounding voice. It was 6:15 in the morning.

"Hi, this is Ray."

"Ray who?"

"Ray Moyer."

"Ray Moyer…? Oh, Ray Moyer." There was the sound of a breath, and the voice suddenly sounded more awake than it had a moment before. "Why, Ray Moyer! I haven't heard from you in, gosh, must be at least fifteen years."

"I'm on my way to Santa Barbara to see Aunt Clara."

"Oh, how is Clara? She must be old now."

"She's 84. Had some problems with her sight — glaucoma, I think — but all in all she's in pretty good shape. She's in a nursing home now, but she can't afford it. That place is sucking her dry. You still got that old room and board place, Norma?"

"Sure."

"Well, I thought I could check it out, see if Aunt Clara could live there."

"Where are you calling from, Ray?"

"The Chevron station."

"Chevron station?"

"Yeah, by the park."

"Oh, you're here in town. It's sure nice to hear from you. I would love to see you. I can pick you up in 45 minutes."

"You have a lovely park here with a beautiful stream. I'll just sit and watch the scenery. Mt. Shasta is beautiful this early in the morning. Besides, I have some papers I need to work on."

Before Norma could say good-bye, Ray hung up the phone. Whistling to himself, he strode back to the bench, sat down, got some papers from his backpack, looked at them briefly, put them back, lay down again, and closed his eyes.

Norma quickly dressed, stepped into her 1979 Chevy, and headed toward Shasta. As she drove into town, she thought about the boy she had grown up with in Napa and the man who had last dropped into her life ten, or maybe it was 15 years ago. Though their families had been close, neither she nor anyone in her family had seen or talked to Ray Moyer for years. She had often wondered what had become of him. It was a little strange to hear from him out of the blue like this, but Norma knew how much Clara had always meant to him. Of course he would want her in good hands.

She parked near the creek and walked along the grass toward the stream. No one was there except an itinerant sleeping on a park bench. She wandered in that direction, thinking she would ask if the man had seen anyone walking around the area.

The Trip

The man sat up on the bench and spoke loudly while Norma was still about 50 feet away. "You sure got a nice town here — fantastic view of Mt. Shasta, and the people are real friendly, too. I met a man on the bus who lived here all of his life. He told me that he wouldn't live anywhere else unless he got paid to. And there was this kid, couldn't have been more than one year old, he was riding all the way from Portland to see his grandma down in Redding."

Norma tried to keep the shock from her face. "Ray, you have changed so much since I last saw you!" The Ray she had known was heavy, but this man was obese. And the clothes he was wearing ... He really did look like a homeless person.

Ray rolled himself up from the bench. "I got a joke for you. There was this terrible boat wreck out of San Francisco Bay, and all the passengers jumped overboard with life vests on. Sharks ate all but one of them, a lawyer. When the sharks were asked why they left the lawyer, they said, 'Professional courtesy.'"

She laughed self-consciously. "So, how are you and Ruth?"

"She believed, thanks to some lawyer, that I had gone astray at Pt. Arena."

Norma was taken aback, but she recovered gracefully. "How did you find me after all these years, Ray?"

"After the lies they made up against me it is no wonder Ruthie divorced me."

She tried to recover again. She didn't know where Ray was going, but she could tell that something was wrong with the man she had once thought of almost as a brother. After so many years, she did not want to rekindle their old friendship on a negative note. This time she spoke a little louder. "So tell me Ray, how did you find me after all these years?"

"If that lawyer hadn't told those lies to Ruth, we would still be married today."

Norma walked to the park bench. They both sat down, Norma towards the end and Ray in the middle. She was not sure she wanted her old friend in her car with the windows rolled up. As they sat there, he talked about his experiences with lawyers who had betrayed him, women who had made up and spread lies about him, and police and judges who had treated him unfairly. Norma felt herself pulling away from her old friend.

He talked about a lot of things, but none of them were connected to the few questions she was able to squeeze in during his rapid-fire monologue. Since Ruth had left him, he had lived in the VA domiciliary in Oregon. He had lived in a board-and-care home in Roseburg. He had run for the local school board to clean up corruption in the school system but lost after a reporter wrote an unfavorable story about him: all lies. He had spent a few months in the Roseburg County Jail after knocking some trash cans down at the home of the superintendent of schools. He proudly announced to a flabbergasted Norma that he had actually been banned from the city of Roseburg by a judge. The reason? "It was because I was onto that lying school superintendent Anderson, and they didn't want the truth coming out."

Everything was He, He, He, but it wasn't funny for Norma. She was starting to get frustrated. Having worked with older residents in her board and room facility, she was used to caring for those on the margins. But this was her old school friend from childhood. She certainly had not expected this. Even though he had dropped in out of the blue during previous visits, even though he had hinted at problems before, she had always been able to have a decent conversation with him.

"Well, Ray, do you want to see the Mount Vista Board and Care Home?"

"Aunt Clara just might like it there."

Norma took that to be an affirmative response. "Okay," she said. "Let's get in the car." She morphed almost effortlessly into the role of professional caretaker. It was her job, and she was good at her job.

They walked to the car, got in and headed for the board and care facility, where she was caring for 17 older men and women. Norma rolled her car window down and turned the heater up to counter the cool early morning air. Ray talked about the CTA/OEA-13 organization he had founded to reform the school systems of Oregon and California. CTA/OEA-13 was a combination of the California and Oregon Educational Associations and First Corinthians 13, the famous chapter in the Bible on love. Having been raised in the same culture as Ray, she knew he was talking about the chapter that began, "Though I speak with the tongues of men and of angels and have not love I am become as sounding brass, or a tinkling cymbal." It ended with, "And now abideth, faith, hope, and love, these three, but the greatest of these is love." Ray was the secretary of the organization, which, he told her, consisted of hundreds of citizens concerned about the decline of morality in the educational system. Perhaps Norma would like to become a member? There were no dues. He would just mail stuff to her. She just listened and tried to make sense of it all. By the time she got home, she was exhausted. She stopped trying to ask questions.

It was such a strange way to reestablish an old friendship. As he explained his misadventures, one after another, he talked as if he were proud of the very accomplishments that any other person would want to keep secret. Norma wondered how Ray could be so sure of himself and so many others could be in the wrong.

"Well, Ray, here we are. Feel free to talk to our guests about the place if you want to. There is an extra bed in this bedroom if you want to spend the night. You must be hot from your long trip. You might want to take a shower here," she hinted. She pointed toward the bathroom. "Here are some towels." Ray didn't take the hint.

Ray told his stories and jokes to many of the residents, most of whom were too old and frail to object to his intrusive behavior. Then he took a long walk in the neighborhood. Later in the evening, after dinner, Norma tried again to engage him in conversation. This time she managed to learn that Ray had found her by calling her brother in Sacramento, but after her discovery of that morsel of information, he launched into another monologue just as difficult to follow as the last. She went to bed early that night.

The next morning, Norma drove him to the bus station. On the way, he told her the one about the time God was checking out heaven and discovered a hole in the fence along the border with hell. "So God called the devil to complain about the hole in the fence and make sure it was fixed promptly. The devil said he wasn't going to do anything about it. When God told the devil he was going to sue, the devil replied, 'Where are you going to get a lawyer?'"

She didn't laugh this time, but it didn't matter. They were at the bus station at last. As he was leaving the car, she asked, "Is there any way I can get ahold of Ruth?"

"Oh, she's in Fresno," Ray said. "Got married to a guy named Dick."

"Thanks Ray," she said as he removed his knapsack, suitcase, and paper bag from the back seat. She watched him make his way toward the bus, then called after him: "If Aunt Clara wants to come here, let me know."

He boarded the bus as if he hadn't heard her.

The charm that she remembered so well in her shy and winsome childhood friend was gone, replaced by an insensitivity that was truly alarming. He seemed disconnected from others in a way that reminded her of some of the residents at the board-and-care home. This wasn't the Ray Moyer she'd grown up with, or even seen at various points in his life. All that talk about religion made her think about his mother, Rose. She'd always been crazy that way. And after coming all this way to look into alternate arrangements for Aunt Clara, he hadn't even bothered to find out how much room and board would cost at her facility.

Only trying to help

The Greyhound bus pulled into Tulare at 7:15 p.m. Ray rolled out of the bus seat and carried his things to a restaurant near the bus station, where he ate dinner. He wandered into the Windsor Hotel. He had never stayed there before, but the price was right. After he paid the 22 dollars to the clerk, he went up to his room and lay down for a short nap. Ray had a habit of not sleeping or staying in one place for too long. For one thing, he had written in his CTA/OEA-13 mailings about certain drug activities of which only he was aware. He was concerned that he, like a certain deputy sheriff of Mariposa County, might also end up at the bottom of a lake with his feet tied to a concrete block.

Too Good To Be True?

At 10:15 p.m., he woke up and decided to take a walk. He took his paper sack filled with assorted things and walked out onto the main street of Tulare. While he strolled in the sultry summer night air, he became aware of feeling dirty. It had been several days since he had cleaned himself. He came to a city park still occupied with late night revelers. He found a men's restroom. He walked in, took off his dirty clothes, washed himself, put on clean shorts and a shirt he had in his bag, washed his dirty clothes in the sink, put the same clothes in his bag, and then headed out the door. Throughout this ritual he was mindless of a parade of visitors through the restroom who watched him and looked at each other, scratching their heads. What the man was doing wasn't illegal — or was it? Whatever the legality, it was strange. Ray walked out wearing Bermuda shorts, a short-sleeved shirt that was not tucked in, and his old shoes.

Three blocks away at the Martinez household, teenager Patricia Martinez lay down in a makeshift bed on the kitchen floor next to her brothers, Roberto and Arturo. Earlier, the family had celebrated Patricia's 16th birthday with a party. Her uncle, Manuel, had brought some melons from the field for the family to enjoy, and the sweet smell of the fresh melons lingered in the room. The little house only had two bedrooms, and tonight Manuel and his wife were guests, so Patricia and her two brothers were sleeping on the kitchen floor. They went to sleep quickly, exhausted from the day's festivities.

At 11:30 p.m., the sound of a door opening aroused Patricia from her slumber. She sensed a presence moving toward her in the dark. She felt paralyzed with fear, unable even to make a sound, not quite sure she was awake. Suddenly a hand touched her shoulder. She awoke fully, eyes wide with terror, a silent scream in her throat. Her brothers slept on.

A voice whispered out of the darkness. "I was out walking, and I noticed that your porch light was on and your door was open. I came in to find a phone so I could call the police, but since you are here I won't have to. You need to keep your door locked and your porch lights off."

As quickly as he had appeared, he was gone. She hurriedly awoke her brothers and parents and told them what had happened. They ran outside. No one was there. Had it all been a dream?

Ray walked on until 4 a.m., when he began to feel sleepy. He returned to his hotel room and lay on the bed. He felt proud that he had warned the girl of the dangers of leaving her door open and the lights on after dark. But he began to worry that the girl might not tell her parents. While waiting for sleep to come, he resolved to go back and make sure the girl's parents had gotten the message.

He opened his eyes at 7 a.m., checked out of the hotel, and bought an afternoon bus ticket to Santa Barbara. He wanted to have enough time to go by the house and talk to the girl's parents. He left his suitcase but took his bag and backpack with him, retracing his steps from the night before. He walked up to the house and knocked at the door. Mrs. Martinez answered.

"Hello ma'am, I'm Ray Moyer. I am on my way to see my Aunt Clara, who's in a nursing home in Santa Barbara. I'm going to find her a better place to stay that won't cost as much. I was out walking last night, and I noticed your outside lights were on, and the door was open. I was afraid that someone could break in, so I stopped to tell someone. At first I was going to call the police that the house was empty, but when I found there were people sleeping, I woke a girl and told her about the door and the lights being on, so I didn't have to call them after all."

Mrs. Martinez, who had been listening with growing apprehension, loudly called for her sons. "Arturo, Roberto!"

Her two teenage sons and her husband appeared at the front door. Patricia followed.

Mrs. Martinez excitedly yelled again. "This is the man who came in the house last night with no clothes on! Call the police!"

"That's what I was going to do last night," Ray explained to Mr. Martinez, "but I didn't have to because I told your daughter, and I wanted to be sure she told you, but I wasn't sure she would, so I came by to warn you that your door was open and the outside lights were on."

Mr. Martinez and his sons grabbed Ray. "Mister, you are going to stay here until the police arrive." Ray tried to pull away, to no avail. In five minutes, the police were there.

One of the police officers introduced himself as Officer Sanchez. He asked Mr. Martinez what happened.

Mr. Martinez spoke. "Officer, last night this man came into our house with no clothes on and woke my daughter. She was terrified. Now he's coming back again."

The officer asked Ray what he was doing there.

With some bewilderment he explained. "I was going to see my aunt, who is in a nursing home in Santa Barbara. I'm trying to find her a cheaper place to live. I was walking past here last night, and I got concerned when I saw that the door was open and the lights were on. At first, I was going to try to find a phone and call you, but then I found that she" — he pointed helpfully to Patricia — "was asleep on the floor, so I told her and left. Then I came back today because I wasn't sure if she would tell her parents about it or not."

Officer Sanchez had heard enough. "Mr. Moyer, you are under arrest."

Ray was charged with sexual battery, attempted rape, and attempted burglary.

The next day in Little Rock, Arkansas, where I had meanwhile returned from our Seattle vacation, I received a call at home.

"Is this Major David Moyer?"

"Yes."

"This is Frank Loza. I'm the public defender in Tulare, California. Your father was arrested yesterday for walking into the home of a family during the night. He's facing some serious charges: sexual battery, attempted rape, and attempted burglary."

"Oh, no!" I groaned. "You've got to be kidding. My father has some serious problems, but he's not capable of anything like that. Whatever he did, those charges are ridiculous."

"He's in serious trouble."

"Obviously, but I know him better than any cop, and whatever he did could not possibly justify charges like that."

"The family alleges that he walked into the house with no clothes on and that he touched their 16-year-old daughter."

"What did he say?"

"He said that he was wearing shorts with his shirttail out and that he went in to warn them because they left their door open."

"So the most they can prove is that he trespassed and may have touched the girl to wake her up."

"Perhaps, but he may not be able to stand trial because of his mental state."

"Listen, I appreciate your calling. I'll do whatever I can. My father has bipolar disorder. He's more a risk to himself than he is to anyone else. I agree that his behavior cannot be tolerated. There's a chance he could get himself hurt, but he needs to be back in Oregon under the care of the VA. He certainly doesn't have any criminal intent and doesn't need to be treated like a criminal. I can't do much from Arkansas. Would it help if I came out?"

"There's nothing you could do here. Until the trial, there will be no findings of fact. Up until then there will be some court appearances to determine if there are grounds for keeping him, and the allegations are enough to assure that, then a hearing where he will plead guilty or not guilty."

"How about if I wrote a letter to the judge explaining the kinds of difficulties he's had in the past?"

"OK, but you'd better make it good, because it looks like the charges are going to stick."

"That would be a real shame. There's no reason for the charges to stick. First of all, Mr. Moyer is not dumb. He has a master's degree in English. He taught high school for years. No one that smart is going to create such a dumb alibi. It's just too dumb to be true, unless it's coming from a bipolar patient who actually believes it. I'm sure that he really meant it when he says he was going in to warn the family. This kind of poor judgment is very consistent with his history. I hope you can get this dropped or at least get the charges reduced to something more reasonable."

"I'll do what I can."

I sent the best character reference I could write. I cited my father's involvement with his church, his employment history, names of his friends who could verify his moral integrity, and then gave a detailed history of his psychiatric illness, describing his eccentric, but harmless hypomanic behavior and his poor social judgment. I described our attempts to get him back on lithium when he visited us in Seattle and recommended he be put back on it. I asked some of our family friends who knew him while I was growing up, and they agreed to write letters verifying his moral integrity. I asked his VA doctors for letters, but they did not want to get involved.

I was concerned, but Ray was not new to the criminal justice system, which had more or less treated him fairly up until now. Well, maybe banning him from the city of Roseburg was a little constitutionally suspect, but his behavior had been a problem for the authorities. His prolific letter-writing certainly hadn't helped. I was confident that once the facts were known, he would either be put in a hospital for a time or sent back to the VA in Oregon for treatment. At the worst, he might have to serve a little time for trespassing, but I figured there were worse places than a jail for him to be. Little did I know.

The pretrial hearing was a perfunctory hearing where the judge decided whether to hold Ray over for trial. According to Ray's lawyer, no findings of fact would be allowed at that hearing. When Ray went to this hearing three weeks after his arrest, he was confused. He couldn't understand why anyone would object to his efforts to help the family. He believed it was his responsibility to walk into a house in the middle of the night to inform the residents that they could be robbed. The defense did nothing but listen to the charges by the DA, and Ray was held over for another hearing to hear his plea. To me, this would have been a good time for Mr. Losa to say, "Sir, there has been a huge misunderstanding." But then I didn't know how the system worked.

Ray was hypomanic, almost as impaired as if he had been psychotically depressed or manic. He had no sense of boundaries. He couldn't accurately perceive himself in a social context. What was in his head was all he could respond to. He was unable to behave appropriately in the real world. The illness that he had was much more than just mood swings. As significant as they were, it also involved judgment-impairing brain damage that increased over time based on the number and severity of his manic episodes.

After the hearing, in jail, Ray angrily refused to button up the trousers that were issued to him. He argued that they were too small. Given his compromised state of mind, he was unable to understand the risk in talking back to the authorities. A guard named Benchfield, in front of other guards, pummeled Ray, hitting him in his stomach and back with his fists. After the beating, more sympathetic guards gave him bigger trousers so he could button them more easily.

Because of his fear of Benchfield, Ray decided he would do what he could to get away from him. Not having the ability to make appropriate long-range decisions, he figured that anything would be better than having to face Benchfield again. A psychiatrist assigned to the task of determining his competence to stand trial wrote the following after he tried to interview him.

> *When Mr. Moyer was brought to the interview room, he came in, sat down, did some sign language, did not speak. He wrote on a piece of paper that he has "Aphasic," and that this had been present for "8 hours only." He wanted to write out things on a piece of paper. I did not want to conduct an interview by having him write out answers to my questions in longhand. I told him that he did not have aphasia and that he could talk. Right after that he did talk in gibberish. At other times during the interview, when he was trying to communicate with me by writing in the air with his finger, he would sometimes say the word softly, but audibly, so that I knew that he could speak if he wished to do so.*

> *I explained that if he were not competent to stand trial, the judge would probably commit him to Atascadero State Hospital for treatment, and he clapped his hands. I then went on to explain that he would still come back to stand trial on the charges against him when he was competent.*

The psychiatrist knew that Ray was putting him on and declared he was competent for trial even though his hypomanic behavior would be a problem. Years later, Ray's explanation for his bizarre behavior was simple. He wanted the psychiatrist to know that the entire episode was a farce that he refused to take seriously. Unaware of the long-term consequences, he was actually angling for incompetence, and in that respect was doubly incompetent.

Apparently, his defense team was able to get a "deal" from the DA if Ray agreed to plead guilty to the "lesser" charges of "sexual battery and trespassing." Ray would have none of it.

Several months later, in December, 1984, at a hearing to plead his case, he shuffled into the court in chains and stood before the judge, who read the charges to him.

"You have been charged with sexual battery, attempted rape, and intent to commit burglary. How do you plead?" asked Judge Allen.

Ray spoke:

> *Hebrews chapter 4 verse 12 says, "Only the Lord is quick and powerful, and sharper than any two-edged sword, piercing even to the dividing asunder of soul and spirit, and of the joints and marrow, and is a discerner of the thoughts and intents of the heart." None of you is able to know what my intent is. In 30 seconds, I am going to do something, and none of you knows what it is. You cannot claim that I intended to rape or burglarize just as you cannot now claim to know my intent.*

He waited a few seconds, then methodically lifted a pitcher of water from the defense table and poured the contents on the floor. The judge asked the bailiff to usher Mr. Moyer out of the courtroom. He slowly shuffled out, chains clinking with each small step.

On December 19, 1984, my father was found to be legally insane and unable to stand trial within the meaning of Sections 1368 et. seq. of the California Penal Code. The statement read as follows: "It was therefore adjudged that Ray Moyer is an insane person. He is to be delivered to the Sheriff of Tulare County to be transported to said Atascadero State Hospital to be cared for as provided by law; and that upon his becoming sane, be redelivered to the Sheriff of Tulare County for return to the above-entitled court." He would remain there until March 1986.

Apparently, in the Kafkaesque world of the legal system, my father was sane enough to rationally consider pleading guilty to lesser charges, but not sane enough to go to trial on the original charges.

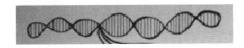

4 - Into the Gulag

Since sending my first futile letter to the judge, I waged a fruitless campaign from Arkansas to get the charges against my father dropped or reduced. Describing Ray's history of difficulties with boundaries when he was hypomanic, and piecing together more information about the incident, I wrote letters to the DA and the judge. I discussed Ray's honorable motives for his admittedly bizarre behavior, trying to paint a broader picture of his character and the incident — in the context of an illness called bipolar disorder over which he had no control. However, my efforts were to no avail. I never even knew if the letters had been read.

When I realized the implication of Ray's being committed, I flew out to Fresno and drove to Tulare, where I had an unproductive talk with Mr. Losa, the public defender. I then retained a private attorney, Mr. Gelding, to represent my father. Mr. Gelding didn't seem too concerned that my father had been committed, nor did he seem to think that a travesty of justice was being perpetuated against him. Though he didn't say it, I imagine he thought that anyone dumb enough to walk into someone's house in the middle of the night deserved to be put away. The complexities of mental illness seemed beyond his comprehension.

I assumed that the legal system was stuck in its own black/white bipolar understanding of my father's bipolar behavior. I wasn't sure who was the sickest: Ray, who did not have the judgment to negotiate a plea to a charge like trespass and simple battery, or the "system" that had erroneously charged him with enough felonies to put him away for the rest of his life. That Ray Moyer's affliction with bipolar illness had impaired his judgment and was continuing to do so was apparently irrelevant. It didn't matter that he was a person with a positive record of civic and community functioning when he was not hypomanic. Because he was deemed incompetent to stand trial, he had been jailed and sent to a state hospital, one that was frequently the final destination for confirmed sexual predators. My father would spend almost two years incarcerated without a trial. During that time, his physical and emotional health would markedly deteriorate.

Going in circles

In 1985, I received orders to move to Castle Air Force Base near Merced, California. Actually, it would be more appropriate to say that our young family received the orders, since they had to go wherever I was sent. That family now included our son, Chris, age 10, daughter Kathy, age 8, and son Thomas, age 4.

The month before we left Arkansas, I phoned the Martinez family to see if I could set up an appointment with them. I spoke with Mrs. Martinez briefly, and she agreed to meet me to discuss my father's situation. Mr. Gelding had strongly objected to my contacting the family, but I wanted to meet them to get their views of what happened and also to explain my father's history and his illness. I did not think they knew much about bipolar disorder.

Late in the hot afternoon of August 18, 1985, the Moyer family caravan turned off the freeway and headed towards Tulare for one last "pit stop" before going on to Castle Air Force Base. I drove our huge rental truck and Gayle drove our Lindy motor home. We parked in front of the Martinez's house. It was an admittedly ostentatious introduction. I would have liked to wear my uniform to enhance my credibility, but Air Force officers had standards to uphold, one of which was to keep a clear boundary between our personal and professional lives, and I was good at keeping things compartmentalized.

I wanted the Martinez family to see that Mr. Moyer also had a family, that he wasn't just some homeless criminal without roots. I wanted them to know that he had grandchildren. I wanted them to know that my reasons for meeting them were important enough that we were willing to make this visit our first activity as we arrived in California to take up our residence. We climbed out of our respective vehicles, and I introduced my family and myself to the Martinez family.

We cordially chatted on the lawn while the kids entertained themselves. We talked about the incident and what had happened to my father up to that point. While speaking to them, I learned that they knew nothing about bipolar disorder. Without such an understanding, they had no way to understand his behavior except in a criminal context. When I explained his story and asked for their permission for me to produce a videotaped interview, they agreed. After we had been at the base for several weeks, I returned and interviewed them with my video camera.

In the interview, I asked open-ended, journalistic-type questions. They reviewed what had happened that night and agreed that, in the darkness, their daughter had mistaken Ray's intentions and state of dress. They proffered that they did not believe my father had any suspect motives for his highly unusual behavior, and they did not want to see him punished. Without the Martinez's testimony, the court had no case. I gave the taped video interview to the District Attorney (DA), bypassing Mr. Gelding, who had strenuously objected to my actions. As a matter of fact, Mr. Gelding had informed me that if I talked to the "victims" to get the story straight, the DA could charge me with interfering with an ongoing investigation.

I had been trying to learn the rules, but the justice system wasn't my world. I incorrectly thought that by hiring a lawyer and illuminating the facts of the case, the court would reduce the charges and my father would get out of the hospital, or at least into a less restrictive environment. However, my plan to sort this out with the Martinez family and the DA did not fit in with how the system worked. I had engaged the services of Mr. Gelding for a $2,000 retainer with the expectation that he would actively defend my father. Instead, Mr. Gelding made a few cursory phone calls and took a single trip to Atascadero State Hospital. He didn't seem at all interested in the fact that the charges were inappropriate for the crime. There was a club, and I wasn't in it. The club consisted of the judge, the DA, and the defense lawyer. I thought that having all the facts on the table would make a difference. I was naive. The DA never got back to me about the tape.

A trip to Atascadero in the fall of 1985 proved equally fruitless. When Gayle and I saw Ray, he was already significantly depressed. The state-employed social worker who I hoped would be open to looking at the facts of the case did not see patient advocacy as part of his job description. After all, weren't all of the patients "innocent"? I reluctantly concluded that my attempts to influence events were futile, and, in the final analysis, what was going to happen was going to happen with or without my efforts.

By April 1986, it had been almost two years since my father had been jailed and almost one year since I had given the DA my videotaped interview with the Martinez family. On April 18, I was in court waiting to see my father again. Through no efforts of my own, he had been sent back to Tulare to face the judge again. There would be no trial because he was in worse shape now than when he had been arrested.

"Ray Moyer case," said Judge Allen.

A thin, frail-looking old man with a beard and long hair cautiously stepped into the courtroom from the side door, his chains dragging along the floor, his eyes furtively glancing around the room. The bailiff pointed him towards a chair. The man appeared confused. He didn't look like my father.

The judge began to speak while the prisoner tentatively shuffled to his chair. "As I understand it, the hospital sent a report back stating that he is not competent to stand trial. They didn't say what they recommended, but I assume they are thinking of a conservatorship."

Ray slowly sat down in the chair. Judge Allen looked at the two lawyers representing Mr. Moyer, public defender Losa and Mr. Gelding.

"Are you both attorneys in this case?"

Mr. Gelding responded deferentially. "Yes, your honor. I am here to assist with a conservatorship if the court chooses to go this way."

"Your honor," said Mr. Losa, "we wish to recommend that the charges be dropped and that Mr. Moyer be transported back to Oregon so that he can obtain inpatient care at the VA hospital at Roseburg. I asked the DA to review the file, but they haven't had a chance to yet."

"Well, we will have to see what the DA says about that," said the judge.

"We also request that he be hospitalized pending final disposition per the recommendation from the hospital."

"I understand it is hard on these patients who are sometimes mistreated by other prisoners, but our mental health people won't admit him for more than a few days. I'll see what can be done. In the meantime, I will ask for an evaluation regarding a conservatorship. We will meet April 23 after the recommendations are completed. Next case is The People versus Peter Johnson."

Nothing I had done had appeared to help. And nothing had been resolved or would be for almost another week at the earliest. I was concerned about the delay and how Ray would manage in jail while waiting for the next court date. The jail doctor expressed concern to me about his weakness and lack of eating, telling me that Ray was no longer able to take care of his personal hygiene.

Perhaps I was an outsider in the world of the legal system, but in the mental health world, I was an insider, or at least enough of one to get a hearing. I lobbied long and hard with the Tulare County community mental health professionals to get Ray into a hospital instead of the jail while we awaited further developments. They agreed that he belonged in a hospital, and made it happen. Two days later, he was transferred from jail to the Valley View Psychiatric Hospital in Tulare.

The family

I awoke early on April 20. The bedroom was dark. I heard a sound in the distance. The only other sounds were of Gayle breathing beside me and the ubiquitous distant sounds of the columns of cars and trucks traversing the North-South route through California on Highway 99. Even the sounds of revving jet engines from the base were absent. I turned over and tried to get back to sleep, but my mind whirled with thoughts, trying to solve an unsolvable puzzle. I heard the sound again. It was the faint sound of an animal mooing. I lifted my head from the pillow and heard it again. I wondered where it was coming from. There were no farms with cattle nearby that I knew of. I heard another moo. Actually, it was more like a bellow. There was a plaintive quality to the sound. I got out of bed and opened the north window and listened. The sounds repeated at intervals of about half a minute. They seemed to be coming from the direction of the local high school. I returned to bed with an uneasy feeling in the pit of my stomach. I tried not to think about what was happening at the meat packing plant just north of Atwater High School.

The morning was a long time coming for me. I couldn't get the image of the helpless animals out of my mind. I kept hearing, or imagining that I was hearing, the faint echoes of their bewildered bellowing. We had lived at this house in Atwater for more than one year, and I had never noticed those particular sounds before.

I tossed and turned until 8:15. Outside the window it was a beautiful spring day. Too nice a day to feel so crummy. Gayle was waking up. I decided to follow the advice of Dr. Bob Goulding, who at that time was a well-known psychiatrist on the West Coast. He had shared a technique at a workshop I had attended. The technique could be used to help our clients, or ourselves to manage or reduce anxiety. He told us all to take a walk in the grass early in the morning and observe the glint of light off the grass, smell the fresh morning air, and feel and hear the sound of our feet stepping through the grass. I didn't have an expanse of grass, but I had a swimming pool.

"How about a morning dip? I turned the pool heater on yesterday, and the temperature is a good 73 degrees."

Gayle turned over.

"OK, I've got a better idea. Why don't you sleep in, and I'll go swimming?"

I put on my swimming trunks, walked down the hall, and greeted the kids, who were watching Saturday morning cartoons.

"Morning," I said with feigned heartiness. There was no response. "I said, 'Good morning.' Anyone want to enjoy a morning swim with me? The pool is up to 73 degrees now."

Thomas spoke up. "No thanks, Dad."

"At least I know that one of you is awake."

I walked out on the patio and dove into the pool. The water enveloped me and I stopped thinking. I focused on the feel of my hands gently slicing through the surface. It was just the water and me. No other thoughts seemed important. After a number of laps, I breathlessly walked up the pool steps and felt the rush of the cool morning air. My version of the Goulding solution had worked ... or so I thought. But as I started to dry off, the precipice-dread returned.

I yelled to Kathy through the screen door. "Don't you have a track meet today? When does it start?"

Fifteen seconds passed. "Kathy, Dad is talking to you," said Thomas.

"This morning," said Kathy.

"When this morning?"

"9:30."

"Well, we'd better get going then. I want the TV off until you're all dressed and ready to go." I walked into the kitchen. Gayle was fixing breakfast.

"Did you know you can hear the sounds of cattle being slaughtered at night over at that meat packing plant by the high school?"

She flipped the pancakes. I wasn't sure if it was our recently announced fourth pregnancy or the ongoing troubles with Ray that was responsible for the silent treatment. Breakfast that morning was quieter than usual. The kids didn't argue over who got the biggest or the most pancakes. Kathy didn't even complain that Chris had put too much syrup on his pancakes, even though the plate was practically overflowing. After the meal, I said to her, "Kathy, I wish I could stay for the whole track meet, but this is the last time I can see the Martinez family and Grandpa Ray before we see the judge again. The Martinez's said they would testify as to what happened. They might help get Grandpa Ray out of jail. Actually, he's in a hospital now, so we are making some progress."

Gayle spoke, "But this is the biggest sporting event of the year for Kathy! You know she's representing Elmerwood in the all-city track meet."

"I didn't say I wouldn't come. I just said I couldn't stay for all of it."

"This has been going on for weeks now, Dave. You don't do anything with the kids because you have to write another letter. You can't help Chris with his homework because you have to call another psychiatric nursing home. You can't watch your daughter run in the biggest track meet of the year because you have to go see your father. And I don't remember the last time we did anything enjoyable together."

"But if I don't help him now, he'll go downhill even faster."

"You didn't make him go into that girl's home. It isn't your responsibility to keep him out of trouble."

"You know as well as I do that he went into that home because he was hypomanic."

"You guys are going to get a divorce," intoned Kathy.

"Kathy, we are not getting a divorce!" I exploded. "OK, Gayle, what do you want me to do? Shall I just write my father off and let them send him back to Atascadero to rot with all the sex offenders there? Or maybe they should send him to some chronic psychiatric nursing home. I guess he could rot just as well there as at the state hospital."

"For all the time and money you've put into this fiasco, you have nothing to show for it except some video of a mother and daughter saying they don't want to press charges, and their original recollections weren't totally accurate. That video didn't change anyone's mind. I doubt if anyone even looked at it. Why do you keep beating a dead horse? The DA is going to do whatever the DA wants to do, regardless of what you do. It's like you don't even live here anymore."

"You know I'll be back after this is over."

"Right, if there's any family left," she said. "So you get the charges dropped and become his conservator, then what? You follow him around for the rest of his life trying to undo all the future messes he makes?"

I tried to point out how badly he had deteriorated. "I don't think he's going to bounce back from this one. He's aged at least ten years. You haven't seen him since he came back from Atascadero. The doctor at Valley View says he can't even keep his clothes dry. There's no bounce left."

"We'll see."

At the meet, I watched Kathy's team come in third in the relay. I left at 12:15, before she ran the 100-yard dash.

The visit

Two hours later I drove into the parking lot at Valley View Hospital for the first time, got out of my car, and walked to the entrance. I pressed the doorbell, and a loud buzzer answered. I pushed the door open and walked inside.

"Can I help you?" asked the duty nurse.

"I'm here to visit Mr. Moyer."

"Please sign the register. He's in the day room, but he isn't talking much. The attendants were able to get him to hit a pool ball this afternoon, though."

I walked into the day room. Chairs were lined up all along the wall. Two long tables were set end to end in the center of the room. Several patients were sitting, all keeping to themselves. I spotted my father sitting by himself in the far corner. He was dressed in hospital clothes with no shoes on. His shoulders and head were slumped forward in the chair. His chin rested on his chest. His hair was long and tangled, and his face had several days of stubble on it. His eyelids were tightly shut.

His picture was on a plastic jail tag on his left arm. There wasn't any of that "FBI's most wanted" look, just an old man, a very old man. The tag identified him as a criminal who, after almost two years of incarceration, still owed society for the crime of walking into a house to tell the residents they had left their door open, or, rather, the crime of being concerned enough to return to the scene to make sure his message had been heeded. I sighed and blinked.

I sat down in a chair about fifteen feet away and watched. What could I say to him? What did we have in common any more? I wished I had stayed at the track meet. I could still leave, and he would never know the difference. I thought of his disorganized, poorly articulated manic plans, which never had a chance to be realized even though he couldn't understand why. I thought back to his numerous letters, his ill-fated candidacy for the school board, his arrest in Oregon for knocking over the trash cans of the superintendent of schools. I thought of all that he had said and done before the police, the DA, and the judge had confined this emaciated Don Quixote to a state mental hospital.

Ray's ideas and behaviors were not normal, but were the needs driving him any different than my own, or anyone else's for that matter? I tried to imagine what he would say if he were hypomanic again, and if he could suspend his mental disorganization long enough to present his thoughts coherently. For a few seconds, I tried to imagine him as he saw himself, addressing his followers who, although they only lived in his head, would, in his eyes, have easily filled a stadium to hear his pronouncements.

I am Ray Moyer. I have a vision. I am going to transform the educational system of California and Oregon so that our children receive a basic education and learn the universal moral values. Through my organization, the CTA/OEA-13, we will encourage teachers to practice the love that is described in First Corinthians 13, love which is slow to anger, seeks to be constructive, is not touchy, and is glad when truth prevails.

Some say I am an idealist. So were the prophets in the Old Testament. And why not? It was Browning who said, 'Ah, but one's reach should exceed his grasp, else what's a heaven for?' There are some who do not understand what we are doing. They are liars and hypocrites, every one, the conniving school superintendent, the bought judge, the lying police. Justice is turned away backward and justice standeth afar off. What Isiah said 2,800 years ago is as true today as it ever was. In spite of this, I shall continue to speak the truth and, in the immortal words of Winston Churchill, shall "nevah, nevah, nevah give up."

We shall go to jail, commit civil disobedience; we will do whatever is necessary to accomplish our goals. Our children are our most valuable resource. We shall not stand by while corruption exists in the school system and our childrens' moral instruction is compromised in words and deeds, even as the crooked officials in Oregon conspire with the Tulare DA to silence me, even if the drug cartel does silence me. Though my voice be silenced, I am a teacher, a prophet, a stubborn old cuss. I am a school board candidate. I am a part of the family of man. I am a part of the whole. I am Ray Wilber Moyer.

I came back to the present, reached into my hip pocket, and pulled out a folded piece of paper that he had mailed to me from Atascadero State Hospital before they made him depressed. I had brought it with me, thinking that it might cheer him up. On it were the words he had written right after he had been declared incompetent to stand trial.

Take his honor off the hook.
The team says Ray M is a kook.
We have goofed; we wish to clear
Our honor, solemn, costly, dear,
Of charges that we made a mess.
But rascal Raymond won't confess
To trespass, so without debate
We'll pack this half-wit with the state.

I put the poem back into my pocket. The man sitting across from me was in no position to be entertained. I walked over to him and touched his shoulder as I pulled up a chair in front of him.

"Hi."

There was no response.

"Do you know who I am?"

After a long pause, he spoke in a whisper. His eyes stayed shut. "No."

I rubbed his shoulders and back, feeling protruding bones.

"Are you sure? Why don't you guess?"

There was another long pause, then another whisper. "Leon?" His eyes still would not open. I stopped rubbing his back.

"No. What did they do to you at Atascadero? Maybe it would help if you opened your eyes."

Ray opened his eyes and looked steadily at mine. I looked into his. No one was home. His eyes were bloodshot, and his eyelids looked too heavy, as if they were somehow weighted with lead, requiring herculean efforts to let in the light. I thought he looked as if he had been crying. Maybe that was why he closed his eyes so tightly — to hold back the flood. He looked down at the floor. What had they done to him?

"Now do you recognize me?"

"No."

"I'm David, your son."

Still there was no hint of recognition. I kept trying to get him to acknowledge me, hoping to elicit some kind of response. When that failed, I decided it was time for 20 questions.

"Do you remember your daughter's name?"

After a long pause, I heard a whisper. "Judy?"

"How about Judy's son?"

There was another long pause.

43

"Eric?"

"Good, how about her daughter."

Silence.

"Do you remember Debby?"

"Yeah, I think so."

I asked if he knew the names of my family members and was pleased when, after some effort, he identified Gayle, Chris, and Kathy. He couldn't remember Thomas's name, but nonetheless I was relieved to learn that he could still think, albeit slowly.

I tried to make small talk. "I heard you played some pool this afternoon."

No response.

"Did you know that you're going to be a grandfather again? Gayle is expecting in October."

"No." He looked up for a brief moment, then looked back at the floor. I continued my one-way conversation.

"I haven't given up getting the charges dropped. I called Mrs. Martinez and asked if I could come by today to talk with her and Pat. I'm going to see if they are willing to come to court to testify that they don't believe you were trying to hurt Pat. Then maybe we can get this whole thing dropped."

I wasn't sure he understood me.

"In any event, we are going to ask for a conservatorship. They haven't got us licked yet."

No response.

A too-cheerful nurse said in a too-happy voice, "Ray, would you like some delicious fried chicken?"

"I guess I'd better go," I said. "I have to see the family before it gets too late."

I shook his hand. I noticed a faint grip as our hands met. "See you Thursday."

On my way out, I was encouraged that he had seemed to be responding a little better towards the end of my visit after that sluggish start. When he had been catatonically depressed, nothing would get his attention. He wouldn't move or talk. But today, he showed some recognition and talked a little bit. Was he depressed? Was he brain damaged? Was he drugged?

I hurried out the door. I didn't want to get to the Martinez family after dark. But suddenly I whirled around in the parking lot and walked back. I pressed the buzzer again. At the desk, I asked to speak to the head nurse. I waited until she appeared.

"Ma'am, I forgot to ask you something. Is there any chance my father is on some medications?"

"Yes, your father is taking 5 mg of Haldol twice a day."

"Haldol, you've got to be kidding! My father is depressed enough without knocking him out with Haldol. No wonder he's so out of it. That's the dose you give to a young schizophrenic. My father is 69 years old and severely depressed. Didn't your doctor read the narrative summary from Atascadero? They took him off all medications before sending him here."

"Well, our psychiatrist thought he looked a little paranoid when he got here, the way he was looking around. So I guess he didn't want to take any chances."

"A confused, scared depressive is a hell of a lot different from a paranoiac."

I began another recitation of my "explain-the-patient-to-the-mental-health-professional" routine. No, Ray never shifted back to manic behavior overnight. No, he had never been dangerous to anyone but himself, unless you consider knocking over a trashcan dangerous. Excessive use of medications was one of the reasons he'd become so depressed at Atascadero State Hospital. That was the reason they took him off all medications before he arrived here. No, he didn't hurt anyone. Yes, the family had volunteered to drop all the charges, and I had them saying so on videotape. And yes, he went into the house, but he did this to tell the family that they had left their door open. Yes, he really did. Yes, he was hypomanic at the time and not taking his medications, but he had been faithfully taking his lithium when he had been briefly jailed in Oregon for knocking over trash cans. And were there any other questions I could answer?

The nurse said she would discuss this with the doctor. I had heard it all before. I was used to it. I was getting less angry about it all the time. I could imagine the note she would write of our visit.

"Patient's son walked up to charge nurse in a hostile, agitated state, claiming his father had been overmedicated with Haldol and demanding the dosage be stopped." They all knew that the apple didn't fall far from the tree.

Why should I have expected a mental health professional to perform an independent assessment of my father's mental status? Ray was a suspected criminal. The tag attested to that. Why should they read the narrative or delve into his depression? I tried to think on the bright side. At least he wasn't in jail getting abused again. The only straightjacket he wore in the hospital was a chemical one.

Crazy making

I arrived at the Martinez home later than I had planned. It was already dark. I parked the Volvo in front of the house. Three young men were sitting on the steps in front of the house. They were speaking Spanish.

"Hi. Are Pat and her mom home?"

"She don't want to talk to you, man." It was Arturo.

"I called and asked if I could come over, and your mom said I could. When I saw her two years ago, she said she would do what she could to help my father. He needs help now because the DA hasn't dropped the charges. They still have him."

"Well, she don't want to talk to you, and she don't want Pat to talk to you. They are tired of talking about your father."

Arturo stood up. So did his friends. I took the hint.

"OK," I said. I started to walk away.

As I was leaving, Arturo said, "And she don't want you to come back."

I got in the car and drove off. When I called earlier, they had given their permission for me to come over. What had gone wrong? Had the DA put pressure on them not to change their testimony? Was the DA covering his tracks to avoid a wrongful imprisonment suit? Did the family now think that Ray was dangerous? Maybe they just didn't want to be bothered. Well, neither did I, but I had no choice.

As I drove north on Highway 99 toward Atwater, I tried to make sense out of my roller coaster day. For Ray, Valley View was not a hospital, but a holding cell, albeit a better one than the jail had provided. In the jail they beat the prisoners who gave them problems. In the hospital holding cell, they drugged them before they could give them problems. The medical staff was acting on behalf of the state for the purpose of socially controlling deviant persons whose behavior didn't fit in.

I thought of all the well-meaning, not-so-well-meaning, and just-plain-incompetent professionals, those at Valley View, Atascadero State Hospital, the jailers, the judge, the police, and the defense attorneys. I was putting the little pieces together and starting to form the big picture. It was all coming together now. They were all parts of the American Gulag, a human processing factory that took human raw material, sorted it, and then disposed of it. The factory provided social control of individuals whose behavior didn't fit into accepted social norms. Compassion, understanding, treatment, and amelioration of suffering were not for those patients who were part of the Gulag. The mental health professionals were keepers of the Gulag as much as the police and the jail guards.

But wait a minute. Wasn't this how my father thought? Didn't Ray see the big picture, too? Didn't he claim that the drug cartel, the corrupt school administrator, and the lying police were all purposefully out to get him? And then hadn't they done just that? But my father was mentally sick, a manic-depressive. Bipolar patients often have paranoid delusions similar to those seen in paranoid schizophrenics. They become paranoid because they have no boundaries or limits. They continually push the limits until they can feel the world impinging on them. Then they feel, often correctly, that the world is not only pushing back but is also out to get them. It was as if Ray had no internal brakes and no awareness of the impact of his behavior on others. I was just glad that I was a mental health professional and therefore able to clearly distinguish reality from fantasy. I just needed to just understand why the Gulag was after my father.

Halfway between Tulare and Fresno, I started to chuckle to myself. The irony of it all got to me. The chuckle turned into a belly laugh, then tears started flowing down my face. I began to feel a combination of anger and deep pain from within demanding to be released. While gripping the steering wheel with all my might and driving down Highway 99 at 80 miles an hour, I found myself screaming a wordless protest to the cordial keepers of the Gulag who were persistently and effectively draining the life from my father as surely as the employees at the meat packing plant in Atwater were draining the life from the bellowing bewildered cattle.

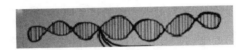

5 - The Burning Man

In May 1986, I was appointed by the court to become Ray's conservator. The conservatorship essentially put me in charge, at least on paper, of his living arrangements and his finances. I would pay for his care, give him money as needed, and try to maintain some sort of vigil over his activities. I never learned what happened to the charges against him; all I cared about was that my father was "free at last." I found a nursing home for him and completed the necessary paperwork.

In the nursing home, Ray stayed on his lithium, but was quickly taken off the Haldol. He rapidly began to improve, too rapidly, in fact. In two weeks, I transferred him to a board and care facility for elderly adults in Merced, where his appetite, energy level, and weight quickly returned to "normal" ... for him.

Back to old tricks

Gayle was right. I was wrong. My father's fire wasn't extinguished yet. As she had predicted, he quickly returned to his hypomanic state even while regularly taking his lithium. Soon Ray was ready to pursue his impossible dreams again. Even though I remained his conservator, four months after his release he left the board and care facility and moved to a shack in the foothills of Mariposa. He had always preferred the foothills to the San Joaquin Valley. Among other things, he wanted to maintain a watch on the drug trade up there. There was no arguing with him. He was impervious to logic, and the deed was already done. He soon came back to new versions of old obsessions. He planned to undo all the wrongs that had been done to him.

In the wee hours of the morning on September 14, 1986, Ray pondered the numerous letters spread out on the table, the bed, and the floor of his small, one-room shack. The forty-watt bulb in the rusty floor lamp given to him by a neighbor illuminated the darkness just enough for him to read. There was the letter to Mr. Garrett, an attorney, soliciting his legal help in suing the cities of Roseburg and Tulare and Atascadero State Hospital. There was a letter to me, his conservator, demanding that I send a $120 check to the U.S. District Court in San Francisco to initiate the lawsuit. There were various letters to state and federal officials estimating the total judgment he sought. The figures ranged from $300,000 to $1,000,000.

Ray had initially demanded that he be paid only for the false imprisonment and mistreatment in the jail and hospital. However, now he was asking that the parties to the suit repay the Veterans Administration for the disability pay he had received secondary to the loss of employment caused by a

49

litany of allegations lodged against him when he was teaching in various high schools. Thus far, the battle had not gone well. At my request, Mr. Garrett had sent my father a written opinion on a number of legal issues in an attempt to help him realize what he was up against. Was there any basis for a suit? No, the justice system can't be sued; otherwise, district attorneys would not be able to act freely against would-be criminals. Was Mr. Moyer financially responsible to pay the $20,000 for his stay in Atascadero State Hospital? Yes, unless he could prove that he couldn't afford it. His guilt or innocence was not at issue as long as the procedures followed had been in accordance with the law. If the city of Tulare or the Police Department could not be sued for false arrest or police brutality, could a particularly abusive jailer by the name of Benchfield be personally sued? No, usually a guard didn't have the funds to justify a suit, and besides, it was the word of the guard against the word of a mentally-ill person deemed incompetent to stand trial. Could the hospital or hospital personnel be sued for precipitating a major depression with ill-advised combinations of psychotropic medications? There was no evidence of permanent disability from this, nor could my father prove that the combination of Haldol and lithium had precipitated his depression. From a legal standpoint, the score was criminal justice system, "10," Ray Moyer, "0."

Ray got out his chess board and started to play a game against himself. In four moves, he had the black queen in a fool's mate. He spoke out loud in an excited tone. "I'll wear them down until they listen to me. I'll get justice through the back door if I have to, but I will get justice. I will light a fire under them to get some action."

He sat down at his typewriter and typed the following words, a new chorus to *America The Beautiful*:

> *Bureaucracy, bureaucracy,*
> *God put some zip in thee.*
> *Reduce thy waste,*
> *Improve thy haste,*
> *Move with alacrity.*

The plan was starting to come together now. He continued typing into the early hours of the morning. When he had finished, he put his work in an envelope addressed to the *Mariposa Herald*. He moved his papers from the bed to the floor and lay down to sleep, confident of the justice of his cause and of his ultimate victory. Waking at the first light of dawn, he skipped breakfast and went right to work. The area around his shack at 3rd and Bullion was overgrown with dried weeds and the stumps of trees that had been cut for the motel that was to be constructed later that year. Ray had wanted to clear the area for some time. It was a fire hazard. Now he could remove the fire hazard and also make a statement that would get his cause the recognition it deserved.

He picked up his hoe from under the foundations of the shack and walked to the front yard. He began hoeing a foot-wide firebreak in the shape of a circle around the yard. He worked diligently for two hours and then stopped for a mid morning snack of hominy grits and beans. After his brunch, he filled two buckets with water and took them down to the yard. He checked the wind direction. A faint breeze was blowing from the Northwest. He lit a match to the grass on the downwind side. Within seconds, crackling flames surged through the grass. Billows of smoke poured from the lot at 3rd and Bullion — right over to the house just southeast of his shack. There Mrs. Ethyl Tetrick was watching "Days of our Lives" when she smelled the smoke and looked out her kitchen window.

"My Gawd, that crazy fool has started a fire! John, call the fire department."

Her husband, John, didn't hear her. He was taking his daily nap.

"John, Ray Moyer started a fire!" The snoring continued.

"Well, if you're not going to do anything, I am. You would sleep through your own funeral!" She dialed 911.

"Emergency response. Is this an emergency?" The voice was very calm.

"Yes, a fire here right next to our house. It's coming this way. Please hurry!"

"Ma'am, I need your address."

"1320 Bullion, right up the hill from the green shack at 3rd and Bullion."

"Is that in Mariposa?"

"Of course it's in Mariposa! Please tell them to hurry."

Sgt. Travis was the first to respond to the call. Ray had been expecting him.

"Morning, Mr. Moyer." By now everyone in the local police department knew Ray Moyer. "We got a call on this fire. You know you have to have a fire permit to burn here."

"I used to be a forest ranger for the State of California. I know all about fire permits," Ray testily responded.

"Then I guess you have a permit."

"Of course I have a permit. I've had it for some time, ever since you gave me that ticket a few months back for trying to reduce the fire hazard around here. You know, if everyone burned the surplus underbrush during the spring, we wouldn't have these huge forest fires in the summer."

Ray handed him the permit.

The sergeant looked it over. "I'm sorry, Mr. Moyer, but I'm going to have to issue you another citation. This permit is only good for the late afternoon."

"I've already taken care of that. I sent a letter to the paper telling them that the worst breezes are in the late afternoon. Told them I was going to start in the morning."

"Sir, they have nothing to do with this. The fire department enforces the policies, and it says right here that you are to start any fires in the evening. I'm going to have to issue that citation."

The sound of fire truck sirens cut through the air, punctuated by the blast of a horn. Two medium-sized trucks drove up and parked. The firemen began their coordinated attack. Within seconds, a hose was in position. The man on the truck, in response to the signal from the man at the nozzle, pulled a lever, and water shot out in a 15-foot stream toward the flames.

The fire had almost burned itself out anyway. Where the grass had been was now ashes. Two tree stumps were still burning. The firefighters quickly put out what was left of the fire. Ray and the sergeant returned to their conversation.

"Here, Mr. Moyer. You need to sign this part of the citation. You're not admitting guilt. You're simply acknowledging receipt of this ticket. You may choose to pay the fine or appear before the judge on the date indicated and explain your reasons to him."

"I won't sign."

"Mr. Moyer, you have to sign. You are not admitting guilt."

"You can take me to jail if you want to, but I'm not going to sign that citation."

"Very well then, Mr. Moyer, come with me."

Ray walked over to the garbage can and picked up the clipboard he had left there, then walked along behind the detective.

Mrs. Tetrick had been watching the entire spectacle from the edge of her property. As Ray rode off towards the jail, she quickly ran inside her house and woke up John to tell him what had happened.

The firemen stayed until the charred stumps stopped sizzling. After he was booked, Ray went to his cell and began writing very intensely. Because he was so well-known to the officers, they allowed him to keep pen and paper.

Once again, I got a call from the police, this time while I was at work at the Mental Health Clinic at Castle Air Force Base.

"This is Major Moyer."

"Sir, we have your father down here at the police station."

"What did he do this time?"

"He started a fire without a permit and wouldn't sign the citation acknowledging receipt of it."

"OK, thanks for calling. Would it be okay if I come up tonight to pick him up? We can keep him at home for a few days." I knew the police of Mariposa quite well by now and had been impressed with their professionalism. Sure, one of the patrolmen had once told me that he could arrest a person for just about anything he wanted. I already knew that. But none of them had tried that with Ray.

Non-Expectation Therapy

When we picked Ray up, he had filled four pages with very small hand written text. Though surprised that they had let him keep a pen in his cell, I was also relieved; it meant they understood that Ray was a harmless eccentric for whom they could bend the rules. Ray greeted Gayle and me by launching into a diatribe about his lawsuit and how he was now, at last, going to get the attention of the authorities. We took him to a restaurant to eat.

By now I was too resigned to be angry. I knew there was nothing I could do about Ray's frequent episodes of irrational behavior. Gayle was not as resigned.

"Ray, you think the whole world revolves around you. There are other people in this world who have lives besides you."

"Yes, but this is the only way to light a fire under them."

"All you can talk about are your feelings. You don't care about the impact of your behavior on the rest of us. You only care about yourself."

"There wasn't one honest person at the Tulare Police Department or Atascadero State Hospital, and I'm going to make them pay for it."

"How, by messing with our family?" Gayle retorted.

I agreed with her, but I also knew how futile it was to try to use logic. "Gayle, you're right, but you know that talking doesn't do any good. Ray has a one-track mind. He isn't going to understand you and respond appropriately. I'm frustrated too, but I just get more frustrated when I start to hope he'll be able to respond to us." I had no problem talking about him in this way although he was sitting across the table; I knew from long experience that Ray was incapable of processing whatever I or Gayle said in any meaningful way. He was as good as deaf when it came to meaningful dialogue, whether it was directed at or around him.

"You know, I think that when I retire from the Air Force, I'm going to found a new kind of therapy," I mused. "I'll call it Non-Expectation Therapy, NET. Maybe I can get permission to use Paul McCartney's 'Let it Be' for the NET's theme song. I can see it now. Thousands are coming to my workshop on NET at, let's see, Madison Square Garden. 'Let it Be' is playing over the loudspeakers as the faithful believers come to hear my words of wisdom. Television cameras are rolling. Tom Brokaw, Dan Rather, even Peter Jennings are there reporting live as it is happening. The credo of my therapy will be: 'Let it be. Let it be. Let it be. Let it be. There will be an answer. Let it be.' I am going to change the world."

53

She rolled her eyes and pursed her lips. Sometimes I enjoyed tweaking Gayle with my own manic fantasies.

Ray's attempts to "light a fire" under the bureaucracy were no more successful than his previous attempts had been. Only he grasped the logic of his actions. His internal reality was so strong that the reality of the external world had no affect on him. Alternative points of view or even negative feedback went in one ear and out the other, or, perhaps they never went in. As his tension increased with each failed attempt to redress the wrongs done to him, his need for action grew irresistible, despite the examples from the past where his behavior had only caused him more problems.

Yet the repeated failure of his frantic, impotent efforts never discouraged him for long. It really didn't matter that no one was listening, or that his lawsuit had no chance of ever being prosecuted. Just like the Man of La Mancha, he had an "Impossible Dream;" it was "to right the unrightable wrongs and fight the unbeatable foe." Only now, after Ray had developed an allergy to lithium, his medication had been switched to Tegretol, a drug similar to Dilantin that is used for control of epilepsy and found to be effective with bipolar disorder. He faithfully continued his appointments at the VA hospital in Fresno and religiously took his medication while merrily continuing on his hypomanic way, leaving those closest to him feeling helpless and frustrated, or increasingly resigned.

Meanwhile, Gayle and I continued raising our family. Our daughter Elizabeth was born. I was promoted to the rank of Lieutenant Colonel. Then, in the fall of 1988, I received orders to Clark Air Base in the Philippines. We considered taking Ray with us — for a few seconds. My father's needs, as important as they were, could not take precedence over those of my family and my career. I did try to block the assignment due to my father's situation, but my request was rejected. Therefore, I had to terminate the conservatorship.

We helped Ray move to Ukiah near the coast in Northern California before we headed overseas. He wanted to move closer to where he had grown up and to be nearer to the ocean. We hoped he would be able to manage on his own for the time we would be gone. Since he received disability compensation from the VA, at least we didn't have to worry about him becoming one of the homeless living on the streets.

At Clark Air Base, I served as Chief of the Mental Health Clinic, where, among other things, I successfully advocated a name change from "Mental Health Clinic" to "Behavioral Health Services." I taught sociology at the Central Texas College extension there and also served as the Consultant to the Pacific Air Force (PACAF) Surgeon, visiting and consulting with clinics throughout the Pacific region. While at Clark, we had to put up with assassinations, earthquakes, and — the last straw — Mt. Pinatubo, whose huge eruption in May of 1991 spread volcanic ash around the world. After almost two and a half years there, I was reassigned to Elmendorf Air Force Base in Alaska, where I served as Chief, Social Work Services.

In our absence, Ray eventually moved to a little town called Philo, California, in the northern coast redwoods, where he rented an apartment. He attended a little community church and made regular trips to the VA in San Francisco for his medicines. Without my oversight of his finances, he was free to spend as much as he wanted on whatever cockamamie schemes fit his fancy, and every last cent and more went to CTA/OEA-13 mailings to friends, strangers, schools, courts, newspapers, congress, and, yes, even the President of the United States himself. He borrowed $8,000 against his life insurance to support his habit. He also contributed to civic projects like the restoration of a crumbling bell tower in the historic community church he attended.

Ray continued to have mild scrapes with the law, one of which, as if to underscore his inability to learn from the past, involved burning without a permit. While in jail, he was diagnosed with adult onset diabetes and was started on oral medications to regulate his blood sugar. I give the justice system credit for that, at least.

In 1994, I was assigned to Beale Air Force Base in California, where I served as Chief, Mental Health Clinic and Family Advocacy. By then, Ray's energy level had declined so much that the acute manic episodes which had plagued him all his life had ceased to occur. He was 78 years old and had lost all of his teeth. Not having the executive skills needed to arrange to get false teeth from the VA, he managed without teeth, until we insisted he get some- and even then he would not use them. I had read that mercury in dental fillings and other heavy metals are one of many sources of bipolar-like symptoms. It was possible that the loss of mercury emissions from dental fillings could have accounted for the reduction of his severe manic behavior. I had also read that for older bipolar patients, the illness tended to burn itself out in response to the aging process.

Whatever the reasons, my father was no longer clinically manic or depressed, and he was off all psychotropic medications. His residual hypomanic beliefs and behavior persisted, however, and found expression in organizational mailings to hundreds of people and agencies. His social judgment remained compromised, but for the most part his eccentricities could be perceived by others as those of an elderly person used to living alone and grown set in his ways.

Not that he was doing well on his own. He wasn't getting arrested any more, but neither was he paying his bills or eating well. We had some fears for his safety on his frequent trips to Ft. Miley, the VA hospital in San Francisco. Once, a homeless person had accosted him and demanded money. My father had barked loudly at him and walked as quickly as he could across the street. He was oblivious to the risks of being alone in San Francisco. His encounter and his response to it disturbed us.

We brought him to Grass Valley, where he stayed for a short time in a board and care home. However, his eccentricities eventually proved too much for the residents and staff to handle. After much discussion, Gayle and I invited him to live with us. With our son Chris gone to college, we had room for him, and we hoped that he would become more grounded through involvement with the lives of our other children, Elizabeth, Thomas, and Kathy, who were at that time in elementary, junior high, and high school, respectively.

As my father settled into his new life with us in the gated, mostly retired community of Lake Wildwood, we looked forward to a time in our lives when we would not have to dread another late night or early morning phone call informing us of yet another bipolar crisis. We could monitor Ray's activities and provide the supervision that he needed to make his golden years comfortable and even enjoyable ... both for him and for us. And maybe, just maybe, we could all move away from the precipice-dread that had characterized so much of my childhood and adult life.

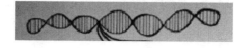

Part II - Perhaps

What we call despair is often only the painful eagerness of unfed hope.

George Elliot

6 - Visit to Another World

When we moved back to California in 1994, we left our eldest, Chris, with relatives in Seattle who saw him off to Whitworth College in Spokane, Washington. Chris enjoyed college and performed well academically. He was active in the college choir and several performing arts groups, having decided on a music composition major. Chris has always enjoyed music. Growing up, he played the piano, the clarinet, and the saxophone. He sang in his high school chorus and, in his senior year, was selected to sing in the Alaska All State Chorus, an experience that was to prove pivotal in his decision to pursue a career in music. He had enjoyed playing on the high school tennis team and acting in a school play, but his real love was music.

Missing the early signs

In September 1997, during his junior year at Whitworth, Chris became obsessed with the stock market, as did millions of Americans at that time. He relied on his own intuition, ignoring reliable sources and, of course, the advice of his father. Sometimes his friends tried to get him to go out with them to enjoy themselves, and he would stay behind to trade stocks online. The more he tried to find the big one that was going to assure his financial future, the more he lost. Ultimately he transformed a $4,000 investment into less than $1,000. Yet in those days of the Internet stock market frenzy, such behavior seemed less unusual than might otherwise have been the case. Magazines and newspapers were filled with stories of traders who had made fortunes doing the very same thing.

Chris experienced some mild depression at the time, not only about finances but over his future as a graduate with a degree in music composition. He was worried about his relationships with women. He felt as though he couldn't relate to others on their terms. Again, such worries are by no means uncommon among college students.

In his senior year, during his last semester of college, Chris met a girl, Joan, with whom he became infatuated. His sister Kathy, by now a sophomore at Whitworth, Darren, his roommate, and other friends advised against the relationship. They thought Joan was immature and manipulative. Gayle and I never met her, but if Kathy said she was immature and manipulative, that was good enough for us. Kathy was a natural-born therapist, with an uncanny ability to accurately read others. But Chris was smitten. He was so happy, it was almost too much. However, shortly after they "officially" began dating, he began losing confidence in himself.

Chris and Joan broke off their relationship just before he went to London for what was called Jan term, an intensive, month-long course of study.

He looked forward to the plays, the musicals, to visiting historical places in England. However, while there he began having trouble sleeping and became depressed. When he returned, he felt that he couldn't talk to his former girlfriend even though they had parted on good terms.

He called home one weekend in early February 1998. "I was on the phone with Joan, and I couldn't even talk. I feel so empty. We had so much to talk about. Now I feel so depressed, I can't even talk to her ... not even about simple things. I can't even talk to Darren any more. I don't know what's going on. I feel like I have nothing to say; like I'm empty. I can't sleep. I keep worrying about what I am going to do."

"What do you mean you can't talk?" I asked.

"I can't be myself."

"How can you not be yourself? Whatever you do is yourself. If you choose to withdraw and not talk, then that is you doing it."

I believed in self-responsibility. I had learned it from psychiatrist Dr. Robert Goulding and social worker Mary Goulding, among others. I thought it was the best model around. People needed to take responsibility for their own behavior and not blame it on something or someone else. It was a construct I had used effectively with many clients. It had become an article of faith for me. The person who believed he created his own world could perform much better in it than the person who believed that his world created him. I had found the concept useful for teaching people who abused their children and spouses. Their behavior was their choice, not a result of the behavior of the victim. My experience had primarily been in outpatient mental health settings where this model had appeared to serve my clients well. I thought the idea of self-responsibility might reduce Chris's anxiety.

"You mean I am in control of myself?"

"Yeah, whatever you are doing, you are the one doing it, not someone else. No one can make you not talk except for you. No one can make you anxious except for you. Now that doesn't mean you aren't depressed or anxious. It may mean that you are not aware of how you are making yourself depressed or anxious. It just means that you are in charge of what you do."

"I feel so empty, like I have nothing to say to anyone."

He proceeded to describe difficulties sleeping, feeling empty, social withdrawal and anxiety, some of the typical symptoms of depression. He was also describing the classic symptoms for a microbe-based brain disease far removed from my current understanding of mental illness, but I didn't know it then. To me he sounded like a college student experiencing some depression as he began to contemplate what would happen beyond the ivory towers.

Chris had always been the intense oldest son. He was bothered by things that didn't appear to bother his siblings. During the summers, I had been frustrated with some of his behaviors like reorganizing my computer and deleting files, but I had simply written this off to the fact that he was headstrong like his father. When I would confront him, he would act as if it was his perfect right to improve my file organization. I do remember a comment by a summer employer, praising Chris for his industriousness. He said that one reason Chris was so productive was that he was always on the go. The word "hypomanic" came to the back of my mind, but no alarms went off. The employer was praising his productivity.

"I don't know if it would help or not, but some of my staff members at work have been taking St. John's Wort for depression," I told him. "One of my co-workers says it helps her maintain a positive mood. It's an over-the-counter herb that is supposed to be helpful in treating depression. I don't know if it would help or not, but you do sound depressed. I tried it for a few weeks to see if it increased my energy at work but didn't see any benefit."

I had worked for the same "company" for 28 years and was nearing retirement. I had been functioning okay at work, but I knew that my heart wasn't in it any longer. I had hoped that taking St. John's Wort might help restore my enthusiasm, but after a few weeks without any noticeable change, I had stopped taking it, assuming that my increasing detachment was a normal part of the retirement process.

"St. John's Wort, eh?" Chris sounded interested. "I think I'll try it and see if it helps."

Unbeknownst to Gayle and me, Chris had started keeping a journal after his return from England. The journal dealt with the usual topics of late adolescence and early adulthood, but with a decidedly bizarre twist. He was writing about new discoveries, "new" religious insights. We were to learn later that he was spending an inordinate amount of time writing in his journal. The world he created there was not the world of a typical student. He wasn't to share that world with us until later.

Caveat emptor: St. John's Mania

Chris bought some St. John's Wort. He took three tablets a day as per the instructions. In three days, I got a call from Kathy.

"Dad, something's wrong with Chris. He isn't sleeping. He's super-agitated and talking about the end of the world. I think you need to come up here."

A thought from the back of my mind surfaced into my consciousness: It couldn't be possible that Chris had inherited that part of his grandfather's genetic makeup that predisposed him to bipolar disorder — or could it? I immediately made the necessary arrangements and flew to Spokane.

On the flight, I tried to calm my fears by sticking to the facts rather than speculating. Chris was manic; that much was obvious. I felt terrible. In my attempt to help Chris better manage what I thought was mild situational depression, had I helped to provoke an episode of mania? Was Chris taking the proper dosage of St. John's Wort? Who was to say what the proper dose was anyway?

I already knew that St. John's Wort had some mild antidepressant qualities and that it was not particularly helpful with major depression. I hadn't read that taking it could provoke mania. I regretted my recommendation, but it was too late to take it back now. Perhaps Chris was just having a bad reaction.

I had never expected that Chris or any of our other children would be afflicted with Grandpa Ray's illness. We had been a stable family. No one had died or tried to commit suicide. No one was a religious fanatic. All our kids were good students and responsible members of society. We were, for the most part, a stable family with no more peculiarities than most families ... except, of course, for Grandpa Ray.

In the imprecise world of mental health, where, in practice, biases were considered about as valid as empirical research and methods of treatment such as Transactional Analysis, Psychoanalysis, Gestalt Therapy, Scream Therapy, Rational Emotive Therapy, Behavior Therapy, and others sometimes appeared difficult to distinguish from religious cults, I did not have a solid grounding in the biology of mental illness. How could I? The problem was "mental," after all. I had a fuzzy understanding that when it came to the mystical connection between mind and body, mind was king. Attitude was everything. Sure, at the margins, there were biological conditions that caused severe mental illness — I couldn't ignore my father's illness — but for most patients there was always that undefinable "stress factor" that provided a missing link. One might say I had my own private delusion. Maybe it helped me to sleep better at night and keep my precipice-anxiety at bay.

When I arrived at Chris's apartment a few blocks from his college, I learned that he had not slept for several days. He spoke of an acute sensory awareness of colors and sounds. He had grandiose ideas related to a prophetic mission and the end of the world. He felt a need to warn the world that the end was near. He said he could smell sulphur.

I took him to billeting at nearby Fairchild Air Force Base, having made an appointment for him the next day at the mental health clinic. During the night, Chris lay awake, shaking. He told me that the demons were shaking his bed.

After a sleepless night, we went to the mental health clinic. I hoped to persuade the doctor to allow Chris to go home with me rather than hospitalize him. I knew all too well what the repercussions of a hospital stay with a diagnosis of mania could be, even if the mania was a reaction to St. John's

Wort. After interviewing both Chris and me, and obtaining the family history of Ray's bipolar disorder, the psychiatrist diagnosed Chris as Bipolar Manic, first episode with psychotic features, and recommended hospitalization.

I said that we could give him the medications at home and that he wasn't out of control or a danger to himself or others. The doctor agreed with me and prescribed 5 mg Zyprexa and 10 mg of Ativan at night. Zyprexa was a new drug, an atypical antipsychotic that was developed for the treatment of schizophrenia but which at that time had been used off-label for mania with great effectiveness. Ativan was a minor tranquilizer in a similar class as the ever-popular Valium. The doctor recommended using as little of the drugs as possible and advised us to seek psychiatric follow-up when we got home.

When I told the doctor that I thought St. John's Wort might have had something to do with Chris's mania, he said that he would send a report about the possible relationship to a medical journal. However, he was unwilling to suggest at present that what had happened was a one-time incident based only on the St. John's Wort. Rather, he believed that Chris's psychotic response to the drug was evidence of bipolar disorder, which would have eventually revealed itself with or without the drug. (In retrospect, given the delusional nature of Chris's journal writing, he was correct.) Still, at that time I did not want to hear this. I did not want Chris to face the rest of his life dealing with the same dreadful illness that had made his grandfather's life a living hell. I didn't want to face the rest of my life dealing with it either.

Chris flew home aboard a commercial plane with me. After a few days on the medication, his acute psychosis resolved, though he continued to experience some of the intense sensory aspects. He reported that colors were more colorful, sounds and smells more vivid. Gayle and I were amazed that his symptoms had cleared up so quickly on the Zyprexa. We assumed that whatever neurochemical imbalance the St. John's Wort had caused was now back in balance.

Two weeks later, a psychiatrist at Travis AFB gave Chris a clean bill of health and recommended that he go back to school. However, he also recommended that Chris stay on the medication. But Chris didn't want to continue taking the Zyprexa. He didn't need medicine, he said, and we didn't object, assuming — or perhaps "hoping" is a more accurate word — that the episode had been a transient reaction to St. John's Wort and not the onset of the dreaded manic-depressive illness.

Back at Whitworth, unbeknownst to us, Chris re-immersed himself in his writings and religious preoccupations. He wrote that the world was going to end soon. He wrote pamphlets and envisioned himself warning the world of the end times. Three weeks later, in March of 1998, he became visually disoriented, but managed to find his way to the apartment of his friend Darren. He told Darren that he wouldn't be around much longer. Darren and Kathy took him to Sacred Heart Medical Center, one of the largest hospitals in

Spokane. He was admitted involuntarily as a danger to himself.

During his hospital stay, Gayle and I maintained frequent phone contact with Chris. By the middle of the second week, he was starting to sound more like his old self. He was moved to a less-restrictive ward, where he composed some hauntingly beautiful music for the piano. However, one day he started talking about the end of the world again, leading us to believe that his psychotic thought processes were returning. I reported the change to a ward nurse, and the next time they gave him his medicines, Zyprexa and Depakote, an anticonvulsant, they discovered that he had been "cheeking" it — that is, keeping it in his cheek and disposing of it later.

Through some strange, little-understood alchemy, Chris's own body was producing drugs that made him "high." He didn't want to inactivate these drugs. He was both a producer and consumer of whatever drugs were churning through his brain, an addict with an unlimited supply. As far as Chris was concerned, the problems in his life were not neurochemicals. The problems were the hospital personnel and his parents who wanted him to forsake his divine revelations and return to normal, ordinary human functioning. Saving the world from destruction was much grander than setting the alarm so he could wake up and go to his college classes. Chris intentionally wanted to stay "high" in spite of the disastrous consequences. He was suffering from "auto-intoxication." The drugs were free, but there was a high price to pay.

The effectiveness of the Zyprexa was proven once again to us. After a two-week stay, Chris was discharged. Gayle and I took him home. His course work was put on hold until a decision could be made as to whether or not he would return to college. This time we made sure that he continued taking Zyprexa and Depakote. Although opposed to this, he complied. When it was clear that Chris could return to school, he arranged with his professors to make up all the schoolwork he had missed, save for his senior recital. He returned to college and completed his studies for the year, "graduating" with his class without a diploma pending the completion of his senior recital. A few weeks after school was out, in spite of our objections, Chris chose to discontinue the medications. He did so, this time, without any repercussions.

Chris was convinced that the St. John's Wort had not influenced his mania and that Zyprexa and Depakote had not influenced his return to normalcy, despite the obvious changes around his "cheeking" episode. He believed that these matters were more related to ongoing personal and spiritual issues than to any biochemical changes in his brain. He was more interested in what was in his mind than what was in his brain. He and he alone determined what he felt and how he acted. I had trained him too well in my philosophy of self-responsibility. And the grandiosity of the illness only reinforced that training.

Looking back, it is possible to see how hasty, seemingly minor short-term decisions can have life-wrenching impact. First, there was my spontaneous suggestion regarding St. John's Wort. I was to learn later that scientific studies of the herb were just getting under way, and because of the lack of regulation for herbal products, there was no assurance that Chris was taking the amount or even the substance he thought he was taking. One ingredient in St. John's Wort is hypericum, a monoamine oxidase (MAO) inhibitor. MAO inhibitors were the first antidepressants, appearing before the advent of the tricyclic antidepressants. They slow the action of cellular membrane serotonin reuptake "pumps," effectively making more serotonin available to the brain. According to the amine hypothesis of bipolar illness, high levels of serotonin, one of many neurotransmitters, are associated with mania and low levels with depression. Second, there was the decision by the doctor at the mental health clinic to prescribe this new drug called Zyprexa. The allure of this powerful drug, which definitely reduced the psychotic symptoms of bipolar disorder, was compelling. We didn't know it at the time, but we had made a Faustian pact with Zyprexa. Chris got his life back, but there would be a price to pay.

In the text that follows, Chris does not portray the chronology of events as I have described, most likely because his psychotic experiences blurred his sense of time and context.

The end of this world

My brain felt as though it were on fire. My body shook violently. After being absorbed in the world of my journal for hours on end, what I had immersed myself in finally caught up with me. It was the most extensive self-analysis I had ever attempted. I had become so enthralled with what I was learning about myself and human nature in general that I had forgotten about going to class and eating. I couldn't possibly quiet my body enough to sleep. The mysteries of my failures in life were being revealed to me through the violent scribbling of a pencil on paper. Thoughts were coming to me faster than I could write them down. But there was something special about these thoughts. I had never esteemed myself a good writer, nor had I ever known myself to be so prolific with words. These thoughts could not have possibly come from my mind, I thought. I am not an original thinker; I borrow other people's thoughts and ideas. Yet before me lay pages and pages of inspired journal writing, interrupted in their composition only by trips to the bathroom and excited banter to roommates, teaching them the latest theories of Chris Moyer in regard to human relationships. No, these thoughts were of divine origin. I was sure of it. God had finally answered my prayers. I wanted to know Him fully. God was beginning to speak to me through my journal, or so I thought. But I should give a little background first.

I met Joan while working at the movie theater. A tall and slender young woman with silky brown hair that fell gently over her shoulders came in one day to apply for a job. Her brown eyes were deep and tender; when I looked into them, I saw a compassionate nature. Something about her excited me. I brought her an application and talked to her about movies while she filled it out. I told her that I hoped she got the job, because I would enjoy working with her. After our brief conversation, she left, giving me a smile as she left the theater. I really hoped she would get the job.

After several weeks, she returned. She came in with two male friends, but she came right up to the candy counter, greeted me, then asked for some water. I gave her some, and we chatted for a while. Although there were drinking fountains in the theater, twice during the film, and once after, she asked me to fill her cup. I happily obliged. On the final fill up, I looked her in the eye, smiled, and said, "I don't think you keep coming here for water; I think you need someone to take you to free movies." At this she blushed, and I could tell she liked me. I boldly asked for her number and had her write it out on a napkin. I felt incredible, like I was on top of the world.

Three days later, I called her, feeling a little apprehensive at first. However, we found plenty of things to talk about, and thus began our relationship. When I was on the phone with her, I felt like I had so much creativity, so much zest and enthusiasm. When I was with her, I felt more alive than I had ever felt before. I never wanted to lose this feeling. Friends and relatives tried to "take away" this feeling by suggesting that Joan was too immature, or too manipulative, or too young, and I should break up with her, but I would not listen to them. She was the first woman I ever fell in love with. The first week of our relationship was smooth sailing, and I felt incredibly close to her. I experienced a "me" I never knew — she brought out the best in me. However, as the relationship continued, I began to fall into self-pity.

I decided to go to London for the Jan Term. The first half of the trip was wonderful, but during the second half I began to feel shallow. I lost my self-esteem and began feeling isolated from others. When I got back to Whitworth, the feeling continued, and I found myself feeling extremely anxious around everyone, even my best friend, Darren. I came to the peak of anxiety one day in the cafeteria while I was talking with a friend. I froze in the middle of the conversation and told my friend I had to leave.

My goal from then on was to try to figure out what was wrong with me, what had plagued me with self-doubt since I was a child. I started writing a journal, and I realized that I could actually learn things about myself through writing. This was a revelation. I became more and more obsessed with the journal, until I became convinced that what I was writing in my journal were the direct thoughts of God, as though he was pouring thoughts into my head.

It was during this time that I was fired from my job at the theater. A customer complained to the manager that I appeared to be on drugs. The truth was that the thoughts continued to occur to me at the theater, and I would rush to write them down on napkins. Mine was a natural high; the chemicals came from my own brain.

Eventually, Joan ended our relationship. I remember as though it were yesterday the conversation I had with her on the day I got back from London. I went to the music building, to the phone right up the stairs from the band room. I had no idea what I was going to say to her, or even why I was calling. I guess I hoped I could start our relationship up again. However, I called, my fingers gripping the phone tightly, and I lost it. I babbled — I don't even remember what I said, but I remember Joan saying something about the government. She was just trying to have a conversation, and that's all I wanted to do myself, but I just couldn't. After I hung up the phone, I lay down on the two-cushion seat, and it felt like the life just went out of me. I felt like my world was over.

This inability to converse did not end with Joan. It was only the beginning. Several days later, I was finding it difficult to converse with Darren. I was terrified at what was happening to me. Finally, one day, I was right in the middle of a conversation with a friend, and I lost it, and couldn't go on. I apologized to my friend and left. I wandered around campus, wondering what I had done to deserve this, wondering how I got into this situation, wondering if anything could make it better. Here is where I began to take my steps into mania.

I got out a spiral notebook and opened my mind and began to brainstorm. I left out no ideas. The ideas started slowly at first, but they progressively got faster and faster, building off each other. Patterns started to emerge, and I began seeing things through new lenses. My whole perspective was changing. My understanding of God was changing. There seemed to be a divine structure to what I was writing, and I literally believed God was speaking to me through my journal.

There were nights that I screamed with sheer pleasure as I came to some incredible insight. There were other nights when I screamed with sheer terror as I felt that the salvation of the entire world lay in my hands. I excitedly lectured my roommates during the day about my findings, and I kept them up at night with uncontrollable bouts of laughter, crying, and screaming. Sometimes in my visions I was saved. Sometimes I was damned. When I was saved, I recognized my own beauty and perfection, and I cried for the souls of others who were damned. When I was damned, I groaned for myself, hating what I had become. Sometimes I would go from being saved to being damned in one day.

For example, when I felt isolated from God because I "knew too much,"

Too Good To Be True?

I thought I was in hell, and I went to see my friends Darren and Mandy and told them so. I lay down on their couch and prepared to die (I had lost much weight from not eating). It took a while, but finally Darren convinced me that I was not condemned to hell and that it wasn't too late for me. Once I recognized the possibility of salvation existed, I bawled and bawled, feeling the "grace" of God overwhelm me. Another time when I was with Kathy, I felt as though I was in a pit, and God was up above, looking down on me. In my mind, I reached out my hand, and God took it in His own. The experience was so powerful that I started crying extremely hard and told my sister the Holy Spirit had baptized me.

There are quite a few other crazy events that occurred during this time. I was so high that I felt I needed to come down. I tried getting in the shower and turning on extremely cold water and letting it pour over my back. I tried suggesting to my sister that she cry, because I could not cry on my own. I wanted to feel real emotions again, and the only way I could feel them was to see them in others. When my sister started crying, I cried, too, and she instinctively patted my back and tried to comfort me. Then I couldn't cry any more. She didn't understand that I wanted to cry. I wanted to have the feeling of crying, because it would bring me down from this hellish high that I was on. I even suggested to Kathy that I wanted to watch something sad on TV so that I could come down, but there was nothing on the tube.

My eyes were probably glazed over from lack of sleep. I started missing classes. Nothing seemed to matter except what I was learning about myself. I came to realize that I had been depending on the reactions of others for my own well-being. When I realized this, my dependency on God to fulfill my wishes was destroyed, and I was faced with the horrible notion that I was entirely alone and responsible for every single thing in my life. I felt as though I was in hell and separated from God. I remember being in the middle of campus, feeling entirely disoriented, not even knowing how to get to my friend Jacob's room. Instead, I found my way to Darren and Mandy's apartment. I told them I had discovered the true power of belief and that I was in hell because I believed it. I thought I would be dead soon. It was then that I was admitted to Sacred Heart and had to cancel my senior music recital.

Sometimes I believed I was going to hell. Sometimes I believed I was going to heaven. Sometimes I was an atheist and didn't believe in God at all. There was no middle ground for me. When I took a call from my parents at Sacred Heart Medical Center, the first call since my manic episode, I felt as Nietzche must have when he went crazy and shouted out in the streets, "God is dead." I was somehow afraid that by telling them my truth, it would automatically become their truth, obviously a sign that I had lost my sense of boundaries. When I told them God was a human construct created in order to magically fill our dependencies, my parents retained their Judeo-Chris-

tian beliefs.

When I came out of the first manic episode, I felt like I was waking up from a bad dream. The majority of the first manic episode was terrifying, and I was glad when it was over and I could go back to "normal" life.

Lull between the storms

During the summer of 1998, Chris sold books door to door along the East Coast for a company called Southwestern. He sold a number of different products, primarily supplemental learning products such as books and CDs to help school children master their subject matter in school. Although his daily diet rarely went beyond peanut butter sandwiches, and he worked from dawn till beyond dusk during the hot and muggy Eastern summer, he had no recurrence of his illness. That fall he prepared and performed his senior recital and obtained his degree in music composition. One of the pieces he performed at his recital was the strikingly beautiful and haunting piano piece he had composed while at Sacred Heart Medical Center.

After getting his degree, Chris worked several jobs. He worked at Whitworth College dining facility and also with a satellite TV installer. The next summer he sold books again, selling twice as many as he had the previous summer and earning approximately $10,000. Again, he worked 13-hour days going door to door, thriving in the hypomanic culture of achievement characteristic of the company.

That fall, on his way back from what he called the "book field," he met a woman, Sandy, through his friend Darren and his wife, and continued a relationship with her via phone and email. They had intense religious discussions. He challenged her conservative views and her conservative life-style. He had difficulty accepting her views and began writing in his journal again about his religious beliefs, challenging traditional doctrine and proclaiming, among other things, that Jesus was a sinner.

For one and a half years, from March 1998 to November 1999, Chris was relatively symptom free. During this time, he refused to take any medication even though we and his doctors had recommended that he do so.

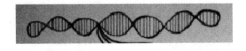

7 - The End of Denial

In the fall of 1999, after Chris returned from a successful summer of selling books, he flew to Puerto Vallarte to celebrate with some of his fellow book salespersons. He then returned to Spokane, where he got a job working in a piano store selling and repairing pianos. Two months into his new job, I received a call from Chris's employer telling me that Chris had acted strangely while delivering a piano to a customer. During the day, he had gotten into a deep religious discussion with a coworker. Later, while installing the piano, he had asked the customer what his "foundation" was. That night in a motel, he did not sleep. In the middle of the night, he started jumping on his bed, laughing. He encouraged his partner to do the same, so both of them could "become like little children" as commanded by Christ. He ran past the motel rooms, knocking on doors and telling people the end of the world was coming. I immediately flew to Spokane, and once again, like the proverbial Dutch boy, tried to put my finger in the dike to stop the floodwaters.

Off to the mental races

When I arrived, Kathy was with Chris. Since she was in the middle of finals and had to return to her classes, she was glad to see me. After she left, Chris discussed the incident with me. While the behavior he described was clearly psychotic, he was able to talk about it in a non-pressured, rational way. Before he went to bed, we had a good conversation about how he was feeling. We talked about his tendency to be overly detailed in his thinking and how this became more acute when he was manic. I suggested that his brain tended to drill down to a few repetitive ideas when he got manic and that medication could help him to break free of these thought patterns. He was open to this. He could converse about several subject areas. He was still "there."

During the night he did not sleep and grew more agitated. His brain drilled down and trapped him in the very obsessive process we had been talking about. In the morning, I started looking through the yellow pages to find a psychiatrist, thinking once again, that I could forestall hospitalization. If I hadn't been in such denial, I would have thought to bring an emergency medicine kit of Zyprexa and Depakote. Now, my denial was in the process of being shattered, but it was too late.

"I'm going to be on the national news, Dad. I have a plan to create peace in the world. People just need to understand and listen to each other."

I found several numbers. But it was 7:45 a.m., too early for a doctor's office or community mental health center to be open.

"I have big plans. There's something I have to do." Suddenly Chris bolted from the apartment, ran across the road, and started walking to his alma mater about half a mile away — in his bare feet. I followed behind.

When we arrived on campus, Chris yelled to some grounds keepers. "The end of the world is coming. Are you ready?"

As I quickly passed them, trying to keep Chris in my field of view, I asked them to call campus security. Chris ran into the dining hall and started speaking in front of the students who were eating breakfast.

Security personnel came, then a police officer. While Chris was talking about the end times to the students and challenging them to prepare, I explained the situation and told him I was hoping we could get him on medications to prevent his being hospitalized again. While the officer took Chris to Community Mental Health, I went back to Chris's apartment to get his shoes and socks.

When I arrived at Community Mental Health, he seemed to have calmed down. We filled out forms and waited and waited some more. The wait was starting to get to him. He began to pace in the patient reception area.

I told the receptionist that we would take a break for lunch, then return. We went to a local restaurant, where he managed to hold it together until after the meal.

"So, tell me, Dad, what is your foundation?"

"What do you mean?" I wasn't in the mood to talk metaphysics while my son was on the verge of a psychosis.

"You know, what is important to you?"

I thought a few seconds, searching for a good answer. Then I tried to defuse the intensity of his query with a flip comment. "Food. Remember that song from the Popeye movie with Robin Williams where Wimpy sings, 'All there is is food?'"

Wrong choice.

He snapped back in a loud voice as heads quickly turned our way. "So you are as shallow and empty as I thought. Food is your God. You are a glutton. You just love biting into those dry, crunchy potato chips or slathering that roll with butter and honey, then letting it slither down your throat."

Customers in the restaurant looked our way. I said nothing. I knew that if I did, Chris would lose any semblance of rationality right there in the restaurant. He talked louder.

"I bet you really get off on eating pie with ice cream on it, or chewing into a big, juicy steak."

I waved at the waitress. "Could we have the check, please?"

She hurriedly brought it over.

I got up to leave, and Chris slowly followed. I was afraid he might make a scene. I could see him pushing over tables or even assaulting me or some of the other "gluttonous" customers. Hadn't Christ done the same with the money changers? I knew from the past that when a thought grabbed him, it wouldn't let go.

If my son had been there, I would have strongly chastised him for embarrassing himself and me in the restaurant. But my son wasn't there. Something had hijacked his brain. My ill-advised comment about food, though far more significant than I could have ever imagined, was the worst thing I could have said at the time. Rather than diverting or diffusing his agitation, my comments had only made it worse. Yet was there anything I could have said that would not have had the same effect? The person I was talking to was not my son, who could appreciate irony and a good joke, but a person with a brain disorder who was incapable of processing information the same way I did.

In the car, I stopped talking, and Chris seemed to calm down a little. We returned to Community Mental Health. We were a "non-emergent emergency," which meant, apparently, that we would be seen only after the more serious cases. But once Chris began pacing and talking loudly in the reception area, we were upgraded. Suddenly, they found the time to see us immediately. Unbeknownst to me, they had already called the police.

We walked into a small office with two staff members. After a short discussion with them, Chris stood up and started to leave the room, saying that I was going to try to stop him. I did try to grab his arm, but I couldn't stop him.

The interviewer's supervisor spoke. "I'm afraid we're going to have to commit your son to Sacred Heart."

This was self-evident. I didn't disagree. The police came again and put him in handcuffs, then took him to Sacred Heart Hospital.

Chris was not combative when he left, but upon arriving at the hospital he became violent, necessitating his placement in restraints and isolation. As the psychotic process enveloped more and more of his brain, he started proclaiming with even greater urgency that the end of the world was coming.

God's palace

The next day, I visited him in isolation. He was smiling a strange, unresponsive smile. His eyes appeared glazed, and he looked feverish. It was as if he wasn't there.

"Hello, my son. I am God, the son of David," he announced as I walked into the isolation room. He wasn't joking. He welcomed me into his "palace," a small room with a mat, four padded walls, and a door with a small window.

We both hugged. I hummed a little tune I had written that I used to sing to our kids when I put them to bed, and he hummed along. We could still relate to each other on a musical level. Chris had arranged the song for four parts and performed it at his senior recital in a mixed quartet, bringing tears to his mother's and my eyes. Many in the audience had also been moved. Yet in spite of this connection, we were no longer in the same universe.

"You seem really confused, Chris."

"No, I'm not confused at all. I am God, the son of David."

"You are my son, and my name is David, but you are not God or Jesus."

We lived in two different worlds. I tried to pull Chris back into mine. The tension was palpable. I had been warned by the staff that he could become more agitated than he already was. With delirious manic patients, they tried to minimize stimulation. The manic patient's brain cells were already firing, as it were, on all cylinders. Additional excitement could overload them. I sensed that if we kept talking, Chris would either get more confused or more upset. I hated to leave him, but I didn't want to make things worse again, like I had in the restaurant. I hugged him and left, saying I would see him later. I had been there just a few minutes.

As I walked out of the hospital, I wished that we had not named him "Chris." It was too close to "Christ," and the name "Christopher" meant "Christ bearer." I regretted sending him to a Presbyterian college. However, his exposure to Christian theology had not made him psychotic; at the most, it had simply influenced the expression of inherent psychotic tendencies. On this particular day, he was God, the son of David. Tomorrow he might be Abraham Lincoln, President Kennedy, even an alien. I was stretching, looking for some explanation and coming up empty-handed.

I remembered reading the classic <u>Interpretation of Schizophrenia</u>, by psychiatrist Dr. Silvano Arieti. He elucidated with great detail and clarity the thinking processes of the schizophrenic. The concept of associational logic conveyed a type of thinking process in which words were linked together based on association rather than logical meanings. It was as if the brain lacked discipline. Instead of processing information along logical lines, it processed it by association. Chris's world was not the same as a schizophrenic's world, but there were similarities when he was psychotic. To his way of thinking, he was the son of David (my first name). According to his religious tradition, Jesus, the Son of God, was also the Son of David, or, in the lineage of David, the ancient prophet and king of the Jews. Therefore the Son of David, Chris, had to be the Son of God, which was the same as saying he was God Himself. It was perfectly logical for a person whose brain was broken.

Over the next several weeks, Chris's psychotic thoughts began to fade. He was moved out of the acute ward and to a ward where he had access to a piano. While coming down from his psychosis, he again composed some beautiful music. His exquisite creativity in response to emotional trauma reminded me of the composer Schumann, who also suffered from bipolar disorder. I had studied his life in a music history course in college. One evening he told his wife that the beautiful music he wrote was given to him by angels. By the next morning the angels had become demons who were damning him to hell. They held him under such a spell that eventually he was to attempt suicide by jumping into a canal. He later died in an insane asylum.

Here is Chris's account. Note that the brackets enclose my comments here and in subsequent chapters.

I'm in heaven

The second manic episode is a whole different story than the first. Whereas the first was dominated by feelings of terror and dread, feelings of being all alone, the second was dominated by pure euphoria and a feeling of inexplicable connectedness. I loved the feelings, except for being in restraints. I was God. I was one of the two witnesses spoken of in Revelations. I was the Perfect Son of God (the Son of David). I felt like I could do anything. This episode began while I was working for a piano company. It started small, by being overly friendly with customers and piano students and asking them rather personal questions, often about religion. One little girl whom I came up to was the sweetest girl, and I talked to her and drew in her coloring book. We sang "Jesus Loves Me" together. Later, when her brother was finished with his lesson, she didn't want to leave without me, and she asked her mother if they could take me home. Then she called me an angel. I began to imagine what it must have been like for Christ. I understood what he meant when he said, unless you are like a child, you cannot enter the kingdom of heaven. I began to understand myself as a child.

I have always been curious to find out the difference between Mormons and Protestants, and going on a road trip with my boss, John, gave me the perfect opportunity, as he is a practicing Mormon. During the trip to deliver a piano, we talked about religion and the end-times.

During the delivery of the piano, I became more and more judgmental towards the fellow for whom we were delivering the piano, as he seemed very materialistic and unconcerned with others beside himself. John sensed this in me and tried to quiet me down, but it was no use. I mocked the fellow for taking tons of pictures of his new piano, thinking how proud this man must be of his new purchase. I made him stay good on his word to take us out to eat, and when we got to the restaurant, I wanted to leave early because my olfactory nerves were working overtime, and I was feeling nauseous from all the odors I was taking in. Plus, my sense of taste was so incredible that I could barely eat what I had ordered. When we got ready to part company, I finally asked the man the big question, "What is your ultimate foundation?" He replied, "Finances." I was confidant that this man was going to hell. I also had a grand vision of separating the wheat from the chaff. I saw a vision of the world where those who had Jesus as their foundation would be separated from those who had financial, self, or other things as their foundation. I imagined going out and gathering numbers of Christian believers, and the way we would know one another would be by asking what each person's ultimate foundation was.

That night John and I stayed at a motel. I couldn't sleep. Thoughts kept running through my mind. I was laughing out loud while John tried to sleep. Finally, I couldn't take it any more. I started jumping up and down on the bed and screaming for joy, shouting that we all have to be like little children to get into heaven. I was acting like a little child. I tried to convince John to be a little child like me, but my behavior made him nervous. I had to share this wonderful feeling. I went out of the room and proceeded to run up and down the hall, pounding on people's door's and telling them that Jesus was coming. I went up to the front desk and found that the receptionist was a Christian, which made me happy. Within minutes, there were policemen there to detain me. I felt like they were on the bad side, sent to protect the "false" peace of the world. I had true peace, and it was my duty to share that with others. And I was prepared to suffer for that truth.

However, more than anything, I wanted to get back home to Spokane, because I had a letter that needed to be sent to Washington, D.C.. I calmed down for the officer, and, after much convincing, talked John into letting me ride back with him in the company truck. John was worried that I would jump out of the truck or do something crazy like that. We made it back safely, and I got in my car and drove home. John called my Dad that morning, and soon after, he arrived. I was convinced that this letter I had written to Washington, D.C. would bring about world peace. I also was suffering under the delusion that if I went to Washington, D.C. in person, the airlines would just let me board the plane, and they would just let me march right into the Oval Office of the White House. I went inside my house with my dad and felt like I had to do something to relieve tension. The tension was building up so high that I couldn't stand it.

Finally, [actually the next morning] I decided to go to Whitworth College and prophesy about the end of the world. My dad tried to stop me, but he could not hold me back. He followed at a distance. In my mind, I was thinking that my dad has no idea what was in store for him and what was about to happen. When I was manic, I always had the belief that something BIG was going to happen wherever I went.

I got to Whitworth and headed towards the cafeteria. I stood at the front of the cafeteria and began to speak to all the students there about how the end of the world was coming, and we needed to all prepare by using our gifts to the best of our abilities. I also began talking about myself, and about how God had been speaking to me. I remembered thinking that *"NOW IS*

THE TIME," *as if people had been doing nothing but sitting around on their butts. I had an overwhelming feeling that I was meant to be a spark to get things rolling, and once people heard my message, they would just leap out of their chairs and start doing good works. Boy, was I wrong. I remember asking what people were doing with their time, and one guy said, "Studying Japanese." When he said that, I said, "Good, then you can take the message to the Japanese people." I guess I sort of viewed myself as an orchestrator of a symphony of Christians, and I would send different people here and there according to their gifts.*

Security guards came. At first they insisted on taking me into another room and dealing with the problem quietly, but I refused, feeling that everything should be talked about in the open. However, I eventually gave in to their demands and went into the side room. When I got there, I began talking to the two security guards about my experience with high school bullies. [Here is another example of how the consciousness of mania is influenced by external stimuli. Chris switched from talking about the end of the world to talking about bullies when two security guards talked ("bullied") him into leaving the cafeteria.] *I told one of the nicer guards, "You remember when they came up to you and pushed you like this and called you faggot, and said you weren't worth shit?" When I did this, I shoved him. However, he realized I was only indicating to him what bullies did, and that I wasn't being aggressive towards him. I had deep eye contact with this security officer, and I told him a time was coming where he would be able to pay back the bullies for the wrongs they had done him. It was during this time that the idea of PAYBACK took precedence in my mind. I believed that Satan had been ruling the earth all this time, and now it was time for the children of God to start kicking some ass over the children of Satan. Back to the bout with the security officers — they called the police, and the police were not quite as nice as the security guards. They cuffed me and put me in the back of their police car.*

When we got to the station, I shoved a security guard to "test" my hypothesis that "peace" officers were evil. I had no intention of doing anything more, but of course they didn't know that. Within seconds, there were about 5 or 6 security guards on me, trying to hold me down. I couldn't believe they were acting this way towards me, and I thought they must have known I did not intend to harm the officer in any way. While they were tackling me, I managed to give one of the officers a good bump on his head with my elbow. Finally they got me down, and I realized the only way to "please" them was to give them what they wanted. I told them I would do whatever they told me to do, and I asked them if that made them happy, and they said yes. They put me in restraints, and the whole time, I was thinking that they were working for Satan. At that time, I was convinced that they were the bad guys, and they were talking about partying and what they were going to do on the weekend. I had a vision that the millennium was the Christians' time to party, and no longer would these "false" peace officers have their way with us. I half expected the door to break down and God Himself to free me from my restraints.

[This narrative illustrates some of the difficulties in trying to reconstruct a psychotic experience where one's normal sense of time and events is impaired. Chris's recollection here is based on a flow of his internal feelings rather than an accurate chronology of events as they actually happened. One policeman initially took him to the Spokane Community Mental Health from Whitworth College. He slowly explained the necessity for the handcuffs, made sure they were not too tight, and was able to solicit Chris's cooperation in taking him to Community Mental Health. I was very impressed with the professionalism of that police officer and told him so. After lunch, Chris's behavior deteriorated to the point that hospitalization was inevitable. At that point, two police officers took him to Sacred Heart Medical Center. The preceding comments actually refer to his second contact with the police.]

When I calmed down, they brought me to Sacred Heart Medical Center and put me in a small room, but without restraints. In this room, thoughts flooded my mind from every direction. At one point, I thought my parents and my best friend from high school, Dan, were in a conspiracy against me. At another point, I thought my mom and dad were two-sided: they showed me love, but then they showed me hate and made it impossible for me to please them. I was the Son of God because I was the "son of David," just like Jesus. In fact, the first time I saw my dad, I greeted him by saying, "Hello, my son." While in the room, I believed 3 to be the "holy" number, so I thought that if I could bend my flexible bed so it had three sides, I could stand on it and reach the ceiling, where I could get out. I also took apart the external covering to the air duct. I was trying to escape by any means. The reason I was trying to escape is that I believed those at Sacred Heart were going to torture me because they were evil and did not want the truth to come out, the truth that only I knew. I went to the door and looked at the glass in such a way that the black lines extended out into the outer room. I tricked my eyes into seeing the lines in three-dimensional space rather than two, and I thought this was some kind of X-ray vision I had developed.

I started thinking that families were meant to stay together, and the reason why we had so many problems in the world was because sons and daughters moved out of their parents' houses to start their own families. I started shouting, "Go back to your family!" I got so into it that I started making a rap to it, and I was looking at people out in the external room and telling them to "Go back to your families." I thought my real dad was God, and when I realized this, I burst into extremely intense sobbing. I knew how good it would be to be reunited with God, and how alone I felt, being separated from Him. I also had an image of my entire family being in heaven together with God, and that brought me great joy.

78

Once I began taking the hospital drugs, it wasn't too long before the incredibly strong perceptions began to fade. However, I still believed myself to be the Son of God, and I still believed that I had a message that nobody in the world knew except for me. This idea of being the Son of God persisted even through my third manic episode, which happened about 6 months later.

To summarize, my time in the hospital was characterized by wild, out-of-control thoughts. Just as I would latch on to one fantastic thought, another mind-blowing thought would occur to me, and my entire paradigm would shift. Logic was nowhere to be found. The sheer force of my emotions propelled my irrational thoughts faster and faster.

The off-road vehicle

When Chris was discharged shortly after Thanksgiving, I took him home with me to Lake Wildwood. He stayed there with us until early December. He continued on the Zyprexa and Depakote. By December 8, he wanted to return to his job selling pianos. His boss was willing to have him come back. His psychotic behavior had cleared up, but he seemed to have lost some of his confidence. We didn't want him to lose his job, so I decided to drive him back to Spokane rather than have him fly alone as we had initially planned to do, then stay with him for a while to be sure he took his medications and achieved some level of emotional stability. I had retired in September 1999, so I had the time to help get him reestablished and support his transition back to the world of work. We didn't think that he was stable enough to be on his own. Fortunately, we had placed my father in a local retirement home and, for now at least, could devote our attentions to Chris. Chris and I left in the early evening in our Subaru sedan. We planned to stay in a motel that night, then continue to Spokane the next day. I decided to go through Reno just for a change of scene.

It was about 8:30 on a cold night as we drove northwest of Reno on Highway 395 at approximately 55 mph. The temperature was below freezing, and there was evidence of snow on the side of the road, but the roads were clear, and though I wondered out loud to Chris if there might be some ice on the roads, I could find no evidence of it. We were looking for motels, which were few and far between in this section of Northern California.

There was very little traffic. As we drove along, we came to a slight incline. All of a sudden, the car began to veer to the left.

"Dad, look out, you're going off the road!" Chris cried.

I tried to correct right, but the car kept going left on the straight road. Hitting the brakes put us into a skid. I turned in the direction of the skid to regain control, but it was no use. We veered off the road on the left shoulder. The car was slowing, and I thought I could get back in control as I braked and skidded along the shoulder. Suddenly I heard a loud scraping sound of metal against rock as the car bottomed out on a rocky bump. We were rapidly approaching an outcropping of rock where the shoulder narrowed. Seeing there was no oncoming traffic, I turned the wheel hard to the right to get back on the road. However, when the right front wheel hit the pavement, the car flipped over, landed on its top, then slid to a stop off the pavement.

I turned the key off. The engine had already died.

"Are you okay? Are you okay?" I shouted, while hanging upside down.

"I'm okay, but how are we going to get out of here?" responded Chris, also upside down.

The roof of the car had collapsed about 8 inches, the windshield had cracked open, and we had little room. The inside of the roof was covered with dirt and snow that had burst through the windshield while we skidded to a stop. I felt claustrophobic. We both released our seat belts, flipped over, and planted our feet on the roof of the car. The windows were closed. We tried to open the doors, but they wouldn't budge. Chris started to hit the car window with his foot.

"Wait a second. Let's figure this out." I turned the key in the ignition and pushed the electric window button. The window on Chris's side slid down . . . or, rather, "up." We inched our way out of the car, crawling on hands and knees over the icy dirt that covered what used to be the top of our car. Just as I followed Chris out the window, I saw the lights of the California Highway Patrol (CHP) and a Cal Trans sand truck coming to sand the road. Never had the lights of a CHP patrol car looked so good to me.

"What a relief to see you," I said to the officer. "We could have spent a cold night out here."

"Too bad we didn't get here a little sooner. My patrol area consists of about 1,500 miles of roads. It's amazing I got here right after your accident."

He explained how, during the day there had been a small rainstorm south of Susanville. A section of road had iced up. A passing trucker had noticed the icy section and had called the highway patrol about it. The CHP and a Cal Trans sand truck had been headed south towards us as we had been driving north.

We examined the wreckage. The right front tire had blown. The top and the driver's side were badly smashed and dented. The air bags had not gone off. The car looked like it had been totaled.

The officer took us to Alturas and arranged for towing our car. We spent the night. The next day, since there were no public buses in Alturas, we caught a ride with a paint salesman who happened to have room in his truck. Eventually, when we got to Bend, Oregon, we rented a car and drove to Spokane. Although our car had been almost totaled in the accident, our insurance company decided to repair it.

Taking the horse to water

I stayed with Chris while he started working again. I cooked meals, visited him at lunch, went with him to church and to Sunday basketball games with his friends, and met with his employer, who was willing to give Chris another chance as long as he took his medicines and had no further episodes. I hoped to connect Chris with support agencies so he could use their services after I left. Part of the support I gave him was to ensure that he took his medications and had a good diet. Left to his own devices, Chris was content to have cold cereal for breakfast, Taco Bell tacos for lunch, and Hamburger Helper for dinner. I made sure that he ate fresh fish, fruits and vegetables, and also that he took omega-3 fatty acids along with his medications, having learned of Dr. Stoll's work at Harvard with bipolar patients and fish oil.

We went to a holiday social event of a local bipolar support group and were introduced to the members. There was a somber, heavy ambience to the meeting. People spoke about their experiences, their medicines, and their psychiatrists. Chris, who was still hypomanic, spoke out with energy and vitality on subjects I would have preferred he not address, but he was accepted. They had been through the same thing; the leader of the group had been George Washington for a time. So they felt no surprise in listening to someone who had been the Son of God, someone who, while no longer claiming the title, still exuded the energy and drive that goes with some prophetic, if ill-defined, mission. At least Chris was one of the more energetic and enthusiastic attendees.

I met a woman there whose bipolar son had killed himself six months earlier. She talked about his many plans to help others. One day he told her that he was going to do something about child abuse on the Indian reservations. She said she just accepted him and didn't try to confront his unrealistic ideas. I thought to myself how sad it was that she didn't try to help her son by fighting his illness more. I still had my own delusion that with enough effort I could make a difference. I expressed my condolences.

I made appointments for Chris to be seen at Community Mental Health. There he was assigned a case manager whose job was to ensure that he took his medications and kept his appointments. I tried to motivate Chris to take his medicines and to become involved with organizations like the bipolar support group, but his heart wasn't in it. He argued that he had much more pressing priorities for his time. I was clearly going to have to stay a while if I was to prevent another episode.

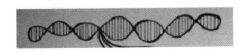

8 - More of the Same Gets You More of the Same

Even though he was no longer psychotic, Chris remained hypomanic. He now had two jobs, his day job selling pianos and his night job, writing a book he called <u>The Bipolar Prophet</u>. This began as a private journal and evolved into a treatise of Chris's new understandings of God and Jesus. He looked at traditional religion from a radically different perspective. He wanted to share with the world his new religious insights, a perspective that essentially contradicted historical Christianity.

It was a hodgepodge of various disorganized religious and delusional thoughts that lacked coherent organization. He challenged traditional Christian teachings, stating that Jesus was a sinner who unfairly attacked the pharisees. He wrote from a grandiose religious perspective addressing his would-be readers as "my little children." He wrote as if he were the prophetic founder of a new religion. He predicted his book was going to be a best seller. The journal was taking him further from reality.

I hoped — there is that word "hope" again — that a dialogue using the discipline of writing would help him to give up in boredom his pathology and return to the real world where I could applaud his real accomplishments. The more time and money he spent on his "book" the less investment he had in the real world. I hoped a meaningful dialogue would pull him down from the clouds and back to earth.

"More of the same gets you more of the same." That was a phrase I had used with clients when I was in the Air Force. I had used it with those who were trapped in futile and even dysfunctional behavior because they hoped those behaviors would be effective. Sometimes the phrase resulted in the "aha" of insight.

Having lived with my father's mania for years I had finally come to accept there was no way I could reach my father. Nonetheless, I now hoped to do with my son what I couldn't do with my father. Hope springs eternal in the human heart, even for a parent who happens to be a therapist. Chris was taking his medications. They were supposed to be helping him. So, on December 18, I suggested that we write a book together to explore some of the issues we had been discussing. He agreed. Here is how it began.

Round #1

Damn this illness. It has a stranglehold on Chris's brain and it won't let go. This morning I shared a dream I had with him. In my life, dreams have contained messages that have helped me solve problems. In this one I was driving down a road in a foreign country with Thomas across from me and an older man and other family members in the back. The old man was talking about some mission. There had been a flood and the mosquitoes had come. I was trying to listen and also trying to find the place where this mission existed. All of a sudden the road, a freeway, turned very sharply and there was no way I could stay on it. The car went careening off into space and there were a few seconds of silence as I saw the ground approaching. All I could do was say I am sorry and wait for the end. I felt sad. My son Thomas looked sad as he saw the end coming. I woke up, sad, but relieved I was in bed and not crumpled up on some road.

Upon hearing the dream Chris triumphantly announced that he knew what it meant. "The dream is telling you to change. It is God talking to you Dad. He wants you to follow him and go off the path you are on." He started shaking as he had in the past when he got in touch with his excitement. I told him that for me it was related to the accident and warned both literally and figuratively of the dangers of going off track and flying into space.

The night before, Kathy had talked to me about a church related mission trip to South Africa she was considering. I said I did not think this was a good idea because of the increasing crime problem in South Africa, specifically rape and AIDS. Also my associations with the word "mission" were none too positive. My father's "mission" to change the educational system in California brought disaster upon himself. Now I saw Chris embarking on his own grandiose bipolar prophetic mission with the same potential for harm. My rolling the car illustrated the pitfalls of ignoring the laws of physics. There was no free way. The natural laws of physics applied. Choosing to ignore the laws of physics did not change them.

Whether low or high, whatever biological process is taking place is literally trapping him in a stream of consciousness around the themes of inadequacy or omnipotence. He goes in and out of blissful psychotic thinking where the answers are clear then into self doubt where he can't do anything right. When I suggested that maybe he would sleep better if he moved to a room away from the traffic noise he stated he is always awake, that his unconscious mind is the same as his waking mind. That's scary. Without sound sleep how can his brain be restored? Chris is a very bright and creative individual. He is a magna cum laude college graduate. But last night when I asked him to read the directions and put medications in a pill dispenser for the week, he couldn't or wouldn't load the pill dispenser appropriately. He is forgetful and absent minded. After all, when you have a pipeline direct to the almighty of what significance are medications, work, girlfriends, friends, food, etc.? Is it the illness, or too much or too little of one medication? We know these symptoms worsened prior to his hospitalization but are the medications helping? It is as if his ability to use his frontal cortex is compromised. His thought processes are so entrenched that no amount of discussion can shake them.

I am trying to show Chris that I am angry at the illness and that I want him to fight it with me. Chris sees me as angry at him and not loving him. He doesn't see that I love the part of him that stays sane and want to know more of that part of him. He doesn't see I am trying to help him return to normalcy. To Chris's way of thinking normalcy is a world in which people act within oppressive social and relational boundaries. For him this is lunacy. He wants me to accept his views and change along with him. He wants me to fly off the road into space where I can find God.

His thinking tends to be very black and white. Maybe when the brain cells are compromised the mind reverts back to a simpler black and white (bipolar) view of reality. All perceptions go through the "good/bad", "right/wrong" filter and are judged and corrected accordingly. He tries to correct any error he sees in my thinking or perception. He gives unsolicited advice to others.

Ahhh! The LIBERATION. The freedom from moral relativism and uncertainty! THERE IS CERTAINTY. GOD IS A CERTAINTY. My father will not accept the certainty of his condition, and that is why he is looking to fix me first before fixing himself. The dream he had is from God. My father is afraid of giving up control of his life and allowing God to do the steering. He had a dream about an uncontrollable event: a flood, and a following mosquito infestation. It could have been an earthquake, or a hurricane, for all that it matters. The point is that there are things in this world we cannot control. And our lives are one of them. We cannot plan out our future, and we cannot even be sure of our present. We could die tomorrow. The point is, unless there is something solid underneath that we know we can rely on, then when things do get "out of control," there is nothing left to do but weep and gnash your teeth. I believe my father has good intentions, but he is more concerned about my "normalcy" in the world than he is with his relationship with the Creator of his life, the one who sustains the entire universe. He is not alone. Many have not found the true path, because they believe all paths are relative. Those who go their "own way" are going the way of the world, which is to work and make money to provide for yourself and your future, and to enjoy a little leisure here and there. This path leads to certain spiritual death, and separation from God, but my father cannot see clearly. He is blinded by his own attachment to money, things, routines, schedules, food, and other such "earthly things." I love my father dearly, and I pray every day he will come to know God by confessing and repenting.

As far as medication is concerned, I only take the medication for the sake of my parents and others. Their worry over my not taking them outweighs my lack of desire to take them. I'm OK as I am, because I have found God, and he has told me HE LOVED ME. This makes me fantastically OK, because I know there is nothing in this life that can cause me to be afraid.

Not even death. My fear of God is much greater than death, because I know death is merely the beginning, when it really gets good for God's children. When one understands the importance of infinity, one can get fuzzy sometimes about current conditions, like sleeping, normal eating, working out mundane details, etc. I agree that I have lost some ability to act with normal "productiveness," but didn't Einstein have that same problem? Didn't he forget how to add up change for the bus fare? His mind was on the universe and the questions of WHY and HOW. This made simple tasks like adding coins seem trivial, therefore it never much concerned Einstein.

I think of the eternal questions of why are we here? Who am I? What will life be like when it's over? What is really true about the universe? When I mentioned this to my dad tonight, he told me that it is not productive to ask these questions because they only lead to more questions. I'm sorry my dad stopped without following the questions through, because many have followed them through and they have found God at the end. Although my father professes to be a Christian, he has a very blurry view of Christ, and he thinks he"ll "find out" about heaven when he gets there. I think it is rather presumptive to assume you are going to heaven just because you call yourself a Christian or just because you go to church each Sunday. I want my dad to understand his presumptuousness, as well as his addiction to the stock market, so that he can have a clearer picture of who he really is at the core. We all have a core. Some are fruitful at the core, and some are rotten. The only way to find out is to search there. Each person needs to search inside his or her heart and find out what is really there. It is never too late to come to God the father, by way of Jesus Christ his son, so long as one can see that one is rotten at the core, and can make the step off of the canyon into hope and real faith. I saw that I was rotten at the core and I chose God. Others will find that they are rotten at the core, and when they find out, it is up to them what to do about it. They can sin freely, with no moral regrets, or they can accept the love of God that is always waiting for them, if they'd only lift their hands up with a heavy heart, and cry out screaming and moaning for forgiveness. They must trust God's way, because all other ways lead directly to hell and eternal damnation. Again, I love my father dearly, and I understand that he wants the best for me, but what he doesn't understand is that I have already found out what was wrong with me, and I accepted my illness, which was sin, with God as my witness. I love him, and I wish for him to know the truth that I know, but doing so requires for him to take a step off into the canyon below, in faith that God will be there. That is all for tonight. Good night.

Round #2

When Chris starting reading this journal he exclaimed, "Dad this is publishable." Later he asked me if I really wanted to continue with it. I said I did. He then warned me that if I did my life might be changed. Sounds like he believes the force of his arguments will change me. I wonder if he sees me as a person with an unstable identity who will be influenced by the power and messages of God coming through him. Sounds like a boundary problem to me. I just wish we could all just stay on the road.

His ability to accurately read others is still compromised as, for example, when he told Kathy that she should have shared negative feedback regarding a friend's behavior. He was unable to understand that Kathy had already checked out the ability of her friend to handle negative feedback and had made an appropriate social judgement. He primarily thinks in bipolar, black and white categories. Any comments that do not meet his litmus test for truth must be corrected. He has no awareness of how "preachy" this feels to others or how people pull away from him when he does it.

Last night he said he was feeling confused. He said he was afraid that others would control him if he gave up his manic thoughts. He sees himself as either controlled or controlling. He doesn't see that he has a whole range of behaviors which he can call upon in a responsible manner once the executive part of his brain is firmly grounded in reality here on earth. He doesn't understand that he can make good decisions in spite of the fact that someone else happens to think he should. Chris spends so much energy fearing control by others when he is perfectly capable of taking from what others have to say and coming up with a decision that is right for him. When he was in stocks he worked long hours and lost $3000. Rather than learn from this he continued more of the same. Recently I suggested that Immunomedics (IMMU) was a good buy and explained the reasons. He insisted that General Magic (GMGC) was the place to be. In the long run GMGC may be a good buy, but in the short run it has faltered while IMMU went from 2 to 5 (later to go to 30 before sliding back). In his stocks he has to make his own decisions and will not seek out other resources.

[As I review the above paragraphs months later I am struck by how my "pull yourself up by the bootstraps" theory still creeps into my thinking. How can the executive part of his brain become firmly grounded in reality when it is not functioning properly? I might as well have been encouraging a schizophrenic person to stop their loose associations. The problem was not that the reality data wasn't there. It was always there. The problem was that his brain couldn't respond appropriately to the data. So, I continued to do more of the same and got more of the same trying to overload him with data from the world of reality wherever I could find it. He was deaf so I kept talking louder. He was blind so I kept turning the lights up.]

Chris commented this morning that he was unhappy about the state of his wardrobe. He needed to iron his clothes. I see this as a positive sign. It shows he is more aware of how his appearance could affect his sales image.

Today I perused a book I found at the Wellness Center, a place where discharged mental patients go for support. It described manic symptoms such as giving spiritual advice to people, being argumentative, grandiose, very insensitive to feelings of others, always moving, unable to stay at one task for a long time, unable to plan effectively. If I had a copy of their book maybe I could better help Chris to better understand his behavior. These folks seem to have a more specialized approach for bipolar patients. They call it a brain disease and they call the patient the "consumer." I like that. The course is very much life style oriented. Regular sleep, regular diet, avoidance of what they call excitotoxins, or substances that can excite bipolar patients are suggested as ways to prevent reoccurrence of episodes.

After reading my dad's last response, I have a better understanding of his position. It certainly makes sense to me, and that is exactly why I feel confused sometimes. The data all seem to be true for me, yet I can look at everything from another perspective, and all the data seem to be false, and a misrepresentation of the ULTIMATE REALITY of God. For the record, I do not believe anyone is trying to control me, as my dad insisted. I said, "fix me" and I believe that statement has quite a different connotation than "control." When I am in "God mode," let us say I see many of the "worries" of life as trivialities. When I hear people making a big deal about my eating or sleeping habits, I get annoyed, because I feel as though I am above it, or that it is not ultimately the point. I hear scriptures in my head that say, "Do not worry about what you will eat or what you will drink." And then I see from my father's own words, and understand his own desire for me to have the "executive part of my brain firmly grounded in reality" here on earth. I do not want my brain to be earth centered. I want it to be God centered, and heaven centered. I want the point to be God. All the time. I want to hear HIS NAME be spoken on everyone's lips, and I want people to understand the importance their creator must have in their lives. The people who are trying to fix others, I believe are the ones who need fixing the most, for it has been said by a VERY RELIABLE SOURCE that those who claim to see are actually blind. They "clean the outside of the cup and dish, but inside they are full of greed and self-indulgence." But then again, to be fair, if I changed the words "trying to fix" to "trying to help" we have a whole other issue. For if one is trying to help, then his heart is in the right place, even if the helping is not perceived that way. So, from the oppositional viewpoint of my own, to be fair, my father is trying to help me in the best way he can, and this involves seeing me get back onto a regular schedule, both for eating, sleeping, and taking medication. He knows no other way to help, so should he be punished for this? Of course not. His intentions are more important than what he actually does. However, there is an important link between an intention and a deed, and usually good deeds flow out of good intentions. When I am in the "GOD" mind set, I view my father as lost, and needing redemption, as well as a deep need to know the character of Jesus. When all he talks about are stocks, money, food, schedule, medications, it makes me see him as very narrow-minded and shallow. When I view my father from my "normal" mind set, I merely see him as my dad, and someone who is trying to help, but not knowing how to get anywhere with me. Then scripture comes up somewhere in my mind that you must hate your father and mother in order to follow Jesus, and that fathers and sons will hate one another, and sometimes I feel I am going through that right now, on the verge of something big. I would never hate my dad, but I can imagine him hating me some day. He would hate me for being "preachy," and for being grandiose, and for embarrassing everyone in the family. I can hear my dad say now, "IF IT WEREN'T FOR THAT DAMN BOOK", when he was referring to the Bible the first time I had a manic "episode," the one where I fluctuated between believing "GOD IS DEAD" and "GOD IS EVERYTHING."

When I was a child, I always trusted those above me, and always thought they knew where they were going. However, as I grew older, I realized these people knew nothing more about life than I did. But I knew I was confused and professed it. Many people are confused in the beginning, but then they stop asking the questions, and stop looking for answers. They accept what others in the "field" are telling them. They accept the shadow, instead of continuing on in their search for truth and reality. They feel the search for truth is a waste of time, and it ends up causing people to ask more questions, on and on, adinfinitum. Personally, I enjoy asking questions to myself about the nature of God, for it was the only way I could truly get to know him. I know more about Jesus Christ now then ever before, and I have a deep conviction in Him, because I kept searching into His character. Even though there were times I thought he was deluded, and times I thought he was vengeful and unfair to the Pharisees, I kept searching because I could not bring together in my mind the hateful, and misguided Jesus, with the loving one my friends continued to bring to me. I knew one had to be true, and the other had to be false, because of who He claimed to be. If you are hateful towards the people that you have created, then you are not a very good God. Jesus as God loved the Jews, though they hated him and killed him. However, he hated their sin, and their proud hearts, and their addiction to money, and their concern over "image," and their blind following of the law, as though blind following could save you. I cannot argue with my father on his terms, because I don't know about the drugs, I don't know what is in them. I just know that where I am now in my life, the drugs neither help me, nor hurt me.

Therefore, adherence to the drugs is more of a schedule and a routine, which I believe would result more in a placebo effect, if I ever were to maintain such a routine.

Today, I had a lot of fun with a little girl, and ended up getting a wonderful hug from her. Her name was Kristin. She said I was handsome, and even beautiful. We colored together for a few minutes in a Sesame Street book. We sang some songs together. She came over to me and gave me a big hug, and told me I was a beautiful angel. I believed her. After her lesson, she wouldn't let me go. She grabbed my hands and tried to bring me home with her. I felt so united with her. I think for the first time, I can understand what it felt like for Jesus when he played with all the children. Jesus loves the little children, all the children of the world, red and yellow, black and white, they are precious in His sight, Jesus loves the little children of the world. It was his abundant love, and abundant personality that drew the little children to Jesus.

Do you know how most kids hate going and sitting on Santa's lap during Christmas? Santa can not offer real love, because he is a conjured up person. A figment of someone's imagination, he doesn't exist in reality. He stands for nothing, except getting things for being good. Christ gives us love even when we are not good. If we are not good, "Santa" will put coals in our stockings. If we are not good, but recognize our lack of goodness, Christ can speak to us in a real way. But so long as we believe inside that we are good at heart, on our own, apart from God, we will deceive ourselves unto our own graves. For without God, no good can come. Without God, we are rotten to the core. But with HIM, and through HIM, we can LIVE, we can LOVE, we can ENJOY his presence, for it is an amazing presence, for those who know him. He fails us not, through thick and through thin. I don't know what any of this has to do with medications, for I feel like I have no need for medications, because God has taken care of all my needs. His presence alone is enough medication for me.

Now, my dad will likely proceed to reject the content of most of what has been written, ignore the fact that his son was able to have a wonderful encounter with a little sweet girl who called him an angel, and will instead see it as breaking the social boundaries, making a mother nervous (though she can be my witness that she was not in the least bit nervous of me), and a symptom of my mania, and something I should not do in the future. I cannot help being kind and loving towards others, and if it draws them to me, it means we are on the same spiritual plane, and have the same spiritual understanding of one another. Children are beautiful. Children are wonderful. I need to see children the way Jesus saw them. That is my goal. My goal is to see all people as little, and even grown-up children, and learn how to get the "childlike" beauty back into their lives. I want to motivate people for GOD. That is all for now. I shall be very curious to see my father's response to what

I have written.

 P.S. HORRIBLE AND INCREDIBLE THINGS ARE ABOUT TO HAP-PEN.

 "Jesus has told us (those who are his true followers), what shall happen before the end of the world as we know it. Eventually ... "you will be handed over to be persecuted and put to death, and you will be hated by all nations because of me. At that time many will turn away from the faith and will betray and hate each other, and many false prophets will appear and deceive many people. Because of the increase of wickedness, the love of most will grow cold, but he who stands firm to the end will be saved. And the gospel of the kingdom will be preached in the whole world as a testimony to all nations, and then the end will come." (Matthew 24: 9-14) I'll leave it at that.

 Good night.

Double KO

 Chris won. Chris and dad lost. So much for the bilateral father-son bi-polar journal. Chris seemed able to understand my point of view. However, he was unable to assimilate any of it into his own thinking. The journal consisted of point, then counter point. He lost by winning. Publishable? Sure, there was no question it was publishable, at Kinko's. They would publish the rantings of a madman for the right price. I knew. A few days before I had tried to run pass interference to enlist their support in preventing Chris from spending his limited resources to "publish" his work. After explaining the difficulties Chris was having I asked for help from an employee.

 "Could you suggest to him that perhaps he could print two, then show them to his friends, then if he found that others want copies he could buy some more?"

 "I'll discuss this with the manager."

 They must have had some discussion.

 That night, instead of sleeping, he completed his book. Today he is $300 dollars poorer, having "published" 20 copies of <u>The Bipolar Prophet</u>. He gave some to friends telling them it would change the world and he would use royalties from it to help the world's poor. The infinite ability of the human mind to delude itself is astonishing.

 Chris says it will "change the world." I have read almost all of it. He told me he wants to "stand naked in front of the world." He does. The usual inhibitions are gone and the exhibitionistic child is coming out. There are some nice poems and narrative in the text. However, there is no overall organization to his ideas. His writings are not unlike those of his grandfather. His statements are overly detailed, loosely associated and confusing. The journal covers a lot of ground. I fear that the more he divulges to others the more they will pull away from him, leaving him with the feeling of being a "martyred prophet," like his grandfather. As I try to attack the illness to reach Chris, he feels misunderstood. He feels attacked when I comment that he is becoming grandiose and that his behavior will lead to negative repercussions.

During this time I continued to be concerned about other behaviors as well. Besides creating an unreal world through his hypomanic writing, he was also exhibiting rocking behavior. He would rock just slightly, not like a Hassidic Jew at the Wailing Wall or an autistic child, but enough that I was uncomfortable with it.[1] When I commented on it, he told me that it made him feel better and continue doing it. Sometimes he would do it in public, as, for example at a restaurant sitting at a table. There are similarities between mania and autism. Neither the manic nor the autistic is able to let anyone else in to his or her life. On the other hand, the manic can share his inner reality while the autistic person can't.

I knew autism symptoms, having given M and M's to Robbie, a teen-age patient at Camarillo State Hospital as a college psychology student. I was supposed to "shape" appropriate social behavior by rewarding eye contact, and extinguishing rocking behavior. We never made it to speech. Didn't make any progress with eye contact or rocking behavior either. I had about as much luck with Robbie as I was having with Chris. Those were the days when B.F. Skinner's behaviorism was in vogue. The behavioral contingencies were important, not the "black box." As an undergraduate psychology student my job was to keep doing the behavioral intervention, or, more of the same, irrespective whether it worked or not.

Chris pulled it together for the holiday season, driving his car to Oregon, and picking up Sandy, his girlfriend from Michigan at the Portland Airport, then celebrating Christmas with our extended family in Salem. I vainly kept trying to make a dent into his impermeable psyche. I tried to enlist family members to confront Chris's hypomanic ideas, but they preferred that his psychiatrist deal with such issues. I still hoped that if I got enough support to challenge his ideas, we could make an impact. He was taking his medications and he was out of the hospital. He "should" have been getting better. I had told my customers for years that "more of the same gets you more of the same." Now more of the same was giving me more of the same. I returned home to the family and Chris returned to Spokane.

The hope that I could reach my son with words was just that, a hope. Regardless of my efforts, I was incapable of having any effect on his thinking patterns or behavior. It was easy to see how bipolar customers become paranoid from increasing isolation from others. People respond to people who respond. The bipolar patient responds to and filters all input from internal processes that are impervious to external reality. I could have gotten angry, but it would have done no good and would have only isolated Chris when he now needed whatever human contact he was capable of.

My "pull yourself up by the bootstrap" approach may have helped some in the Air Force whose brains functioned normally, but it was useless for customers who had a brain disorder. Did the journal help Chris? No. Did it help me? Yes. It helped me to realize that what I was dealing with here could not be influenced by reality therapy, cognitive therapy, journaling, or any other symbolic interactions. His basic reality was not his to choose, nor mine to influence. His biology thrust it upon him. Fix the brain disorder and the rest would follow. To paraphrase Bob Dylan, "there was no success like failure and failure was no success at all." It didn't matter if the communication was spoken or written. Talk was cheap.

Sliding downhill

After Christmas he was let go from his piano job. He got a job selling cell phones at Alert Cellular and within several months was the top producer in the office. However, in the spring he began having intense religious discussions with fellow employees and again began obsessively writing in his journal. He had stopped his medications once again, in spite of our reminding him of the importance of continuing to take them.

Kathy called again, this time to warn us of Chris's increasing hypomanic behavior. He wasn't sleeping again. She and her roommate watched him while Gayle and I drove up to Spokane. We set up an interview with his psychiatrist. The psychiatrist agreed that Chris should not return to work. He recommended that he should start on the medications again and go home with us. He resisted, then agreed.

At home, he was not psychotic, but remained hypomanic. He was excessively friendly and enthusiastic with kids, saying that he preferred the spontaneity of kids to the lack of same in adults. He took Zyprexa and Depakote under our supervision. He remained hypomanic.

Chris decided he wanted to sell books again. We had misgivings but he insisted that was what he wanted to do, and he agreed to stay on his medications. In June he was to drive to Nashville to attend sales training.

Meanwhile, having gotten bored with day trading, which as of March, 2000 no longer held my interest, I was offered and accepted a real job, albeit a temporary one with Nevada County Behavioral Health Services. I would be working with high risk youth.

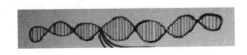

Notes

1. An interesting and perhaps not insignificant footnote here is that in Jerusalem, one of two depressed patients (50%) are bipolar while in Sweden, one in five (20%) are bipolar. While purely speculative, the potential significance of this, is nonetheless very interesting. Are there environmental or genetic predispositions that promote bipolar illness in Jerusalem? Is Jerusalem a magnet for some individuals whose thinking processes, and, even perhaps religious delusions are comparable to those found in bipolar disorder?

Belmaker R.H., van Praag H.M., (eds.), <u>Mania: An Evolving Concept</u>, Spectrum Publications, New York, 1980, Introduction.

9 - *Flipping out in the Matrix*

During the summer of 2000, we didn't want Chris to return to his job selling books on the East Coast. The job required a hypomanic temperament. The successful salesman had to be willing to work 6 days a week for 13 to 14 hours a day. That was the last thing we wanted for him. However, since he agreed to stay on his medications, that was the best we could expect. Beside, we had no alternative. He was going. We couldn't force him to stay home. His student manager also had reservations, but he agreed to allow Chris to return to selling books if he would promise him he would continue on his medications. He promised. Before he left we made sure he had enough medication to last the summer.

Hypomanic school

He had a very intense training experience in Nashville. While in training he called home and spoke in a very detailed monologue about a particular meaningful group meeting he had attended. He told me everything was fine and he was looking forward to "big things" this summer. He began having sleeping problems during the training and either stopped taking or inconsistently took his medications. After leaving Nashville he and his team headed for Connecticut, the book-selling territory where they had been assigned. Chris began getting grandiose again. Chris's student manager was informed by his teammates of Chris's condition. He offered Chris the choice of taking his medications or going to the hospital. Chris threw the pills on the floor and told them to take him to the hospital. They took him to the University of Pennsylvania Medical Center in Hershey Pennsylvania where he was admitted.

Upon admission he was briefed on his rights as a patient. One of those rights was to obtain legal counsel if the patient thought this was necessary. He tried to call Bill Gate's lawyers to find out what they could do for him. When the operator told him he needed a credit card in order to call long distance, he requested one from a patient with a Visa card that had been discontinued due to bad credit. Chris didn't think it would make a difference, and insisted that the patient give it to him. He became more agitated as staff tried to make him stop and threatened to do flips if he didn't get what he wanted. He was physically restrained and placed in seclusion where he was observed on a video camera. At some point in this process he said he would cooperate and the staff removed his restraints, while keeping him under observation in the seclusion room.

The Matrix was one of his favorite movies. He had seen it several times. I saw it once. That was enough for me. I didn't like the juxtaposition between reality and fantasy. Chris liked that. He already knew how to construct and live a reality that was not limited by the laws of logic. Shortly after he was taken out of restraints, he ran up a wall and did a flip like he saw in "The Matrix." He landed on his hands and feet. It was a stunning performance, considering he was on 10 mg of Haldol. He felt so emboldened by his first success he tried it a second time. This time he landed on his right kneecap, breaking it in several places.

I could understand the anger of those parents of vulnerable children who protest the effects of the media upon their children. I could also understand the anger of parents whose psychotic children cut off body parts as directed in the Bible. In Chris's manic state he could defy the laws of gravity. He probably could have dodged bullets as well.

He was consulted to an orthopedist who operated on his knee. The doctor drilled two holes vertically in the kneecap and inserted two-inch long metal screws, connecting the top and bottom of each screw with wire to assure a constant tension between the kneecap and the screws. Then he inserted a pin laterally to keep the rest of the pieces together. After a two-week period of hospitalization, Chris flew home.

Magical mystery tour

This is the first manic episode that actually interfered with my work life. Before, they were limited to affecting my family and friends. Now they were beginning to affect my potential career. Chad Beuhler and I had lunch at a bar and grill, and at that time, Chad wanted a solemn commitment from me that if they noticed that my behavior was out of line, or I was beginning to get manic, I would take my meds. I agreed at the time, thinking that if it ever happened during the summer, I would have the willpower to take the meds.

Sales school was more intense for me this year than any year in the past. I was "fully" into it, and I felt like I was bonding and connecting with people in a way that I never had before. I felt as though I "belonged" and I was a part of something bigger than myself. My vision had extended from my own personal goals, to the goals of others around me. This year, my motivation came from within, rather than from other students and managers. I felt as though I was on par with the top salespeople in the company. However, by the third day of sales school, I was not sleeping, due to intense thoughts I was having at night. I was beginning to have apocalyptic visions of the end of the world again. I started believing that God had much more in store for me this summer than just selling books. I became consumed with the book I had started writing during the year entitled, "Jesus Christ Condemned," and instead of sleeping at night, I would go into the bathroom and jot down ideas I was having that I could not contain. (It is ironic that at the beginning of the summer I was convinced of Christ's sinful nature, and believed him to be nothing more than an ordinary, sinful man, but after a few days of mania, I was convinced he was the Son of God and would be returning to judge the world.) I started believing that I was a special prophet who would warn the world of God's coming wrath. I would help to separate the sheep from the goats, in the sense that everyone who was open to Southwestern books would be the sheep, but everyone who was closed to the Southwestern books and rejected me, were the goats. In my mind the sheep were those who accepted God and would have a place in heaven, but the goats were those who rejected God, and therefore were condemned to hell. With all these thoughts raging through my head, I could sense that I was beginning to lose control, so I started taking my Depakote again, but I think it was too little too late. The lack of sleep started to wear on me, and I began getting manic, and coming up with wild schemes.

Among other things, I walked up to the President of Southwestern and told him that things were going to start happening in Connecticut as a result of me. I had a very strong feeling that a major revolutionary movement would take place in Connecticut, and I would be the one to start it. I believed that the residents of the city where I was working would view me as either a prophet of God, or a deluded madman. I believed people would take sides regarding me. Some would be followers of me, and would prepare with me for the return of Christ, others would be haters of me, and would clearly be on Satan's side. Just how would Southwestern fit into that? As I said before, those who were on my side would buy Southwestern books, even if they had to borrow from other people to get them. If they couldn't afford them, I would have a network set up where those who were financially well off would donate to those who were less fortunate. All these ideas were in my head as I got in my car to head out to the territory, beginning a long, long drive.

In my car I had a lot of time to think. These thoughts became more and more real to me, until I could practically visualize how things were going to happen in my head, like watching a video. I became extremely emotional. I would listen to music, and get so into the music I began sobbing uncontrollably. I began writing a book in my head, a book called Heaven. In the book, I imagined all the wonderful things heaven could be, and I experienced them first hand. I could visualize what it would be like to fly, and to ride on the backs of dinosaurs, and have sex with whomever I wanted (because after all, God made us all beautiful) and to be able to create things with your mind, and be able to be a part of one huge wonderful and loving family, where everyone is considered your brother and your sister.

As I was thinking along these lines while driving, Kris and Holly pulled over. When I got out and asked them why they pulled over, they told me that they had seen sparks flying out from under my car. I looked under the car to see if anything was dragging, but could find no evidence of anything that could have possibly been dragging. I started laughing hysterically, and told them it was a sign from God. I began feeling very powerful at that point. I was sure the sparks were a sign from God. What else could have caused them? (After I drove again, and the sparks stopped, Holly and Kris rationalized that it must have been reflections from the street light or something to that effect. I wasn't convinced).

Now that my confidence was so high, I began talking to complete strangers about how things were going to happen in Connecticut. I told them to watch for news in Connecticut. Big things were going to happen there. When we finally found a motel for the night (I wanted to keep driving all night because I had abundant energy plus I was anxious to get to Connecticut), I became psychotic in the middle of the night. I needed to tell everyone about how a revolution was going to start in Connecticut, so I thought the best thing to do was go to the news stations. I went to the Motel office and spoke with the clerk there and he told me I could use the telephone. I used the Yellow Pages, and called numerous television stations, but no one answered. So I finally called Fox News. When the answering machine came on, I started at the beginning and told them I was God and was going to change the world, starting with Connecticut. I told them everything about me, including what clothes I was wearing, what my posture was like as I sat in my chair. I told them about how I came to earth to experience all the joys and sorrows of humanity, and now it was time to gather up the believers. I must have left over one hour of recorded message on their tapes. Each time the answering machine went off, I took it to mean that the tape ran out, and people who were working at Fox News were scrambling to find another one, so anxious not to upset me, as I was, after all, God. Every time, I asked if someone was brave enough to pick up the phone, and every time, no one did. I thought it to mean that they were intimidated by me and were afraid to. In reality, it's probably because no one was there. However, in my mind, I visualized dozens of reporters gathered around the answering machine, awaiting the next prophetic message from God.

After I left the messages, I thanked the concierge and went back to our room. I so much believed that my message was heard at Fox, and was marveled at, that I thought they would instantly air it on TV, despite what was on. I turned on the television and woke up Holly and Kris. They told me to turn off the television, but I told them I had to watch something. They didn't understand, I thought. They don't realize the significance of Who I am. I turned the volume way down, and continued defending my right to watch TV in spite of both girls telling me to turn it off. Finally, I came to the conclusion that Fox News wouldn't have had enough time to air the story right away, because they would have to do some work with the film first before it was ready to be aired. I realized I would have to wait until 8:00 for the "news."

Flipping Out in the Matrix

At 8:00, I turned on the news, but there was no mention of my revolution. I was rather beside myself. Although I longed to keep going at night, in the morning time, I didn't want to go, but I wanted to stay at the Motel. I hatched another idea that everyone should stay at home and watch TV. This was God's divine plan. So when Dead Poet's Society came on, I watched with so much intensity, it almost hurt. I cried when they cried, I laughed when they laughed. I was fully engaged in the movie. Kris and Holly were concerned about me, so they called my parents. My dad instructed Kris to get the drugs I had promised to take. However, when Kris came back with the Depakote, I refused to take it, telling her that it would just sit in my tummy, and go out the other end. She insisted, and I hit the bottle out of her hand, spilling the Depakote all over the floor. I had no idea at the time of how insensitive and rude I was. All I was aware of were my own thoughts and my own motives, and those motives did not include taking medication. I felt so good, that I did not want to lose the feeling by taking a drug.

Kris and Holly were stuck and didn't know what to do, so they called Chad. After we watched TV for awhile, Chad arrived at the motel. He reminded me of the conversation we had at the beginning of the summer, about how I would take the meds if I started getting out of control. I had made a solemn promise to Chad that I would take them under such circumstances. However, my "plans" were too big to include medication at the time, and when Chad gave me the choice between taking the meds, or going to the hospital, I said, "To the hospital we go."

When we got to the hospital, and went up to the main check-in counter, I was asked many questions, and I answered them as truthfully as I could, under the influence of my psychosis. I told them I was the Son of God and had been sent to start a revolution. After the questioning, the man left in a hurry, as if to get some back up. They brought out a security guard, who I believed represented the "false peace" of the world, and I poked him all over and ridiculed him, telling him that soon he will be very afraid of me.

They put me in a confined room, where I continued having my delusions. Chad came up to the window and said he was sorry, but he had to leave me there. I understood. When they finally let me out and allowed me to walk around the ward, I walked into another person's room, and used their bathroom. I took a shower, and, imagining a large group of people were listening in right outside the door, started to prophesy about what I was going to do and how the world was going to come to an end. Finally, when I was done with my shower, I put on someone else's shoes and opened the door, shouting simultaneously. Nobody was there. I walked out into the main ward and I tried to call Bill Gates, so I could have his lawyer help me out of this mess. When I got on the phone and said, "I'd like to make a collect call to Bill Gates," the operator wouldn't let me do it and said I could make a long distance call if I had a Visa Card. I asked if anyone on the ward had one. One man did, but he said it wouldn't work because he had bad credit. I said it didn't matter, but then one of the nurses on staff told me not to ask for his visa card anymore. I sincerely thought I could get Bill Gates's lawyer to help us all find places to stay during the summer, and that could be the way to continue my summer and get out of this mess.

I don't remember specifically what caused my next confinement. All I remember is that it took about 7 or 8 guys to hold me down. I was in full-blown mania at this point. When they put me into a solitary room, the mania continued, and I tried to imitate Keanu Reeves in the Matrix or Jackie Chan, and I attempted a back flip off the wall. The first time I succeeded, landing on my hands and feet. The second time, I landed first with my knee and fractured it. The hospital took care of the injury, even though it still gives me pain to this day (4 month after the operation). After that, things quieted down. It's pretty difficult to be active when you have a cast over your entire right leg. After 2 weeks, I returned to California to be with my parents.

[Actually, he was restrained prior to his flips. He told the staff he would control himself, they took him out of restraints, then he did the flips.]

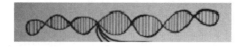

10 - "There Is Not Enough Room in My Mind ..."

When Chris returned from the hospital in Pennsylvania in August of 2000 he was taking 10 mg a day of Zyprexa and 150 mg a day of Depakote. He continued this dosage from June through August. However, while the medications prevented psychosis, they had no effect on his hypomanic behavior. He was also taking 1,000 mg of omega-3 fatty acids a day.

He accompanied us to basketball tournaments to watch his sister Elizabeth compete. On these trips he exhibited heightened energy with her teammates. At times, when laughing and joking with the girls, he came across with enthusiasm. Other times, when he spoke loudly, or seemed too personal or too friendly he appeared hypomanic. Gayle and I hoped that Elizabeth and her friends would see the enthusiasm. We feared they would see the hypomanic behavior. He was just a little too friendly, too talkative, and too loud. At a team dinner in a restaurant in Reno after one tournament, he sat with the junior high girls, saying he preferred the company of spontaneous young people to the company of stodgy old adults.

Act before you think

He was frustrated over not having a job. So he decided he would provide piano lessons for kids. He wrote an advertisement.

LEARN TO PLAY PIANO BEAUTIFULLY

*Have you always wished to be able to play music? Have you longed to touch those wonderful savory keys of the piano, only to have your longing crushed by difficult assignments, teachers who didn't care, and parents that forced you to play? Don't let fear plague your life. Experience Joy through the Piano. You do not need to "feel" competent. You cannot lose at this. There are no "wrong" notes in music. This is not a system. It is an experience. You will experience songs in a way you never have before. You will learn note by note, until you can actually feel the music within you. You will learn songs that you love, and be able to play them within seconds. You will experience no judgment from me. I will never tell you that you hit a wrong note or did something the wrong way. There are no wrong notes, there are no wrong ways in music. Feel one with music. Feel at peace with yourself. Give the gift to yourself, and to your children. Music exists in our souls. **LET THE MUSIC BEGIN!!!***

There are no fees for these lessons. I want you to enjoy this experience with no thought of money. However, donations will be accepted graciously.

We tried to discourage his advertising in the community and instead suggested he ask our neighbors if their kids were interested in piano lessons. He reluctantly agreed. But things were not developing fast enough for Chris. He said he missed having a place of his own. He viewed Gayle and me as holding him back from accomplishing his projects.

We had an unfinished single room structure behind the house where we had put a ping pong table and some worn carpets we had recycled from the family room. There was drywall on the framing, but it had not been taped and there was no ceiling. Some of the drywall needed to be replaced. There was a workbench and a pegboard to hang tools and plenty of storage space in the cupboards. We had discussed remodeling it, adding plumbing and making it into a guest room, or even a father-in-law's quarters to allow my father (and us) increased privacy. That had been the extent of our discussion. Gayle and I had never been sure what to do with it. Chris knew.

He felt he needed to be doing something. He was clearly getting frustrated simply playing the piano and doing other activities around the house. He wanted to paint the back room. In response to repeated pressure from Chris, I bought some tape and plaster, showed him how to tape the dry wall, and then helped him and his siblings tape and plaster it. After taping the majority of the dry wall it was clear that some of it needed to be replaced. But Chris, whose interest in spiritual foundations was all consuming, didn't want to wait until the proper physical foundation was in place. He insisted on painting the room and painting it now, not later. I tried to point out to him that he was getting manic again. He was already unable to listen. Chris's emotion propelled him to action. It would have been futile for me to try to stop him. Rather than allow the situation to escalate, Gayle and I decided to let him go ahead and paint the room. Over several days he not only painted it but also added colorful messages on the walls and doors. It was his room. Permission was not necessary. He got Elizabeth and some of her friends to participate in the project.

By the time they were through there were four different themes on the four different walls of the room. Starting to the left as one walked in there were sports themes with paintings of tennis rackets, balls, baseball bats. Then there was the nature theme. He painted a series of mountains on one wall with a cross on top of the tallest and a sun rising from behind the mountains. The large sun was surrounded by bright red projections that reached out far from what one would expect from the sun's corona. They looked like tentacles. The next section was religious with phrases such as "Seek and Ye

Shall Find." And "Only God knows why?" On the pegboard the words "Heaven" and "Hope" were written in yellow in foot-high text. Finally there was an abstract theme with strange evocative shapes above the workbench. The outside door contained large letters printed in white.

PEACE LIES WITHIN

During this time we continued to assure that he took all his medications. And again they did not appear to be helping him with his hypomanic behavior. Around the first of August he was out of Zyprexa. We wanted to wait until the psychiatrist could give us an opinion as to benefits and risks of continued long-term use of this drug. Also we were waiting for his Medi-Cal to be authorized. A month supply of Zyprexa cost $170. But we had a prescription and we could get it if we needed it. Zyprexa was likely to be approved by the FDA for short-term treatment of acute mania but it was not designed to be a long-term drug for this disorder.

Five days after he ran out of Zyprexa, he saw a TV commercial for a plastic egg cooker and tried to buy ten. Thomas and the phone representative talked him into five. One day later he got up early in the morning and began moving the TV and stereo from the house into the room, refusing to stop when we asked him to.

"But I want to open a youth center where kids can come and have fun."

"Chris, you are getting manic again. Don't you see it? You are starting to look like you did when I visited you at Sacred Heart and you told me you were God." I was getting frustrated. Once again logic was not changing his mind. Later I asked his brother Thomas to put the entertainment items back in the house. He did and Chris did not try to stop him.

Chris wrote the following in response to my concerns over his wanting to open a community youth center in the room behind the house. In that statement he hit the proverbial nail on the head.

Dad was arguing with me about how he could see the "signs" of mania coming out once more. He mentioned the "confident" voice, the deliberate speech, the oppositional behavior. He said that I couldn't "see" it in myself. He feels threatened, and I have no way to relieve him of that experience, except to be aware of how I am coming across. This is particularly challenging for me, because in the heat of the moment, all I feel is the searing impulse throbbing inside me. I can't perceive my dad's feelings because all I am aware of are my own. It is as though there is not enough room in my mind for awareness of both of us. This is why I feel cut off from the world. I am not in tune with others. I feel empty."

Zyprexa to the rescue?

Gayle and I agreed now that Chris needed Zyprexa, regardless of my long-term questions. We had the prescription filled and made certain that Chris took the medication. That night he went berry picking with the family and behaved in an appropriate manner. That was the last we would see of his intense hypomanic behavior for some time. Zyprexa had saved the day again, preventing another episode of full-blown psychotic mania.

The Zyprexa also dulled his personality, increased his weight, masked the expressiveness of his face. When he walked or moved he exhibited a rigid stiffness. As a trained professional who had seen many patients on medications, I could easily see he was on something. To an untrained person, he probably appeared to lack spontaneity. That was the price he would have to pay to keep himself out of the hospital. He wasn't yet ready to come off the Zyprexa. It looked like Zyprexa was going to be an indispensable life jacket to keep Chris from being sucked down into psychotic waters.

I wasn't sure if the Zyprexa was treating the mental disorder, or if withdrawal from Zyprexa was causing or aggravating the mental disorder, or if both were true. I knew that Zyprexa bound with histamine, dopamine, and serotonin receptors, and that taking it effectively lessened the impact of these neurotransmitters. Maybe the Zyprexa was necessary to regulate this excessive production. I was still bothered by nagging questions however. What if Zyprexa was creating an iatrogenic "black hole" which would continue to require more Zyprexa to fill? I recalled his first doctor warning us against using too much of it. If the action of the Zyprexa led to communication within his body that he was running short of histamine, dopamine and serotonin receptors, then what would prevent his body from manufacturing more? A mere 5 mg of Zyprexa was needed to stop his psychotic behavior the first time. Now he needed 10 mg to maintain when he wasn't psychotic, and still he was hypomanic.

I knew that when abusers of speed stopped using they suffered severe depression as the brain rebounded from diminished neurotransmitter production. Flood the brain with speed and the brain slows production of neurotransmitters. Could a reduction of Zyprexa create a flooding of his brain by activating more receptors? If one blocked the neurotransmitter receptors would his brain make more? What if his body produced more neurotransmitter receptors in response to the "deficit" caused by the antagonistic effects of the drug? To put it in more technical terms, long-term blockage of dopamine receptors could cause them to upregulate. Such upregulation could cause tardive dyskinesia. What would be the impact of this? Could there be a greater need for Zyprexa for the same effect? That seemed to be Chris's experience.

I had seen Attention Deficit Hyperactivity Disorder (ADHD) children coming off their Ritalin and Adderal and it was not a pretty sight. A medical professional would conclude that the underlying ADHD is very disabling. But could an observer using a different model conclude that the withdrawal from the medication was just as disabling, if not more so as the ADHD? Whether Zyprexa was or was not the long-term answer for Chris, there was no question that without it he was headed toward mania and beyond. We needed to find a psychiatrist who could help us.

Psychiatric care

His first hospital bill, about $20,000 had been covered by our health insurance since he was still our dependent then. The second bill — for $19,000 — had been reduced by Medicaid in Washington state, then forgiven by Sacred Heart after he was hospitalized again in Pennsylvania. His third bill, about $25,000, was also forgiven. Perhaps the hospital in Pennsylvania was generous ... or perhaps they wanted to forestall a lawsuit over his broken kneecap. In any event, at least Chris did not have the concern of how to raise approximately $45,000 over the next few years, but he essentially had no money.

Chris completed the application for Medi-Cal and was approved. We could have made 15-minute medication appointments through the Nevada County Behavior Health for free or, since I happened to work there, we could opt for a more in-depth albeit costly alternative that guaranteed (for the moment at least) our privacy would be protected. We chose to pay for his psychiatric care directly and to use Medi-Cal to help with his medications.

We met with a colleague of mine, psychiatrist Dr. Lund, in his private office on July 25. He recommended increasing the Depakote to 2,000 mg a day, stating that this would help manage his hypomanic behavior and allow him to eventually come off the Zyprexa.

It worked — sort of. Chris's hypomanic behavior ceased. However, his ability to perform tasks was now even more compromised. He expressed frustration that he was unable to accomplish relatively simple tasks. At our next appointment Dr. Lund recommended continuing the higher dosage of Depakote and also recommended Wellbutrin, 100 mg at night. By August 14, Chris, while still not demonstrating any hypomanic behaviors, appeared listless, depressed, and unsure of himself. The increased Depakote appeared to be solving one problem and creating another. I wrote the following to Dr. Lund.

> *He complains of memory problems, seems at times listless,*
> *depressed. Verbalizes a lot of negative thinking about his*
> *future, etc. We don't know if it is the Depakote or Zyprexa*
> *that is making him seem so tired, but he definitely seems less*

clear mentally, asking directions over and over again and not remembering recent events.

He has decided to try selling books here and also has a job offer for some telephone sales work from a new acquaintance. Initially his plan was to return to his phone sales job in Spokane after the end of the summer, but now he wants to stay here longer before moving back to Washington. We would like to see him return to his old self before he leaves us and are concerned that the medications may be making him overly tired. We prefer this to his hypomanic behavior, but would like to see him returning to his old self.

On August 14 I spoke with Dr. Lund about Chris's depression and tiredness. He suggested taking him off the Zyprexa. I said that with his history of psychosis after withdrawal that maybe we should slowly reduce the Zyprexa. He said that he didn't need the Zyprexa because he was no longer psychotic. He wanted Chris to come off the 10 mg of Zyprexa "cold turkey." I disagreed. I reduced the amount to 10 mg every two days for a week, then 10 mg every three days for another week. The Physicians Desk Reference (PDR) reported an average half-life of 30 hours, so I thought that by tapering off slowly Chris's body could better adjust to the changes. I didn't want to defy Dr. Lund's orders, but he remained unaware of the potential problems with his coming off Zyprexa. Even though I gave examples of the risk, I couldn't get through to him. After all, Chris's symptoms from Zyprexa withdrawal were one of the reasons we took Chris to see him in the first place.

Since Chris began cutting back on his Zyprexa, events seemed to be moving in the right direction. He appeared to be improving. He became more outgoing and socially involved with others. He enrolled in a course at his church. He took nightly walks with me. He said he was sleeping and, in spite of his depression, was making efforts to improve his life. He wrote an email to his sister apologizing for some previous hypomanic email.

On August 25, during the retirement party for the departing executive director of Nevada County Behavioral Services, I ran into Dr. Lund. "How is Chris doing?" he asked.

"Better in some ways. He seems to have more energy and doesn't seem quite as depressed. I didn't take him off the Zyprexa entirely because of his history of going psychotic when he comes off it. I started giving him one every other day for a week, and then one every three days."

"He is not psychotic. I would go ahead and stop the Zyprexa entirely. If he gets manic again we can increase the Depakote."

"The last time we stopped the Zyprexa he starting getting manic. He has gone psychotic twice after stopping Zyprexa. Are you sure you want to stop the Zyprexa?"

"Yeah, he will be okay." I hadn't read, and, apparently neither had he, a small typed statement in the Physicians Desk Reference (PDR) under the subtitle, "Dosage and Administration" that reads as follows. "Further dosage adjustments, if indicated should generally occur at intervals not less than one week since steady state for olanzapine would not be achieved for approximately one week in the typical patient. When dosage adjustments are necessary, dose increments/decrements of 5 mg QD are recommended." Yet, even if we had read this, it may not have registered to either of us as important given that there was no description of what could happen if one exceeded the recommended decrement dose and there were no warnings about any specific dangers associated with stopping the drug. There was no warning box saying, in large capitalized letters, "CAUTION! SUDDEN WITHDRAWAL OF THIS DRUG HAS BEEN KNOWN TO PRECIPITATE WITHDRAWAL AKATHISIA, REBOUND PSYCHOSIS, AND/OR SUICIDE!"

This was a social occasion and I didn't want to argue. Dr. Lund clearly had more faith in Depakote than I did. Yet we had been increasing the time between doses for two weeks and Chris's energy level clearly had improved. I assumed that the higher dose of Depakote would help prevent any problems Chris might encounter coming off the Zyprexa.

Although he seemed to have more energy he still complained of poor concentration. He had obtained a temporary job but felt he wasn't doing a good job for his employers. He couldn't do simple tasks and was furious with himself for not being able to perform. He still felt anxious about the future.

Different friends called with job offers and suggestions. One offered him a place to stay. His former employer offered him his old job back in Spokane. One friend suggested that Chris consider graduate school. Chris downloaded application information from the Internet on the University of Washington School of Music, even emailed author Danielle Steele, whose web site encouraged musicians who are bipolar to apply for scholarships through a foundation she had developed in memory of her son, Nick, whose bipolar disorder had led to suicide. However, when he saw the complexity of the application process he got discouraged and didn't think he would be able to fill it out. His identity seemed to be on hold. When he spoke with someone suggesting a solution, he declared his new intentions. He made and changed his plans depending on whom he talked to.

Beware of helpers

In contrast to when he was manic, when he would not listen to anyone, now he would listen to everyone, and change his views accordingly. Chris told me how all his life he had relied on other people for directions and wanted to know if he could change that. I said that he could if he wanted to. I tried not to be a "helper" but it was difficult.

Gayle, Elizabeth, and Thomas had left to take Thomas to college so Chris and I had a lot of time together. We walked nightly together. During one such walk, I talked to him about the dangers of "helpers." I shared a quote from Gestalt therapist Fritz Perls, a psychiatrist who achieved a name for himself during the '60s. "Beware of helpers. Helpers are con men who offer something for nothing. They keep you dependent and immature." I warned him that he would have to live with the consequences of any decision he made and that relying too much on others, including professionals, friends, even me, regardless of how sincerely we were trying to help, might not be best for him. Little did I know.

On August 26, following my conversation with Dr. Lund, I went over the medications with Chris. I took out the Zyprexa.

"Shouldn't I continue with this pill?" Chris said.

"Dr. Lund says that you don't need it any more. He is concerned about possible long-term side effects. Since we have been cutting back without any major problems he wants you to stop it now entirely. "

Earlier, we had discussed Dr. Lund's recommendation for abrupt withdrawal versus my alternative of a tapered cutback, and Chris had agreed with my plan. He agreed now as well. I was helping the helper, Dr. Lund, to help. Chris didn't argue. At this point in his life, he was a depressed compliant patient. When he was high he knew everything and we knew nothing. But now that he was down, he idolized his mom and me for our capabilities while denigrating himself for alleged inadequacies. The pattern wasn't entirely unlike the idealization/devaluation phenomena seen in borderline personality disorder, a chronic lifelong disorder characterized by, among other things, unstable identity, mood swings, and impulsiveness.

On August 27, he attended church and later signed up for a six week class offered by the church. That evening he spoke with Sandy and even joked about how if he ever got his act together he might call her "10 years from now and propose marriage." Sandy later said she had not heard him sounding so positive for a long time.

By August 28, he appeared to have improved even more. On our walks together he talked about his decision to take the Alpha course at our church. Alpha was a class for those who were interested in exploring basic Christian beliefs. Chris talked about how he needed to get back to his earlier religious identity and away from some of the far-out thinking he had expressed in his journal. I supported that decision.

I opined that there had been no suicides while I was stationed at Little Rock AFB in Arkansas and three when I was at Castle AFB in California. I then wondered out loud if the underlying Little Rock culture had values that were closer to a Judeo-Christian perspective and whether that had anything to do with the lack of suicides when I was there. In my own mind, I immediately questioned myself as to whether I should have even mentioned the word "suicide," let alone mentioned the suicides that occurred when I was stationed at Castle AFB, but it was too late to take it back.

The concern wasn't over the lack of scientific validity to my ideas. I knew I couldn't scientifically defend what I said. For all I knew the difference in suicide rates could be explained by coincidence, or, if there were some relationship, it could be noise levels, command cultures, or even demographics. I thought Chris would understand the point I was making, namely that returning to his historical cultural roots might be stabilizing for him. It was only small talk, but the precipice-dread oozed into this area as well. My concern was simply that I had talked about the issue of suicide.

Suicide was a topic Chris and I had discussed before. He reported having suicidal thoughts, but he had always denied any specific intent or plans to harm himself. The closest thing to a plan was a fantasy of being with an old girlfriend, taking an overdose and dying in her arms.

On the evening of August 28, three days after he stopped the Zyprexa, I asked him a question while he was cooking Hamburger Helper. Chris looked blank and stopped stirring the food.

"When you asked me that I can't answer it and do what I was doing."

"Are you feeling anxious?" I asked.

He answered, "Yeah."

He seemed incapable of multitasking. I thought that he was coming down off the medication and was starting to feel things again. "Would you like me to help you tomorrow with some relaxation exercises to help you with that?"

"OK."

I didn't give it a second thought. I remembered a phrase I once heard from Dr. Rollo May. "Anxiety is pain in the narrowest place." Chris could learn to utilize his anxiety to help trigger his growth. I found the constructs of the trade to be helpful. They helped explain events and created a world with some predictability and control, at least for the therapist. As long as the anxiety was not "psychotic" anxiety Chris would be fine. I had no reason to believe otherwise now that he was on more Depakote and his doctor had said he would be okay ... or so I told myself.

We had an uneventful evening and we went to bed.

By the next morning, Chris had written a schedule of activities and some personal goals for himself.

I was surprised and concerned to see him up at 6:30. Normally he slept in and when he didn't it usually meant he had been up all night. That was not a good sign, since one night of not sleeping had either provoked or been reflective of manic behavior in the past.

The first thing I asked him when I greeted him was if he slept the night before.

"I had a hard time getting to sleep, but did OK once I got to sleep. Dad, I decided last night to write down a schedule and stick to it. That way I can get more done and not just waste my time." He showed me the schedule.

CHRIS MOYER'S LIFELINE SCHEDULE
9:00 Work on knee with various exercises
9:15 Breakfast
9:30 Swim laps in the lake.
Keep track of laps
10:00 Jog/walk

I was concerned over his problem getting to sleep, but was encouraged that he had made a schedule to put some order in his life. I knew from previous experience that as long as he was getting some sleep, the likelihood of old demons awakening was slim.

"Today I am going to Steve and Debbie's to work. She's coming to pick me up."

It had been exactly four days since Chris had stopped taking 10 mg of Zyprexa every three days.

"OK, have a nice day."

A half-hour later I walked out on the deck on the way to work. The weather was different, a change from the previous three weeks of swimming-in-the-lake Indian summer. It was a windless, cold, overcast day with clouds in the sky. I felt that subtle, but palpable foreboding that I had felt before in my life, though I could not connect it to anything significant. I thought of the rain, the cold that would be coming soon, heralding the end of the summer season. I thought of Alaska where the "termination dust" (snow) would soon be creeping down the mountains surrounding the Eagle River Valley. I thought of our house near Chugiak State Park where we used to live and to which I still hoped to return one day. Folks in Alaska would probably have snow on the ground in a month and a half. There wasn't any reason to be depressed. We were in California. We wouldn't have to look forward to the sunless days, the long winter nights, and the 20-below-zero draft coming through the bottom of the French doors. We might have some rain and fog, but our winter here would be very mild compared to what it would be in Alaska. There was no logic to my sense of foreboding, but it was still there. It was just that kind of day. Maybe it was my precipice-dread.

I didn't know it at the time, but Chris had not been honest with me. He had, in fact, been up all night. He had written a second file as follows:

THINGS I AM AND CHOOSE TO BE

Warm
Loving
Tender
Kind
Thoughtful
Considerate
Gentle
Compassionate

THINGS I AM NOT AND CHOOSE NOT TO BE

Impulsive
Imprudent
Rude
Discourteous
Hateful
Jealous

"I admire the gifts of God in others. And I thank God for the gifts he has given me. He has given me the gift of music; he has given me the gift of compassion and love. He will help me to be tender if I seek it. I must always meditate on God's love for me and others, lest I forget who I am."

Had I known of this file, I would have not been overly concerned. I would have thought that Chris was at work deciding the kind of person he wanted to be by establishing positive goals for himself. I would never have suspected that those positive words were the "good Chris" attempting to placate the demons of the "bad Chris." I would not have guessed that the demons in his brain had been waiting for just the right pretext to spring into action. Nor would I have known that the tyranny of bipolar, black and white psychotic thinking had already begun. Chris's mind was getting so small there wasn't even enough room for him in it. He had already started alternating between the "good Chris" and the "bad Chris," in the fashion of Dr. Jekyll and Mr. Hyde. His ability to synthesize the thoughts, feelings, and behavior in his brain disappeared as the "good" and "bad" wrestled for control. I wouldn't know it until later that night.

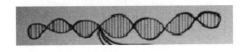

111

11 - Running Amok

Webster's Dictionary defines "amok" as a "psychic disturbance characterized by depression followed by a manic urge to murder." The term is from Southeast Asian culture.

Trying to work

In July, Chris had accepted a job with a couple, Steve and Debbie, whom he had met through some mutual friends. Chris had much in common with Steve, who was also a musician. The couple was starting up a business selling artificial turf, and they needed a part-time person to do telephone screening of prospective customers and also to help with administrative tasks. Chris was a perfect fit for the job. He wanted part-time work and could sell just about anything.

The work would not normally have been difficult for him. He had done far more complex jobs and done them well. His tasks involved calling prospective customers who had expressed interest in the product at the county fair. He asked them if they were still interested in knowing more about Perma Green Grass for their homes. He would point out the advantages of having green "grass" all year long without having to fertilize, water, or mow it. Then, if the person were interested in having a home visit, he would write down directions and agree upon a time for Steve or Debbie to pay a call.

Yet ever since he had started, Chris had felt inadequate in the job. He put himself down verbally whenever he made a mistake, no matter how small. He had particular difficulty getting directions down accurately, and he blamed himself for this. He wouldn't consider the possibility that his medications or his illness were slowing down his mental processes. He wouldn't accept that depressed bipolar patients have reduced blood flow and associated low metabolism in the left frontal cortex and other areas of the brain. All he knew was that he had graduated from college with a magna cum laude degree in music composition. He had made $10,000 one summer working 75-hour weeks selling books door to door. At the end of that summer, he'd gone back to every household that had ordered books and delivered them. If he hadn't been able to find the houses, he would not have been paid. Yet now he couldn't talk to a customer and write down directions to their house without making a mistake. It had to be some fault of his. He assured his employers that he would eventually overcome these problems.

While Chris blamed himself for not being able to meet his own expectations, Debbie had noted his difficulties, and, having had experience with ADHD children, was careful to break his tasks into small, easily defined pieces. She made sure that he understood what he was supposed to do. Chris liked both Steve and Debbie, but Steve was more of a taskmaster.

Chris was getting it, but it had been slow. After we cut back on the Zyprexa in August, he hadn't complained as much about his difficulties doing the job, leading me to believe that the medications might have been limiting his functioning in some way and now, with less Zyprexa, his performance had been improving.

Verdict? Guilty! Sentence? Hell!

I got home from work around 6 p.m. on August 29 and noticed that Chris wasn't home yet. He had been late before. The employer-employee relationship was fairly ill-defined. Steve and Debbie, besides being his employers, were also his friends. Sometimes he would stay and talk. Sometimes, he would play their piano. So I didn't give his absence much thought until about 9 p.m., when he still hadn't shown up. I didn't want to call Steve's home to ask if Chris were there. After all, Chris needed a few places in his life free from the influence of his parents. I knew he wouldn't like me checking up on him. We had supported his need to get a job and have a life away from his family, especially because he had expressed concerns over feeling more dependent on us.

I wondered if Chris had decided to walk home. I thought he might be lost as he frequently told me he had difficulty with directions. So I finally decided to call Steve's house to see if he had left. I dialed the number.

Debbie answered, "Hello."

"Hi. This is Dave Moyer, Chris's dad. I was wondering if he had left your place yet because he hasn't shown up here."

"He isn't here. I assumed he had gone home. Steve went into Sacramento. I don't think he took Chris with him, but he might have. I thought he left this afternoon and that someone picked him up."

"No, my wife is in Seattle taking my other son to college, and I didn't pick him up."

"When Steve gets home, I'll ask if he knows where he is, but I thought he left this afternoon."

"Can you tell me how he was today?"

"He looked kind of white and ashen all day. Had a hard time getting into the work. He was supposed to put address labels on envelopes, and he seemed to have difficulty concentrating on this. I think at one point he was playing the piano, and he woke Steve up. Then he just left. He said something to my son about not wanting to miss this opportunity when he left and that he apologized for not finishing the work. We thought he had a ride. Is there anything going on with Chris?"

"I don't know if he told you or not, but he has bipolar disorder. His psychiatrist recently took him off some of his medications. I wasn't sure if Chris told you about his background or not, and I wouldn't have told you myself except that we need to figure out what is going on."

"No, he didn't tell us that, but he did tell us once that when he was in college he had the experience of feeling like he had demons in him and that he totally lost his own sense of where he was."

"Well, he says he has trouble with directions, so I was concerned he may have decided to walk home and gotten lost. I'm going to drive around just to see if he's walking along the road, then I'll call back later when Steve is home."

I felt afraid. Chris had been on his own for more than six hours. My mind raced back to every conversation we had over the preceding days. He had not voiced any suicidal plans or intent. He had been reaching out more to others. He seemed to have more energy. He had started playing the piano on Saturday nights at the Lake Wildwood clubhouse and had seemed to enjoy the positive feedback and the tips. Yet I also knew that when a person comes out of depression is often the period of highest risk for suicide.

I ran downstairs. I checked Chris's pill dispenser. All the pills were there. I checked the entire house, looking for a note. I found none. I went to the room that Chris had designated the "Community Youth Center" just to make sure he wasn't there. I kept telling myself that he couldn't have killed himself. He had too much going for him. He probably just got lost. I even contemplated the possibility of foul play.

I drove for 45 minutes up and down country roads around Steve and Debbie's home, feeling like I was in a bad dream that I would wake up from at any time. As I remembered the walk across the Golden Gate Bridge with my father, the multiple times I had feared for his safety, the precipice-dread started to turn into a precipice panic. The roads were empty and dark. When I returned home, I called Steve's house. He was back.

"Hi, Steve, I'm Chris's father. Can you fill me in on what happened or where he is?"

"He left here about 4 p.m. He was supposed to be putting address labels on envelopes, but wasn't getting much done. I tried to take a nap, and he started playing the piano. I got up and told him I was trying to sleep. Actually, I told him I was 'trying to fucking sleep.' Chris apologized then went into the garage and opened a pack of cigarettes and took a couple. I was going to get him his check, but he walked out. He didn't tell us good-bye. I assumed he had called someone to pick him up."

"So you're saying he's been on his own for about six hours?"

"Since you called, my wife and I checked around the house and didn't find him."

"I don't know what's going on, but I think I'd better call the police and see if anything has happened to him."

"I'm sorry that this happened. We knew Chris was having some problems. I hope you find him."

It was now 11 p.m. I called 911.

"Hello, is this an emergency?"

"I'd like to report a missing person, my 25-year-old son."

"Please explain the circumstances."

"He left from a home near Highway 20 about a mile down from Pleasant Valley Road at approximately 4 p.m. We haven't been able to find him. He's bipolar and had some recent medication changes. He's been depressed but was not actively suicidal."

"We haven't had any calls on a Chris Moyer — no — wait a second. About ten minutes ago we got a notification of a young man who was found on Highway 20 in Yuba County. If you'll give me a few minutes, I'll check to see if it's him and then call you back."

Yuba County? That was west toward Marysville, not east toward Penn Valley. I hung up. A few minutes later the phone rang.

"Sir, the police have picked up your son on Highway 20, about seven miles from the home you are describing."

I breathed a sigh of relief. "Is he okay?"

"I am going to give you the number of the Yuba County policeman who was involved with this and he can tell you what happened."

"But is he okay?" I asked, a little louder now.

"I think so, but you need to talk to them. Here's the number. You'll want to talk to Officer Hulsey."

She gave me the number. I called immediately and asked to speak with Officer Hulsey.

"Sir, can you tell me what happened to my son? I understand you found him on Highway 20."

"Yes, we had several 911 calls from drivers who saw your son walking down the highway with blood all over his head and shirt. We sent out an ambulance around 8 p.m. He appeared to be hiding in the bushes, but we found him. He had severe lacerations to his head, deep cuts on his wrists, and two cuts on both sides of his neck. He told me that he had committed an unpardonable sin and that he deserved to go to hell and that he wanted to die. He said he found some broken glass and started cutting himself, then he grabbed a rock and hit himself on the head several times."

I switched into quiet and clinical. I had learned to manage my feelings during a crisis, having been through similar situations before in my life. Just before Chris was born, I had received a call that one of my patients had cut his wrists and was in the Emergency Room. I had gone out to assess him, and when I returned Gayle was in labor. I had experience in being quietly clinical.

"Did he say he was trying to kill himself?"

"He said he didn't want to live any more."

"Are his wounds severe enough for him to be in danger now?"

"When we picked him up, he appeared to be starting to go into shock, but I think they have him stabilized now. He's in the ER at Rideout Hospital. I can give you the number there if you want to find out how he's doing now."

He gave me the number. There was a pause.

The officer said, "Do you need anything else?"

Did I need anything else? Where would I start? I wanted to know why. I wanted an explanation. I wanted some hope that Chris wouldn't eventually succeed in killing himself. I knew the officer had reports to write up, other crises to attend to, and that he had no more of a clue than I did. I thanked him for his help and called Rideout ER. An orderly put the doctor on.

"This is Dr. Zoll," said a woman's voice.

"Hello, Dr. Zoll. I'm Chris Moyer's father. Can you tell me how he's doing?"

"We've sutured up his wrists and his head lacerations and one of the neck wounds. However, we need to have a specialist, an ENT doctor take a look at the left neck wound. It's still oozing badly, and we want to make sure there are no other injuries before we suture this injury. He doesn't appear to have damaged his tendons or his larynx and fortunately he missed any arteries."

"The officer told me he was starting to go into shock. Are his injuries that severe?"

"When he came to the hospital, he had lost a lot of blood, but his platelet count was normal. He was covered with blood mostly from his head wounds. Apparently he repeatedly hit his head with rocks and that caused most of the bleeding."

"Should I come down tonight and see him or wait till tomorrow?"

"I would wait till tomorrow. He is very tired and may be having surgery on his neck tonight."

I gave her a brief overview of Chris's history, including the medicines he had been taking. She thanked me for the information and said she would relay it to the consulting psychiatrist. I thanked her for her help and told her I would be in to see him the next day.

By now it was 12:30 a.m.. It was too late to call Gayle. If I called her now, she would be up all night upset. I decided to try to sleep and call her in the morning. I went to bed. My mouth was dry. I could feel my heart pounding in my chest. What did Debbie mean that Chris was white and ashen all day? What had I missed? Had he tried to kill himself? Was he trying to release the demons that were flying around in his head? Had he reacted impulsively to Steve's anger? Had withdrawal from the Zyprexa caused this? Was his belief that he had committed a so-called unforgivable sin the reason for his actions or simply the best psychotic justification he could come up with?

I couldn't get the events of the past few hours out of my head. My mind was spinning out of control with random thoughts. I wondered what it must be like to have thoughts racing out of control with no way to control them. Was this what life had been like for both Chris and my father? I tossed back and forth in my bed waiting for sleep that never came.

Trying to identify with what Chris was going through, I thought back to a time 30 years earlier when I was in graduate school. I was abruptly awakened from sleep as moth wings flapped against my eardrum with a deafening sound. The moth had somehow flown one way down my ear canal while I slept. The sound of the flapping caused me to jump out of bed, hit my head hard with the palm of my hand, and run around the room like a crazy man trying desperately to stop the noise and pain in my head. I somehow was able to drive to an Emergency Room where a doctor eventually extracted it. Having seen patients hitting their heads against objects before, I could now see an inner logic in their attempts to make the pain inside go away, logic I had not afforded to them before, even while showing the empathy I had been trained to display.

There is a German phrase I picked up years ago, "Er hat Vogel im Kopf." It means "He has birds in his head." Moth wings, birds, thoughts — they were all the same when they are flying around inside your head and there is nothing you can do to stop them, except the self-infliction of more pain ... or death.

Each time Chris's illness had struck, we had all lost something. First there was his timely graduation from college. Then there was the loss of an optimistic, industrious worker who had been ready to face the world with no limits. Then there was the loss of an athlete who could run, walk, and do flips whenever he wanted to. And now it was the possible loss of a son to death by his own hand. I started to mourn the possibility that either the illness or the treatment of it could cause me to lose my son forever.

After a night of sleepless tossing and turning, I got up at 6:30 and called Gayle. As bad as the events of the previous night had been, the entire experience still seemed unreal, almost dreamlike to me. I hadn't seen Chris. I hadn't shared the news with anyone except my father, who, by this time was living with us. I dialed the number.

"Hello," a sleepy voice answered. It was Ga (sounds like "God" without the "d"), Chris's grandmother. On that side of the family, the first-born of the next generation renamed their grandmothers with the first sounds with which they addressed them. For example Ga's mother was "Ning," as named by her granddaughter.

"Ga, I need to talk to Gayle."

"OK, just a minute, Dave. I'll get her."

I took a deep breath when my wife picked up the phone. "Hi, sorry to call you so early in the morning, but I didn't want to wake you up last night. Chris is in the hospital at Rideout."

Muffled sobs at the other end.

"Apparently he was playing the piano at Steve's instead of working, and Steve got impatient with him for keeping him awake. Then he left early and started walking down Highway 20. He picked up some broken glass and cut himself on the wrists and neck. Then he grabbed a rock and hit himself on the head."

"Why would he do something like that?" she cried.

As my clinical mask dissolved, the events from the night before became more real. Between sobs I told her, "The cop told me that Chris said something about committing the unpardonable sin and that he deserved to go to hell. He said he was trying to kill himself, but if he really wanted to he could have jumped in front of a car. I think he was trying to relieve the pressure in his brain. It has to be from that damn medicine. I think he became psychotic in response to coming off the Zyprexa. I'm going to visit him today. I'll tell you more when I see him."

We talked about whether or not she should come home right away and then hung up. She still had to take Thomas to college.

Later I called the hospital. The surgery on his neck had been uneventful, except for the fact that he refused to sign the permission slip to get anesthesia for the operation on his neck. He said he wanted to feel the pain because he was going through some kind of dress rehearsal for hell and wanted to be prepared. They gave him anesthesia without his permission since he was too psychotic to provide informed consent. He was recovering now with one-on-one supervision. He seemed pretty out of it still. They wouldn't transfer him to a psychiatric hospital until his wounds had healed.

Sorting it out

I drove down to Rideout and walked into the Intensive Care Unit. Chris was lying in bed. His neck was covered with a bandage. His face was pale. A nurse was watching him.

"Chris, what did you do to yourself?"

"Dad, you shouldn't be here. You don't know me. I am evil."

"I thought you were feeling better."

"I didn't sleep and I felt there was no sense going on."

"You told me you had trouble getting to sleep, but that you did sleep soundly once asleep."

"I didn't want to tell you because you would think that the change in

119

medicines was causing the problem. I didn't want you to win." Chris in his mind remained the "captain of his ship, the master of his soul" and he didn't want any facts to spoil his beliefs. I wondered how I could help him if he was so oppositional that he would lie about something so basic as whether he slept or not.

Chris described the events of that day. He spoke of his frustration as he sat with his mind racing and tried to put address labels on envelopes. He spoke of his playing the piano and Steve's anger at being awakened from his nap. He said he became so upset over his insensitivity to Steve that he stole some cigarettes from him and just started walking down Highway 20. He said he didn't know where he was. He said he felt he was lost and knew he was going to hell. There was that psychotic associational logic, again. Being physically lost was the same as being lost eternally, or, damned to hell.

Chris talked about walking for hours on Highway 20. He bit branches on trees and lay down in the dirt and rocks, attempting to prepare himself for the terrors of hell. Since he was going to hell, he wanted to inoculate himself against the suffering he would soon experience there. He wanted to kill himself because he had committed the unpardonable sin and God could never forgive him. The Bipolar Prophet that represented his new thinking about God and Jesus had now doomed him to hell. He feared killing us and "reasoned" that killing himself would save us. He picked up a piece of broken glass along the road and cut his wrists and neck. He hit his head with a rock when he was unsuccessful with the glass. I had never heard such ideas during our long discussions with each other prior to the events of August 29. How could one emotional event kick off a psychotic break? It had to be withdrawal from that damned Zyprexa. Chris had run amok.

I didn't stay long.

That night when I went to bed I worried about what was going to happen next. Chris would get better or worse. In the long run he would either live or die. There had to be a way to find something positive in this tragedy. I remembered a decision I had made years before during Peace Corps training when I heard a speaker talk about coping with life's stresses. He shared a decision he had made that no matter what challenges life threw at him, he would find a way to prevail and to grow through the experience. It was an attitude, not of invincibility, but just a quiet confidence that whatever life throws at you, you will handle it. To the extent you can make a difference you conquer it or find a way to grow through it. I had decided during that talk that I would do the same. That decision had been very helpful during other crises in my life. I would find it helpful for this one too.

Throughout my life I had tried to the extent possible to keep the family secrets secret. As a youth, as a college student, even as a professional, I had compartmentalized these secrets, revealing to others only what was absolutely necessary. Even our friends knew little of Ray's history. Once the door to the secret compartment was opened there was no telling where it would stop. We did not want neighbors to know that the man with the unusual behavior next door had spent two years at a hospital for the sexually perverse. When Chris started having problems, I stopped sending our usual upbeat annual Christmas poems to our friends. Each Christmas we received news of exciting trips and school accomplishments of their children. They heard nothing from us. We figured this was better than telling them that our son had been in a psychiatric hospital. I did not want our family to carry the stigma that goes with "mental" illness. A brain tumor or a car accident we could share. Mental illness was different. There was an elephant in our living room and we had been trying to live as though it didn't exist. We couldn't continue to ignore it. Now we were going to have to face it head on.

I finally slept. I dreamed I was at the edge of a long, narrow frozen pond in the midst of a snow-covered forest. The ice was thick near the edge, thinner toward the middle. I saw people lying face-down on the ice near the center. I couldn't tell how many. My focus was only on the ones nearest to me. They were still; I thought they were dead at first. But then I noticed indentations in the ice from the warmth of their bodies, and I knew they were alive. Alive, but terrified that if they moved so much as a muscle, they would fall through. I couldn't get out to help them without breaking the ice myself, so I turned and trudged as fast as I could through the thigh-deep snow until I found a long branch poking out of a snowdrift. Slowly, breathlessly, I dragged it back to the pond. Someone else had come along while I was gone. He stood on the opposite side, gazing at me helplessly. I carefully pushed the branch across the ice to him. When both of us had a firm grip, we slid it toward some of the people and yelled for them to reach out and grab hold. They hadn't stirred while all this was going on, and even in the brief time I'd been away, the heat of their bodies had melted more of the ice. Yet for a long time, or what seemed like a long time, no one moved. Then, without lifting his half-frozen face from the ice, a man raised his right arm and carefully, blindly, swept it back and forth through the air, searching for the branch we were shouting for him to grab onto. Just as his hand touched the branch, I woke up.

Hell

When I returned home from The University of Pennsylvania I still was not completely over my mania. I believed that in order to enter the Kingdom of Heaven, one must become like a little child. I began relating more to the kids than to the adults. I also began acting very childlike. I came up with the idea of having a clubhouse for children where they could come, play games, and worship God.

I also planned to teach piano lessons out in the clubhouse, but to do so by "feel" rather than the traditional way of using workbooks. My thoughts were extremely flighty, and one minute I would talk about working for a soup kitchen, the other I would talk about becoming a Big Brother. I also considered taking speed-reading classes at Sierra College.

In getting the clubhouse "prepared" I argued with my parents. I wanted to paint it a certain way, and my father wanted to make sure I did the job the "right" way. There were arguments as I took the television out of the family room downstairs and brought it into the clubhouse, rationalizing that since I had bought it in the first place, I could do whatever I wanted to with it. I opened my boxes and brought the contents into the room, thinking that the kids could play with the Transformers, and look at the rocks and shells inside. I brought my baseball cards into the room as well, thinking I could offer baseball cards to children when they had a good piano lesson. I swam late in the pool with Elizabeth and her friends, and when mom said it was late and time to get out, I argued with her, unconcerned that the noise would bother the neighbors.

After a while, things started to calm down. I began to make strides to improve my life. I called the Wildwood clubhouse, and was able to secure a job as a piano player, playing once every other Saturday. I got a job working for a company called Perma Green Grass, and was involved in setting appointments for Steve and Debbie, the owners. Just when things were starting to look great on the outside, they were looking bleak on the inside. I lacked confidence in my job. Every day I went to work, I got down on myself, thinking that I was going to screw up, thinking I wasn't doing a very good job. Even when Steve and Debbie assured me I was doing fine and told me not to be so hard on myself, I became even more hard on myself. I began feeling as though I couldn't function in life. At this time I was taking the meds and so I knew it was a problem with myself.

I started talking with my dad about my problems. My dad taught me about the child/adult/parent relationship, and after I learned it, I began to realize truly what a child I was and how dependent I was on everyone around me. When I analyzed my life, all I could see were "childish" decisions. I realized I had made adult decisions in the past, but now, those times seemed far removed and distant. I would never become a mature adult, I thought. College was over, Southwestern was over, and the best and most productive times in my life were behind me. These were the thoughts that led to what happened next.

[Note that in his narrative the crucial decisions involving the Zyprexa are not even mentioned. He can only relate to his personal feelings and has little awareness or appreciation of the context in which these events occurred.]

When I left to go to Steve and Debbie's, I had a feeling that something bad was going to happen. I didn't know what, but I was feeling very apprehensive that day. I didn't know how I would relate to Debbie or Steve. Debbie *arrived to pick me up, and she brought me over to the house. The task ahead was relatively simple, and brainless. I was to put address labels and stamps onto postcards. I was relieved that the job was so easy, because I wasn't sure I could have handled calling people, in the state I was in. I started the task, as Debbie worked on something else. Debbie began speaking to me, and all I could think of was that my mind was blank and I had nothing to say in response to her. I felt so empty. I wasn't even doing a very good job at putting on the address labels and the stamps. Debbie showed me a simple procedure for cutting more address labels at a time, and I felt stupid because I didn't think of it first. Debbie left several minutes later, and told me she'd be back in a couple hours. I worked silently over the next few hours, but my mind was screaming with all different ideas, most of them negative. The tension inside was building more and more as I began to despise myself more and more. Finally, I had so much tension, I felt I had to relieve it. I walked over to the piano and began playing loudly. Unfortunately, Steve was sleeping at the time, and I woke him up. He was rather upset, and when I asked him, "Oh, I'm sorry, were you trying to sleep?" He responded, "I was fucking trying to."*

At this I was horrified, and couldn't believe what I had done. I left abruptly and told their son to tell Debbie that I apologized for not completing the task. As I left their house, I saw in their garage a package of unopened cigarettes, and in my desire to calm myself down, I opened the pack and took a cigarette with me. After doing this, I felt even more horrified, feeling like a criminal. Not only had I rudely awakened Steve, but I had also stolen one of his cigarettes. I had so much tension building up in me, I didn't know what to do. So I started walking. I don't even know where I was walking to, I just thought if I kept walking, things would get better. But they didn't. I lit my cigarette, knowing in the back of my head, that it might be the last small joy of my life. After the cigarette was gone, all that was left was me and the road, a road that led to nowhere. I felt extremely lost, both physically and spiritually. I watched cars scream by and contemplated jumping out in front of them. The more I walked the worse my tension got. I started to think about why such a terrible thing was happening to me, and I knew it must be because God was punishing me for being such a terrible person. After all, I had claimed to be Him, and then, what is even worse, I condemned His Son Jesus Christ to hell. How could I ever escape the fires of hell, I thought? I began feeling as though I was extremely evil, as though God would not allow me the option of repentance, for it was too late. I tried repenting, but the feeling of evil ensued. I began to truly think I was the Antichrist, and not a good one at that, but a horrible man who craves evil things.

I began feeling that hell was going to be my eternal home, and I became extremely aware of the evil that existed within me. I pictured myself going home and slaughtering my family and whoever else was around. These im-

ages were so terrifying, I knew I had to kill myself, so I wouldn't risk bringing about such a horrible evil. I looked around for something to hurt myself, and I found the top to a broken beer bottle. I shoved the glass into my left wrist, and pulled it across my wrist. Blood began spurting out. I thought that would be enough. I went off the side of the road to the edge of the forest and lay down, hoping none of the cars would stop to try and save me. I waited a few minutes, hoping to start losing energy, expecting to soon rise out of my body. It appeared to me then that death wouldn't be as easy as I thought before. I put another slice into my wrist, so now I had two bleeding wounds. My whole life was appearing in my conscious mind. I remembered saying that I could beat up God as a child. I remember saying in church at the age of 4 that my Mommy made me rather than God. I saw how selfish all my actions were in life. Even the "good" things I had done I saw as selfish deeds done to boost myself up.

The whole time I was hurting myself, I knew that things would only get worse. At first, I thought death could be peaceful, and I would quietly lose energy and fade out of existence. At least I hoped this was the case. However, the more difficult attaining death became for me, the more I became aware that hell would be much worse than anything I could imagine. In fact, while I was hurting myself, I became aware that in hell, people would experience the greatest conceivable pain forever. However, I was trapped. If I stayed, and died, I would experience this incredible pain. However, if I went back home, I would surely go out of control and inflict incredible pain on the people I once considered family and loved. There was no way out for me, either way, so I decided to do the best thing, and kill myself without inflicting pain on others. It was my last ounce of good.

As time went on, and the blood continued flowing, it wasn't fast enough for me, so I took the beer bottle top and stuck it into my neck on the left side, and made a cut. Blood ran down my neck and over my chest. Then I made another cut on the right side of my neck. I figured that would be enough. But it wasn't. I still felt the tension building and could not get it to stop. I picked up a large rock and started pounding my head with it. All I wanted was to not feel anything. I lay down by the side of the road, and waited to die. It didn't happen. Probably half an hour later, I decided to continue walking down the street. After several minutes, I came upon a police car and an officer who was shining a light out into the darkness. The officer beckoned me, and reluctantly I came forward. Within half an hour I was in an ambulance headed toward the hospital. The fears of hell did not go away right away, but it took days of being in the mental ward in Sacramento before they began to fade.

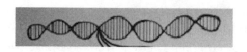

12 - High Anxiety in the Cuckoo's Nest

In spite of my best efforts to keep family problems isolated from my professional life, this was no longer possible. Chris was on Medi-Cal and could not afford to pay for his fourth hospitalization.

Chris was admitted involuntarily to Live Oaks Hospital in Sacramento, with some help from Dr. Lund and the crisis team at Behavioral Health. Apart from a few cursory conversations with Dr. Lund, who said, he had never seen anything like this before I no longer confided in him or trusted in his opinions.

Off to a bad start

My first visit, not good. I walked in, and Larry, a tall, hefty staff member with one earring, said, "You can visit him briefly, but if I see he's getting agitated, I'm going to have to ask you to leave."

Well, duh, I thought to myself. I've only been in this business for 29 years. Didn't say anything.

Walked into a crowded visiting, snack, and/or recreation room where several patients were watching TV and talking. Chris was lying on a couch. He had bandages on his wrists and both sides of his neck. He did not look well. When he saw me, he said "hi" and sat up. Out of the corner of my eye, I could see staff members observing the goings-on from behind a window. There were no staff physically present in the room.

We returned to the subject of what he had done and why he had done it. He started talking again about the unpardonable sin that had damned him to hell.

"Chris, you probably won't believe me, but I think you had a reaction to withdrawing from the Zyprexa." Although he didn't say anything, to me he appeared to be tracking what I was saying. While we were talking, one of the staff walked out of the inner sanctum and intruded on our conversation.

"He won't be able to process what you are telling him for several days," she said.

She probably thought she was trying to help. The message I heard was that they were in charge, and that I was in their space. They would determine the interventions, and I was not to interfere. I asked Chris if he could repeat what I had said.

His responses were slow and tentative. "You think this has to do with my coming off the Zyprexa?"

I looked at the woman.

She returned without a word to the place behind the window where the staff lived during their shift. Chris did not become agitated. I was allowed to stay. He didn't have much to say except for his recitation of what would become an obsessive litany regarding his belief that he had committed an unpardonable sin and didn't deserve to live. Something had happened in his brain so that he now looked back on his grandiose prophesies and believed he had blown his chances with God.

On my way out, I wanted to ask the charge nurse if there had been any lab work that would give any clues as to the basis for this episode. I stood in front of her at the nursing station where the sliding glass window was open and waited several minutes for her to acknowledge my presence. She appeared to be involved in paperwork and was not subtle in giving nonverbal cues that she would not mind in the least if I were to leave. I wondered if all parents were treated this way or just the parents of an indigent, which, at this point, my son was. She finally looked up wordlessly, resigned.

"Hi, I'm Chris's father. I wanted to ask you if there was any lab work done that would help us to understand what happened. Four days before Chris cut himself, he stopped taking Zyprexa on his doctor's orders. I wondered if you had any way to know if withdrawing from Zyprexa contributed to his decompensation." I hoped that using the lingo would give me greater access.

She responded in what I perceived as a defensive and belittling manner. "We always do a routine screening on our patients. He does not have a medical condition that would cause this. I mean, he has a psychiatric disorder."

Oh, that explained it, a psychiatric disorder. I repeated my concerns about his coming off the Zyprexa, and, when I realized I was talking to the air, thanked her and left.

As I walked into the elevator, I wondered what the difference was between a medical condition and a psychiatric disorder. I thought Chris had a biologically based brain disorder, but according to the nurse, he had a "psychiatric" disorder. The word "psychiatric" was derived from the Greek word "psyche." "Psyche" means soul or personality. No wonder Chris blamed himself for not being right in his head. He had a "soul" problem. He wasn't in control of his "psyche" as he should have been. Words such as "mental" and "psyche" were not just words. They conveyed basic assumptions about the nature of Chris's illness. These labels explained everything ... and nothing. I decided from that day forward, if only for the maintenance of my own psyche, that I would privately christen the helpful charge nurse as "Nurse Rachet." I was in a damned Cuckoo's Nest.

Considering Chris's condition and the "vibes" I received from the hospital staff, it was no wonder that my first visit was such a downer. I decided I would bring my guitar for subsequent visits. Chris was profoundly and morbidly depressed and obsessed. His thoughts kept returning to the same place. But one thing that had always been present, whether in his most manic or depressed episodes, was his love of music. Perhaps music could reach him now and offer him a way out, a path back to the world, or at least a lifeline to hang onto in his current limbo. A little music might do the rest of the "psych" patients some good as well.

Creating our own milieu

The next visit went much better. Chris and I strolled down the main hall, away from the eyes behind the window. We sat on the floor, I took out my guitar, and we started singing folk songs, pop songs, some old hymns, and some songs I had written over the years. It was strange to see him enjoying this so spontaneously and freely. When he talked, he would talk about his thoughts of killing himself, his mom, or me. When he shared his writings, he would read a dialogue between the "good" and "bad" Chris where the bad one was winning. These kinds of thoughts are called automatic negative thoughts, or ANTS. I had seen the pattern often during his psychotic episodes. His brain drilled down to one thought or cluster of thoughts only and became trapped there. Yet when he sang, he not only got temporary relief from the ANTS, but seemed to enjoy himself. So we sang a lot and talked a little.

Patients wandered down the hall to listen and join in. Many of the patients sang along with us. Some of them cried, including me when I tried to sing James Taylor's "Fire and Rain." "Just yesterday morning, they let me know you were gone ..." was tough to get through. The chorus was especially troubling. A woman and a man sobbed openly when we sang "Amazing Grace." It was Okay. There were no pretensions, just a lot of shared pain that found expression in the music we sang. I felt closer to the patients than to the eyes behind the door.

They introduced themselves. Mary, the depressed woman in her fifties who had sobbed through "Amazing Grace," was very appreciative of our music. Sharon was a woman in her twenties who looked much older. She told me that her husband had divorced her because of her bipolar disorder. She was also the mother of God, and her special powers allowed her to "read" others. Her kids were in another country with the ex-husband, and she had been living in a group home. When she spoke, I noticed severe extrapyramidal side effects such as involuntary grimacing and unusual tongue movements. I thought she might have tardive dyskinesia, a permanent neurological disorder characterized by grimaces and muscle spasms that can occur as a result of long-term use of antipsychotic medications. Jan, in her forties, was a very friendly, spunky, and delightful lady with schizophrenia. Her associations were loose, making it difficult to understand her. Based on her comments, she had been either the CEO of her company, the president of the union, or maybe someone who worked there. Tim was an 18-year-old experiencing his first paranoid schizophrenic break. He was always moving in and out of social interactions, never staying long enough to talk. Dwight was a senile older man, hard to tell how old. His vocabulary seemed to consist only of phrases pertaining to Elvis Presley. He appeared to have had a pretty hard life, judging from his physical state and the tattoos covering his arms. I surmised he was brain damaged from abusing drugs or alcohol.

One of the patients told me they had enjoyed hearing Chris sing a song he had composed in college earlier in the day, a song I remembered from his senior recital. It was entitled "Got To Get a Date," a humorous jazz song and rap. I had a hard time imagining Chris singing a solo a few days after injuring himself so severely. To obsess about killing himself and to perform a light, humorous song was just too incongruent. It was as if the singing and the destructive obsessions were from two different people.

When Chris focused on the activity at hand, he seemed perfectly appropriate. But if he focused on his internal reality, he would share his continued homicidal and suicidal ideation, and his fears that he was going to "blow." He said he was afraid to come home because of fantasies of killing family members, fantasies he had never hinted at before. He described a fantasy of coming at his mother with a knife and protecting her by running outside and eating an oleander plant; we had these poisonous plants all around the front yard and the pool area.

Chris insisted that he should be sent to jail or a ward. He could think of no reason why he would want to hurt anyone, except that he kept thinking about it and couldn't get it out of his mind. In his manic state, Chris had obsessed on the greatness of his insights and ideas. Now that he was depressed, he obsessed on fantasies of saving his loved ones from his own violence by killing himself.

I asked a nurse if Chris could continue on the omega-3 fatty acids he had been taking before his hospitalization.

"We'll have to ask the doctor."

"OK, just tell him that a Dr. Stoll at Harvard did a double-blind study on treating bipolar disorder with omega-3 fatty acids, and the results strongly support their use. Here's the article, and here are the pills." I handed her a copy of the article I had downloaded off the Internet. "It would be great if he could continue with this while he's here."

We were on the sidelines now. We could suggest all we wanted, but the fact was there was nothing we could do about his care.

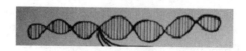

13 - Too Good To Be True!

Like his fateful seven mile walk on Highway 20 from Penn Valley towards the Yuba River Bridge, Chris had been going downhill for too long. He had been through four hospitalizations, three for mania and one for depression, the latter of which was most likely caused by excessive medications and exacerbated by withdrawal from Zyprexa. He needed — we all needed — to find another road. Zyprexa and his other drugs were powerful ... maybe too powerful. What if he met another doctor who said that if he took more Depakote or some other drug, he wouldn't need the Zyprexa? What if he decided on his own to discontinue taking the drug? It hadn't even been tested for long-term maintenance of bipolar disorder, yet that is exactly what his psychiatrists had been using it for, not because they knew what it was doing, or how, but because his behavior deteriorated whenever he went off it.

While Gayle took Thomas to college and Chris languished at Live Oaks, I spent most of my waking hours trying to learn more about bipolar illness and its treatment. Immediately upon learning of his hospitalization, I had asked for and received two weeks off to deal with this crisis. My supervisor also approved my request to work part time for several months once those two weeks were over since I was going to need to be fully involved in Chris's medical follow up. In keeping with my decision to make the most of whatever life threw at me, I began an intensive Internet search on the subject of bipolar disorder — everything from causes to treatments. Actually, it wasn't so much a beginning as an expansion of research I had already been doing. Since working for the county, I had already filled several notebooks with information about ADHD, bipolar illness, allergies, nutrition, and other related topics.

The search

After two days of intensive searching on the Internet, my right shoulder started to hurt. I moved the mouse and pad to the left side of the keyboard. With my left arm and my trusty but slow 28.8 modem, I laboriously traveled through the universe of the Internet.

I was looking for answers to questions I hadn't even thought of yet. In my previous life as a lieutenant colonel in the Air Force, I had spent many hours at the keyboard writing practice management software so that my staff and I could focus our efforts on clients instead of bureaucratically directed administrative requirements. The software allowed us to let the computer take care of the redundant paperwork. That was when the pain in my right shoulder had started. Back then, I could always quit until the pain went away. The automated forms could wait. Now I couldn't afford the luxury of waiting

129

or quitting.

I visited a few chat rooms where participants claimed that Depakote caused them or a family member to become more depressed. I did not pursue this in any depth since my main focus was on Zyprexa which, I had learned, was more effective than Depakote for acute manic episodes.

The Zyprexa conundrum

I reviewed a study sponsored by Lilly Research Laboratories on the use of olanzapine, popularly known as Zyprexa, for the acute management of bipolar mania. In this study, researchers compared the effectiveness and safety of Zyprexa against a placebo, a pill that has no biochemical action. They randomly assigned acute bipolar patients to a Zyprexa group and a placebo group. Those who had been on other medications were slowly tapered off their medications, after which they were placed on either Zyprexa or the placebo. The results showed that the patients taking Zyprexa were significantly improved on the Young--Mania Rating Scale (Y-MRS). Patients treated with Zyprexa demonstrated a higher rate of response (65% versus 43%, respectively; p=.02) and feelings of well-being (61% versus 36%, respectively; p=.0l) than placebo-treated patients. [1]

On the down side, the group taking the Zyprexa gained an average of 2.8 kilograms while the placebo group gained an average of .43 kilograms. Approximately 38% of the Zyprexa group had a problem with sleepiness while about 8% of the placebo group had this problem (p=.001). The article only addressed the use of Zyprexa for acute mania, not for long-term use.

The conclusion read as follows: "Olanzapine demonstrated greater efficacy than placebo in the treatment of acute bipolar mania and was generally well tolerated."[2] I already knew that. Zyprexa had brought Chris back from psychotic mania. It had been less effective in reducing hypomanic behavior.

According to an article in the *Journal of Clinical Psychiatry*, during the Zyprexa clinical trials with 2500 participants, there were 20 deaths, 12 by suicide and two of the remaining eight from aspiration pneumonia, considered by FDA reviewers as possibly related to the Zyprexa. The same review showed 22% experiencing a serious adverse event such as akathisia, hypotension, diabetic complications, and white blood cell disorders.[3] Akathisia is an inablity to sit still, a symptom that can be associated with agitated depression, as well as taking or withdrawing from certain psychotropic drugs.

I found another resource with some disturbing comments about the drug. The article, a *Boston Globe* piece dated November 17, 1998, was posted on the Internet. The author was medical reporter named Robert Whitaker. He reported on the drug trials of four new antipsychotic drugs: Zyprexa,

Resperidol, Seroquel, and Serlect. His article claimed that among 12,176 patients enrolled in the drug trials for these four drugs, there were 88 deaths, including 38 suicides. The suicide rate for the clinical trials was two to five times greater than the annual suicide rates for schizophrenia patients. While the annual death rate for these patients ranged from two to five deaths per 1,000, the death rate of those involved in the trials (including deaths up to 30 days after the trial) were 10 per 1,000. Whitaker claimed that financial incentives had motivated psychiatrists to enroll patients whose medications should not have been changed. He believed these incentives may have led researchers to terminate working drugs for the testing of new, unproven drugs. The article also claimed that evidence was emerging that sudden withdrawal from antipsychotic drugs could lead to a rebound psychosis more severe than if the patient had never been treated with the drug at all. Of particular interest to me was a quote attributed to David Cohen, then a professor in the Social Work Department at the University of Montreal who has done extensive research on drugs such as Zyprexa. "They [the doctors] don't tell them [the patients] the kind of suffering it will entail. They don't tell the patients how severe these symptoms may be, and that they could be life threatening, and that they could be driven to kill themselves."[4]

Kill themselves? The article stated that withdrawal from certain medications designed to help alleviate the symptom of acute mania, Zyprexa among them, could lead people to kill themselves.

I returned to the computer and moved the mouse. The colorful plumbing pipe screen saver disappeared, and in a few seconds I found my way to a chat room. People were writing about their experiences with Zyprexa.

> *Hi,*
> *I have been suffering from depression for the past three years. I have been on Zoloft for two years but found that it was no longer effective. I have been on Paxil for two weeks with some improvement. Today I have been put on a new drug that is supposed to augment the Paxil. It is called Zyprexa. Has anyone had any experience with this stuff? It is designed to treat Schizophrenia.*
> *Wanttofeelgood*

> *Wanttofeel,*
> *Many docs prescribe Zyprexa for people with severe depression that has psychotic features — i.e., I know everyone hates me — I have no friends — I'm ugly — I'll never amount to anything, etc. Often, these terrible feelings are the root of the depression. Be prepared to be very tired at first — also*

very hungry. After a while, these side effects will ease up. Best wishes!
MD2000

Want,
Hi! I was on Zyprexa for 6 months last winter. I was being treated for post traumatic stress disorder. It helped a little bit but not as much as they suggest. It puts a lot of weight on ya. I gained about 100 pounds within the first three months ...YIKES! which I am just now starting to lose. They also kept upping it on me even though they admitted that there were not enough tests on it to show how it affects the body after 25 mg. I think it was the worst drug I have ever taken, and I would advise anyone NOT to take it! Right now I am doing good on Elavil — no side effects to complain of. I would ask around and do more research on this before you take it. Good Luck:)
IowaRanch

Hey Gang,
Don't take it. It is an awful drug and an antihistamine.
Ramblinrose

Wanttofeelgood,
I tried Zyprexa for about a month. Once it kicked in, I felt better than I ever had with any medications (I have tried the whole spectrum). I also have Tourette's syndrome along with manic depression. The only problem was what the other people are saying. I started putting on weight very fast. That was very unfortunate because it did work well. My doctor told me there was a very high success rate with w/ Schizophrenics, but their quality of life was so poor they didn't care about the weight gain. The manufacturers say it does not promote weight gain, but I think it alters the part of the brain that controls your appetite because it is the same region where you have the chemical imbalance that causes the depression. When I would sit down to eat, the feeling you get when you're full just wasn't happening. I hope they can fix this drug.
greenhornet

I had a different perspective now. The posters seemed naïve to me, as naïve as I had been. I hadn't realized we had been playing with fire. They didn't seem to either. Besides, I was looking for discussions on what happens when people stopped taking these drugs, not when they started. I had raised the issue in several chat forums and had received no useful responses. With the exception of the article by Whitaker, most of the references to the atypical antipsychotic drugs I had found pertained to starting, not stopping the medication. Why was there so little about what happens when a person comes off one of these drugs, particularly when it appeared that the risks were so high?

I found the following in a 1998 letter from a Dr. Loren Mosher announcing his resignation from the American Psychiatric Society: "At this point in history, in my view, psychiatry has been almost completely bought out by the drug companies ... . We condone and promote the widespread overuse and misuse of toxic chemicals that we know have serious long-term effects: tardive dyskinesia, tardive dementia, and serious withdrawal symptoms."[5] I found an article stating that children taking risperidone or olanzapine (Zyprexa) may be prone to a profound discontinuation syndrome unless the dosages are tapered very gradually. One professional stated, "If you go cold turkey, you're going to have fireworks. The staff quakes in their boots when [children] go off atypicals."[6]

What were the long-term consequences of taking psychotropic medications? I found one article, based on rat studies, stating that proliferation of glial cells and hypertrophy (swelling) of the prefrontal cortex is "a common response to antipsychotic drugs" and may "play a regulatory role in adjusting neurotransmitter levels or metabolic processes."[7]

If chronic use of these drugs did this to rats, what did they do to humans? I didn't know much about glial cells, but I knew what hypertrophy meant. It meant that these drugs caused a swelling in the prefrontal cortex. Maybe I was biased because of my experience with my father, but I wouldn't like the idea of some drug swelling my son's prefrontal cortex, let alone mine.

Downer,
You might want to check out Truehope.com. They have a different way to treat depression.
Stilllooking

Truehope?

I typed in the Uniform Resource Locator (URL) and a page slowly revealed itself on the screen. To the upper right were the words, "The Synergy Group of Canada." Below that was a picture of a family dated 1989 with a caption stating, "The Stephan Family in 1989, finding true hope in despair. Depression and suicide takes a mother of ten." This guy sounded like he had tried to turn a tragedy into a triumph. I could relate to that. I was trying to do the same. Then at the bottom of the page were these words:

> "*Synergy, a nonmedical research group dedicated to finding answers to the CNS Disorders of Schizophrenia, Bipolar Disorder, Depression, ADHD, Panic-Anxiety Disorders, OCD, Tourette's syndrome, Autism and the disorders of Fibromyalgia-Chronic Fatigue Syndrome. The Synergy Group of Canada Inc. is a research partner and consultant to the largest university research consortia ever to utilize a nutrient protocol for CNS research purposes.*"

Wait a minute here. OK, enough already! It looked like they were lumping psychiatric and neurological illnesses into CNS disorders. And what was this about the Synergy Group being a "consultant to the largest university research consortia?" Did that mean "only" university research consortia? If it did, then it probably meant that no other "university research consortia" would be interested in promoting such claims as this.

Had I been seduced by the story about the wife's suicide? These people must think the public was pretty simplistic to buy their claim that a simple nutritional protocol could treat bipolar disorder as well as so many other "CNS" disorders. Maybe this guy also had swampland in Florida or beachfront property in the Mojave Desert for sale!

As I clicked on some of the links, I became angrier. After this guy's wife had allegedly killed herself, this guy, a real estate property manager and another guy who owned an animal feed consulting business came up with a vitamin and mineral supplement that not only resolved his three children's bipolar disorder but the childhood schizophrenia of the other guy's son. The idea for the supplements came from the fact that vitamin and mineral supplement are used by farmers to cure ear and tail biting syndrome, an often-fatal disease in which pigs attack and kill each other. Something wasn't quite right. Whoever heard of the same treatment for schizophrenia, obsessive compulsive disorder, depression, bipolar illness, and, of all things, fibromyalgia, a neurological disorder characterized by muscle pain throughout the body? And the solution to these diverse illnesses was founded on a vitamin and mineral supplement for *hogs*? I had been a mental health professional for 29 years. I had served as an executive director of mental health clinics from Little Rock Air Force Base in Arkansas to Clark Air Base in the Philippines. I had presented papers and workshops — even published papers — on a variety of mental health treatment issues. And I had dealt with bipolar disorder throughout my life both personally and professionally. I knew there were no easy answers. This was just too good to be true!

I looked through the site for some explanation as to how this approach supposedly cured such disparate illnesses. I found nothing except case reports with impressive looking graphs. I knew that case reports alone could not establish efficacy. Besides, who was to say the reports were truthful, or, for that matter, that the guy even had a wife who had killed herself? There were thousands of shady operations on the Internet. Truehope was starting to look like TrueCon to me.

Before I decided to reenter the work force with a temporary job working for Nevada County Behavioral Health Services with high-risk kids, I had enjoyed and profited from day trading. It was fun to go for the long shot once in a while, like the shares I bought at 15 cents a share and sold for almost two dollars a share. Other purchases had bombed. I couldn't afford to invest in a speculative treatment when it meant I could lose my son.

Truehope had a discussion group link where people could share their experiences with the Synergy approach. I logged on and read all the discussions in each of the chat rooms, including Depression, Bipolar Disorder, ADHD, Schizophrenia, Fibromyalgia, and even Tourette's syndrome, a disorder in which the patient has uncontrollable physical ticks and utters obscene statements. To me it looked like a typical chat room with lots of different, often-unconnected threads. There were positive comments about the supplement approach and also negative comments from those still having problems. There were many comments just offering support to each other and not even talking about the supplements. From the chat rooms, it certainly did not appear as if the Synergy supplements were the last word on mental disorders.

Normally I would not even have bothered. I would have moved on to something that appeared more promising. But I felt angry at the implied promises I had read on the site. I suspected this was a case of unscrupulous characters peddling false hope to suffering patients and family members. I resented those who had almost seduced me with "true" hope. I titled my comments "Too good to be true!"

I am very skeptical of the over inclusive claims of this company. I see no scientific basis for them. The company lumps together disorders such as bipolar illness, fibromyalgia and schizophrenia and then claims that nutritional supplements can help patients suffering from all of them. I even doubt if the developer of this supplement had a wife who died of suicide due to her bipolar disorder. My son is in the hospital right now. I think he is there because we followed his doctor's orders to discontinue one of his medicines, a drug called

Zyprexa. We already made one mistake, following his doctor's orders. We don't need another. As desperate as my wife and I are to find answers, we are not desperate enough to become laetril parents.

There, that should help some hapless parents from getting sucked in, I thought. I remembered the story of actor Steve McQueen going to a clinic in Mexico to get laetril treatments to ward off his pending death from cancer. My writing the note was what those of us in the trade would call "ego dystonic behavior," that is, behavior of a kind one would not normally engage in. Chris's running amok had blurred my usual professional and personal boundaries. I could feel for the hapless searchers like myself, who, like Odysseus, the main character in Homer's Odyssey, had to steel himself against the siren sounds of seductive mermaids to keep himself from jumping overboard in their pursuit. I felt their desperation. I felt a need to warn them. Having accomplished that, I moved on to more useful research. I started searching to learn the effects of Zyprexa withdrawal, the biology of bipolar disorder, new alternative treatment approaches, and long-term management of the disorder.

Several days later, I decided to return to the Truehope site just to see if anyone had responded to my statement. Someone had. The person responded non-defensively and seemed to identify with how difficult it was to understand the logic of using supplements to treat these different illnesses. He described some biochemical processes I couldn't understand that take place in order to supply the brain with tryptophan, one of many amino acids essential for proper brain functioning. He included a link.[8]

I clicked on the link to find an amazingly complex array of biochemical processes involved in the production of tryptophan. By clicking on the chemical names, I saw a breakdown of the genetic structure of each of the chemicals involved in the process. I recognized the basic DNA building-blocks of adenine, thymine, guanine, and cytosine, but the rest was too complex for me. I wondered how pharmaceutical companies and psychiatrists could accurately correct "chemical imbalances" by inserting psychotropic drugs into the brain when the process of creating just one substance, tryptophan, was so complex. How could the right selective serotonin reuptake inhibitor (SSRI) or the right antipsychotic drug correct the proper defective pieces, and only those pieces, of this complex biochemical puzzle? It seemed logical to me that any agent that either enhanced serotonin or blocked it would have multiple effects on multiple processes. The simple logic of supplying sufficient nutrients so that the body could create the substances needed for proper brain functioning seemed more intuitive than trying to give the brain the exact substance needed to correct the imbalance or imbalances.

The simplistic model I had been operating under, and one I had shared with my clients, was that certain psychotropic medications reduced serotonin for manic states and increased it for depressive disorders. It was a simple, easy-to-understand paradigm wherein certain reuptake pumps in the brain's cells were tweaked by the particular medicine to correct some "chemical imbalance." Returning to the chat room, I wrote the following:

> *So if I understand you correctly, you are saying that adding a specific medication to such a complex interrelated system could throw it off balance, but that providing a nutritional foundation to help compensate for whatever foundational deficiencies or genetically caused metabolic errors would be more effective. It sounds like you are saying that on a biological basis these illnesses simply represent different ways the body tries to deal with inadequate nutrition or genetically programmed inadequate metabolic processes. And if you front-load the system with the necessary ingredients, then the brain can better establish its own well-functioning homeostasis.*

I wanted to know more. When I started my search, I had tried to suspend my preconceptions even though I knew I would not be able to easily jettison 18 years of education and 29 years of practice in the mental health field. These ideas certainly challenged my preconceptions. When I suspended my disbelief, the idea of nutritional supplementation for CNS disorders was intriguing, though not compelling. Was it science or snake oil? The only way to find out was to get more information. I would play along and pretend to give them the benefit of the doubt. I wrote an email to the president of the company, Anthony Stephan.

> *Sept. 9, 2000*
> *Sir,*
> *Would you please send me information regarding your supplements for bipolar disorder? Are you looking for clinical trial subjects? Are you selling the supplements outright? Do you have information on what is in them and what, if any, side effects could be expected? Do you have any information on the logic used to select certain vitamins and minerals for the supplementation? How many bipolar patients have taken them and what have been the results? Is it possible to talk to a person treated with the supplements? What*

do doctors think of your approach? I assume you cannot claim cures since, in the US, the FDA would strongly object unless there were clinical trials supporting "cures."
Dave Moyer

The next day I received a response:

Sept. 10, 2000
Dear David,
I read with interest your email as well as your discussion board submission.
I am the father of the family described on the web story whose wife took her life because of bipolar disorder.
http://www.Truehope.com/aboutus.html
I would like to help you.
Please email me with your phone number and I will call you at my expense.
Regards,

Anthony Stephan
President The Synergy Group of Canada Inc
Research Consultant for the faculty of Medicine
The University of Calgary

I read the email and wept. I had looked for hope before only to find more pain. Hope was being offered to me again.

A cure for bipolar disorder?

The day after I received the email message from Anthony Stephan offering to help, I called information and asked for the number for a company called Synergy Group of Canada. I didn't want to wait. I dialed the number. A voice-answering machine answered.

"Hi, this is Dave Moyer. You sent me an email yesterday. I was asking questions about your supplements." I gave my number and asked him to return my call.

The same questions popped into my mind again. If the president of the company was willing to call me, he must be either very compassionate, not very busy, or hard up for business. What was going on here? I began to have doubts about pursuing this. I wasn't sure if I had an open mind or an empty head.

That afternoon, I got a call from Anthony Stephan. He introduced himself and explained how his first wife and her father had died by suicide, and how his pregnant second wife had left him because his son was threatening to kill the baby she was carrying.

"Every night when we heard him move in his bed, we would both tighten up."

He explained how he went from psychiatrist to psychiatrist looking for answers. One showed him passages of DSM-IV describing bipolar illness as a chronic, lifelong illness. All the psychiatrists could offer was a management approach that would reduce the acute manifestations of the illness. They couldn't offer long-term hope.

Tony had talked with his good friend David Hardy, owner of an animal feed and nutritional consulting business. David kept returning to the subject of nutrition. He told Tony about similarities he saw between bipolar-disordered behavior and behavior exhibited by pigs with ear and tail biting syndrome. He said that modern production methods have taken pigs away from an environment where they would normally pick up essential nutrients and enzymes from the soil. David told Tony that veterinarians have treated this syndrome successfully for years with vitamin and mineral supplementation. He sold supplemented feed for hogs to the Hutterite farmers in the area to prevent the syndrome.

Tony said that when he heard this story, "It touched me close to my heart." He and David began researching the processes by which the human body creates the essential elements for proper brain functioning. At first, they gave four commercially available products to Tony's son. Tony said he started acting normally for the first time in years. Later, when there were some quality-control problems with these products that negatively affected his son, they worked with a nutritional supplement company and came up with their own formulation to which he responded positively. In 1996, all three of Tony's children started taking the supplements and became symptom-free. Two years later, one of David's sons had a psychotic episode later diagnosed as schizophrenia. His son began taking the supplements and his schizophrenic symptoms ceased.

Tony continued. "On October 4, Dr. Bonnie Kaplan from the University of Calgary will present a poster session on the Effects of Nutritional Supplementation on Bipolar Illness at the Canadian Psychiatry meeting in Vancouver, British Colombia. She will present 10 case studies, bipolar patients, all of whom are now symptom-free. The first footnote in the presentation is a reference to the work of Dr. Ann Marie Meyer, an author who has noted how modern farming methods have reduced vitamin and mineral content in our food supply. A number of studies are suggesting that the rates of bipolar disorder and other mental disorders are increasing in response to these methods."

He described unsuccessful attempts to enlist the support of physicians and other academics in the community to study the supplements. At last they had approached Dr. Bonnie Kaplan, a psychologist and professor in the Department of Pediatrics at the University of Calgary, to help them research the supplements. They explained the logic behind the supplement approach and the number of patients with different disorders who might be helped. At first she told them she did not do research on speculative therapies and was not interested. However, she did agree to talk with parents and children who had allegedly been helped by the supplement program. After talking with a number of parents and children with diagnoses ranging from ADHD, oppositional defiant disorder, bipolar disorder, and even Asperger's disorder, a developmental disorder characterized by autistic social behavior as well as high academic achievement, she agreed to participate in a formal assessment of the supplements. The parents and the children reported improvement on the supplements. Her task was to find out if there actually were demonstrable changes that justified their enthusiasm.

I was taking notes as fast as I could. "Are you accepting patients for trials? What about your FDA equivalent? How do they feel about your operations? Have you had any bad outcomes?"

"The equivalent to the FDA in Canada is the Health Protection Branch (HPB). They have already threatened to close us down. If they did, there would be such a huge response from people who are doing great on the supplements that it would provide even more publicity for our work. We have to be careful to let people know that we are not giving medical advice. All the case studies on the site are true, and there are many hundreds more. The reason the academic community is interested now is because the results are so promising; I don't anticipate any problems with the regulatory agencies. For example, if you asked me about your son, I could only tell you what we did with our son and what others have done. I would not give you direct advice. Actually, we prefer that you would work through your own doctor."

"Where is a person to find a doctor who would work with a bipolar patient on supplements?"

"I know it is hard. They are not trained to see the benefits of nutritional approaches to illness."

"You know it would only take one bad outcome to undo all the work you have already done. We get bad outcomes all the time from psychiatry — look at my son's situation. But psychiatrists are licensed to create bad outcomes and you aren't."

He told me about a woman who had called him about her bipolar son. She said he was getting worse. He was afraid and anxious on the seventh day of the supplements. Tony asked if he had been better at all during the seven days. She responded that on the third day he had done very well. Tony explained that the problem was that the boy should have either stopped or reduced his medications.

"The rule is that the faster the recovery, the faster the withdrawal, and visa versa. Selective serotonin reuptake inhibitors and antipsychotics are like sledgehammers to the brain. When the brain tries to establish its own homeostasis, the symptoms reoccur because the balance gets thrown off again. Many doctors don't accept this."

"That reminds me of that story about ulcers," I said. "Remember the doctor in Australia who proved that ulcers were treatable with antibiotics? He said they were caused by some bacteria called *H. pylori* (*Helicobacter pylori*)."

"Yes, and did you know that veterinarians have been treating ulcers with antibiotics for years?"

"I didn't know that!" I exclaimed.

"There are a lot of medicines that are used by humans that started out being used for animals."

Somewhere in the back of my mind I had a recollection that Thorazine had first been used for horses with infections. I could identify with Tony, and I felt that Tony could identify with me. Our families had both suffered after getting the best that psychiatry had to offer.

"Are you saying this is a cure for bipolar disorder?"

"Dave, I don't think there is a cure. But as long as people stay on the supplements, they will not experience bipolar symptoms. If they take antibiotics orally, their symptoms may reoccur because the antibiotics kill bacteria which are needed for proper digestion. For our family, I consider my three kids to be cured as long as they stay on the supplements."

An eventful decision

"Can I get the supplements for my son? How much are they?"

"They are not available to the general public, but if you want to participate in an informal trial, I can assign you a number and call Evince International to order them. They are about $50 a bottle and each bottle contains almost 450 pills. Normally we recommend 32 pills a day for bipolar patients until their nutrition situation improves, then we recommend a maintenance dose of about 16 a day."

"OK, let's do it."

He gave me a number and got Evince International on the line for a conference call.

"How can I help you?" answered a voice.

"Hi, I have a dad here who wants to order some supplements," Tony said.

"I would like to order four bottles," I confirmed.

"Would you like to pay for that with a credit card?"

"Yes."

With an admixture of hope and cynicism I pulled out my credit card and haltingly read the number over the phone. To think that this might change the course of Chris's illness, that it might actually help my clients, was too much. The promise that his suffering could be alleviated by something as simple as a vitamin and mineral supplement was powerful. While I owed it to my son to give him that chance, I also needed to carefully guard my own needs for hope. I would critically assess this approach knowing I could always return to Non Expectation Therapy. Tony gave me his personal and work phone numbers and invited me to call him at any time during the process.

The next day, Gayle returned home from taking Thomas to college. Chris had been in the hospital for eight days. We started visiting him daily. During these visits, it was difficult to be physically near him for any period of time. His body and his breath exuded a metallic smell, a consequence, most likely, of the medications he was taking. When we talked, the subject matter continued to regress to themes of suicide, murder, the "good Chris," and the "bad Chris." We continued to choose to sing rather than talk. It was more fun, and his breath wasn't in our direction when he sang. The hospital was allowing me to do primal sing therapy, right in their own hallway.

As an outpatient therapist, I had explored with clients their thoughts and fantasies. Exploring their inner reality sometimes helped them to be more aware of and in control of their behavior. But looking for dynamic meanings or constructive awareness in Chris's consciousness was a nonstarter. His brain was broken. It was as simple as that. There were no oedipal conflicts to explore, no unconscious hostility to discover, no repressed memories to exhume.

Medication: the opiate of the mentally ill?

Others on the ward were not doing so well either. Jan was becoming more of a social outcast, increasingly unable to relate to others in any positive or meaningful way. The craziness was still there, but the drugs she was taking muted her spunky personality. During one of our visits, Mary screamed at Jan. Jan was hard to talk to because of her loose associations. Sharon, the bipolar patient, appeared to be having more extrapyramidal symptoms (EPS), so much so that after one visit I advised Nurse Ratchet that she appeared to have significant EPS. As we were leaving, I told her of a recent lawsuit where a bipolar patient had won a judgment of $7 million from a physician in Philadelphia for allowing the patient to develop tardive dyskinesia. From an objective professional point of view it was, to be blunt, none of my business. My comments were a violation of professional boundaries. I really didn't care any more. I cared more that Sharon had severe symptoms of EPS, and possibly tardive dyskinesia, because of the medication she was on. I realized then that I had ceased to think of myself primarily as a mental health professional. I was a parent who was becoming increasingly disappointed in the system that was supposed to be treating my son and all the men and women on the ward.

We brought Chris books and Internet pages on bipolar illness. We brought him information from the Truehope Web site. We shared my conversation with Tony and the personal interest he had shown in helping us. During one of our visits, Chris said he would like to take the supplements when he was discharged.

During one of these visits, we discussed the supplements with him in the presence of a group of patients who had been singing with us. I shared some of the Truehope downloads with them. We had a spirited discussion about medications. Most of them had strongly ambivalent feelings. Then there was Jan. She chimed in loudly with ideas that some might call schizophrenic insight and others loose associations. "The psychiatrists are nothing more than atheistic dope-peddling Nazis!" It was strange but gratifying to hear a group of mental patients laughing and welcoming Jan back into their circle, even if only for a few moments. She had been clear enough to make a cogent comment about medicines and psychiatrists, even if it was inapprpriate.

Sharon had only positive words for her psychiatrist and her medications. She had learned that the best she could hope for was to live in a group home where her needs could be met between acute exacerbations of her illness. Previously she had advised her best for Chris, suggesting he get on disability and go with her to her group home. Her "special powers" given by God would have to compensate for the loss of her husband and her children, her lack of opportunities for employment, and her inability to care for herself. She appeared unaware of her slurred speech, the strange involuntary movements of her tongue, face, and hands.

After this visit, while driving back home on Interstate 80, I said to Gayle, "You know, it is really hard to imagine that those supplements could help many of these people. I have been in the business too long to really believe that, and yet that is what Truehope is claiming. It seems so 'pie in the sky-ish.' I wonder what would happen if they all starting taking the supplements?"

"That's something you won't have to worry about," she responded. "You can't even get them to give Chris omega-3 fatty acids. They would never go for nutritional supplements."

"I agree, but I think they will eventually approve the salmon oil. When

I asked his doctor about it, he asked me to write and sign a statement that we would hold the hospital free of liability if the fatty acids caused any negative outcomes. So I wrote a statement and signed it. They probably have to clear it with their legal counsel before they can give it to him."

"By the time they get all that done, Chris will be out of the hospital."

"Maybe they think we'll be unhappy if Chris gets fish-breath. That was one of the side effects in the study at Harvard."

"I noticed his breath is pretty bad now. It has a metallic smell to it."

"His breath couldn't get any worse than it is now. He's not diabetic, so we don't have to worry about any blood coagulation problems. I'll admit it is strange. Some bipolar patient in Philadelphia gets a $7 million settlement because she gets tardive dyskinesia from Risperdal, and these guys want me to clear them legally so Chris can take 3,000 mg of fish oil. Hell, Chris could get neuroleptic syndrome, tardive dyskinesia, severe ketoacidosis or status epilepticus from the drugs he's taking, and we need permission to give him fish oil that he could get eating a few helpings of salmon."

"I'm impressed."

"Hey, I've been doing my homework. I found articles where people have died from all those illnesses, except for tardive dyskinesia, and if Chris had that, he would probably want to die. The chances are rare that any of these disorders would occur, but they could, and they could be fatal. Psychiatrists can take those risks. They are licensed to give people these medicines. Anyway, I agree with you. We could never get his psychiatrist's blessing to allow Chris to take the supplements on the ward. But we could bring him some vitamin and mineral snacks."

"I don't think that would be a good idea. What if he had a bad reaction to the supplements?"

"Let's see what happens."

By day 13, Chris was taking 150 mg Wellbutrin, 1,500 mg Depakote, 900 mg lithium, and 20 mg Zyprexa. On day 16, Chris told us that his doctor and the court had extended his commitment for 30 more days and that the amount of Wellbutrin had been increased to 300 mg a day. Chris was not progressing well enough to join the others in the dining hall. He continued to express suicidal and homicidal obsessional thoughts. I asked him why he would feel like hurting others.

"Just because I know I could do it."

"In other words, because you can think it, you would do it?"

"Yeah."

"So having the thought is the same as doing the deed."

He responded in a flat affect, "Yeah."

Gayle spoke. "Chris, you once said you sometimes thought about pushing people down the risers during a choir concert, but you didn't."

"Yeah, but all I think about now is hurting myself or others. My mind isn't involved in anything else."

On the way out, I asked the charge nurse what was happening with our request that Chris take omega-3 fatty acid tablets. It had been approved. Chris would be taking 3,000 mg a day. His psychiatrist would later address this issue in his narrative summary with the following: "The patient's father was quite intrusive in the treatment and worried that his son be given omega-3 capsules. The patient was started on that, but it was explained to the father about the risks and benefits of giving non-recommended FDA-approved treatment."

Driving home, I felt frustrated. "You know, the only thing the hospital is providing is a safe place and drugs, and I don't think the drugs are helping. The fatty acids might help, but I think we should start giving him small amounts of supplements. I can bring in four pills a day in my guitar case. They would never inspect it. You could bring some other snacks along with water, and he can take them while we are down the hall from everyone else." Gayle, while not enthusiastic, didn't disagree.

Healthy snacks — peanuts and pills

The next time we visited, the nurse asked to see what we were bringing in. I showed my guitar, and Gayle showed a sack filled with nuts and candy, a bottle of water and some books. Then we went down the hall to our singing place, away from prying eyes.

"Okay, Chris we brought you some supplement snacks. You need to take them now and quickly, with the peanuts." I opened my guitar case and took out the pills. Chris swallowed them. From then on, we brought him four supplements almost every day.

Shortly after he started taking the supplements, during one of our visits, I noticed that his hands were shaking. He was manifesting Parkinsonian symptoms. He denied it, but Gayle and I both noticed it, and so did other patients. I told Nurse Ratchet that he was developing extrapyramidal side effects from taking 20 mg of Zyprexa, and I emphatically recommended that they lower the dose. They lowered it to 15 mg per day. His symptoms stopped. Later I was to learn that the supplements potentiate the effects of psychiatric drugs; in other words, giving Chris the supplements while he was still on his medication increased the potency of the medication.

I called Tony to ask about the effects of four supplements on top of regular psychiatric medications.

Tony responded, "A partial supplement won't make him tired like the full 32 pills would. If you are giving this to him while he is in the hospital, he will be ready to be discharged in a few days and the doctors will think that the increase in the Wellbutrin is what caused it."

Sure enough, on September 23, six days, after starting Chris on peanuts and pills, Chris's doctor called and reported that he had improved sufficiently that they would be looking at discharge soon. They weren't going to need the extra 30 days they had authorized after all.

On September 27, Gayle, Chris, and I met with the social worker and discharge planner, a woman named Ginny. She asked each of us what our concerns were. Gayle shared her fears that Chris wouldn't tell her how he was feeling. She told him she really wanted to know what was going on with him, even if he was feeling suicidal. Chris talked about his thoughts.

"I was thinking that if the bad Chris started to get the upper hand, I might put a knife to Mom's throat. But if I did that, the good Chris would take over, and I would run outside and eat an oleander plant."

Gayle later told me she regretted her conversation with him years ago about some Boy Scouts who had died after roasting marshmallows on oleander sticks.

I asked Ginny, "How do your understand these thoughts?"

She responded, "It sounds like he still has some delusional thoughts, thoughts of saving his mother from his own anger. We have bipolar patients who have all sorts of delusional thoughts, and sometimes these thoughts don't go away, but with medication and support they learn to manage them. Do you feel like acting on these thoughts, Chris?"

"No, not now, but before I came in, and in the hospital, if I had the thought, I felt I had to act on it."

I shared with Chris my fears over the possibility of more unpredictable behavior. When I told Ginny that we were going to use the supplement program, she expressed reservations. She said she had seen a lot of bipolar patients who had been able to manage quite well when they found the right drugs for them. I said that Dr. Lund had told us that a medication such as lithium, while effective for acute management of mania, is not as effective in preventing episodes as had commonly been thought. I also said we planned to continue using the omega-3 fatty acids pills that Chris had received on the ward.

"I didn't know we gave that here."

"You didn't, but I asked that he continue on it, and his doctor agreed. I had to sign documents absolving the hospital of any responsibility for untoward outcomes. They did a double-blind study at Harvard showing the effectiveness of omega-3 fatty acids for bipolar patients."

Ginny spoke. "If everything goes well, we should be discharging Chris on Friday. I hope it goes well for you."

I responded. "Thanks for talking to us."

On the way home, I felt a sense of anxiety as well as excitement. We were heading down a new path, and we didn't know where it was going to go. I thought about a conference that Gayle and I had attended in Tel Aviv,

Israel in 1975, the year Chris was born. The week long conference was entitled, "Stress and Adjustment in Time of War and Peace." I had the privilege of hearing the noted therapist and author Dr. Rollo May give a presentation on anxiety and values. In his presentation, he described how anxiety, which literally means pain in the narrowest place, can be very restrictive and disabling. It can cause us to cower and hide. Yet it can also propel us to growth and discovery. The key is our values about anxiety. When we see anxiety as a friend rather than an enemy, then we can use it to discover new possibilities. Dr. May put anxiety into a different perspective for me. He reframed it as the "dizziness of freedom." I liked that concept then and still like it now. We would not withdraw in fear. We would leave one paradigm and explore another.

Anxiety, the dizziness of freedom

When we got home from the Hospital, I called Tony.

"Hello," a woman answered.

"Hi, this is Dave Moyer. Is Tony there?"

"Hi, Dave. Tony has been wanting to talk to you." What a kind voice, I thought. Must be his wife.

"Hello?"

"Hi Tony, this is Dave."

"Dave, can you call me back on the land number? This is my cell phone number."

"Sure." I called back to his home phone. I remembered Tony telling me earlier that he got anywhere from 20 to 30 calls a day.

"Thanks for calling back. Things have been pretty busy around here. I've been working with Dr. Kaplan on her presentation, and tomorrow I am going to be interviewed on Canadian TV. We have several major news releases coming out shortly."

"We sure appreciate your willingness to help us with this. Chris is being discharged Friday, and he wants to start on the supplements."

"Good, I will be glad to walk you through this."

"We are thinking about reducing his medications first then starting the supplements. If he is going to get an Acute Drug Reaction (ADR) in a few days, wouldn't it be better to slightly lower his drugs first, then start the supplement?"

"You should only cut the medication if he is overmedicated now. The problem is that if you withdraw the drugs before providing a nutritional foundation, you run the risk of provoking the original symptoms."

"OK, so we need to start with the supplements and go from there. I don't know the amounts, but he's going to be taking Zyprexa, Depakote,

Wellbutrin, and lithium. I read Dr. Breggin's book, the one about coming off drugs. It's called <u>Your Drugs May Be Your Problem.</u> He says you should take 10% off of one drug at a time for 7 days before continuing to take another 10% off. Also, I read that lithium should be withdrawn slowly over a long period of time. Some have had seizures when they withdrew too quickly from the drug."[9]

"Dave, Dr. Breggin recommends withdrawal without the support of any supplementation. We can reduce the amount faster because the proper nutrients will be in his body when we withdraw the drugs. Generally, I recommend withdrawing about one-fourth of everything, not just one drug, because some drugs may counteract the others. For example, if you pull the lithium and Depakote and continue with Wellbutrin, there is a possibility of provoking a manic attack."

"Tony, you sound so confident with this. Don't you ever have fears that something could go drastically wrong?"

"No, I have done this with hundreds of folks. I can think of one case that didn't go well. I was invited by the National Association of the Mentally Ill (NAMI) to speak in Idaho to a bipolar support group, and while I was speaking, a nurse kept interrupting me with questions, claiming that patients would go psychotic on this program and have all sorts of bad outcomes. I looked at the audience and saw an elderly woman I knew who was missing her middle finger. I asked her if she would be willing to stand and tell her story. She told of her struggle with bipolar illness for years, of numerous hospitalizations, suicide attempts. She explained how she cut her finger off because the demons told her to. I told the nurse that I buried my wife whom I still love after she killed herself because of this illness. I said that some might consider me to be a fanatic, and then I asked the audience if the existing treatments were working for this lady.

"The woman decided to use the supplement program, but it wasn't successful for her. Her doctor was willing to try it because he knew nothing else had worked. But he was more conservative than I would have been, lowering her medications by one-eighth after the first ADR. When he called me to say that she was in bed and severely symptomatic, I told him he needed to increase the withdrawal from the drugs. But the woman, who had been taught for so many years that she must stay on her medication, refused to allow her doctor to lower the amounts. I had to tell him to discontinue the supplements because it was unethical to keep her on them without slowly removing her psychotropic drugs."

"Have you had experience in working with people who have had a cocktail of medications? Chris has a lot of medication in his system."

"I met the husband of a 62-year-old woman at a meeting in Alberta. He said that she was taking 11 different medications, including Ativan. He introduced me to her, and she wanted to try the program. She started it, and when she had her first ADR she began having seizures and had to be hospitalized. Her nurse thought Ativan addiction might be the cause, so she gave her a small shot of Ativan, and her seizure activity stopped. We had to move slowly with the Ativan because of the physical addiction. We withdrew her from the other medications in the usual manner. She is now symptom-free and off all medications."

"You know, if your program helps Chris, I'm either going to have to change our system in the county or quit. I won't be able to sit there..." My throat tightened and I stopped in mid-sentence. I thought about a client of mine, a 10-year-old boy whose body had been shaking two days earlier after running out of Ritalin.

"It's easier to work with lay groups and less easy to work with professionals," Tony said. "They've been trained to see things a certain way and have trouble adjusting to the idea that nutrition could play a role in mental disorders."

Tony went on talking, but I wasn't there. Since Chris had cut himself, I had been what we in the trade would call "emotionally labile." My emotions were right at the surface. I still was thinking about the 10-year-old boy, who was no longer shaking. I had arranged for him to see a psychiatrist, who had started him on another drug, Adderall, which he touted to the boy and his parents as being superior to Ritalin. I returned to the conversation.

"Okay, so how effective is your program with ADHD, and what is the difference between ADHD and bipolar?"

"None. They are the same thing. It's just a matter of degree."

"You know, I've been thinking that there is a strong similarity between ADHD and bipolar ever since Chris's employer told me that she used techniques she has used with ADHD kids with Chris when he was working for them. You're the first person I've ever heard say that the two are the same."

"I have a garden that does not produce very well. I'm having to build up the soil so that it will not only produce, but also produce nutritious food. No matter what chemicals I add to the plant, unless the soil can supply the proper nutrients, my garden will fail or produce crops that are inadequate."

I found the analogy to be appealing, even if it was only a metaphor.

Chris returned home on September 29, exactly one month after he had run amok. When he got home, he continued with his psychiatric medications and started taking 32 pills a day of the nutritional supplements, a total of 42 pills daily.

Gayle and I wanted to believe that the supplements had helped him to be released earlier, but we couldn't be sure. It could have been the Wellbutrin, or a decision from managed care gatekeepers that he was well enough to go home because he had exceeded the allowable days. Chris might have gotten bored with telling his psychiatrist that he felt like killing his mom and dad or himself and simply told them what he knew they wanted to hear.

However, we had noticed that Chris was less morbidly preoccupied with ANTS and better able to focus on other issues after he'd started his peanuts and pills regimen. He could share his thoughts and feelings, and Gayle and I would not feel depressed and helpless as we had before. He commented on TV shows he had seen. He shared his experiences with fellow patients in the cafeteria and exercise room. He also talked more to us about relationships he had formed with other patients. He talked about the 25 pounds he had gained while on the ward. He had weighed 175 pounds before his episode. Now he was up to 200.

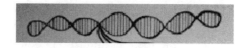

Notes

1. The smaller the "p," the more significant the findings, so a small "p" meant that the Zyprexa was actually more effective than the placebo. In most research, a "p" of anything less than .05 is considered significant. That means that the findings weren't just coincidental. The probability (p) that the result was due to chance was only 5 out of 100.

2. Mauricio, Tohen, et al., "Efficacy of olanzapine in acute bipolar mania," *Arch Gen Psychiatry,* 57:841-849, 2000.

3. Conley, Robert, "Adverse events related to olanzapine," *Journal of Clinical Psychiatry* 61, supplement 8, 26-30, 2000.

4. Whittaker, Robert, "Lure of Riches Fuels Testing," *Boston Globe,* November 17, 1998.

5. Mosher, L.R., "Famous Psychiatirst L.R. Mosher Resigns from American Psychiatric Association," December 4, 1998.
http://www.bhagd.com/media/mosher.htm

6. Bates, Betsy, "Atypical Antipsychotics: Watch Side Effects in Youths," *Clinical Psychiatry News,* 27(1):20-21, 1999.

7. Selemon, L.D., Lidow, M.S., Goldman-Rakic, P.S., "Increased volume and glial density in primate prefrontal cortex associated with chronic antipsychotic drug exposure," *Biological Psychiatry,* 46:161–172, 1999.

8. Institute for Chemical Research, "Tryptophan Metabolism," *Genome Net* WWW Server, Koyoto University, 2000.
http://www.genome.ad.jp/kegg/pathway/map/map00380.html

9. Breggin, P.R., Cohen, D., <u>Your Drug May Be Your Problem</u>, New York, Perseus Books, 111-131, 1999.

14 - To Research or Not to Research

If Chris improved on the supplements, there should be a corresponding improvement in his brain functioning and there should be some way to assess that improvement. If the supplements worked with Chris, they might work with many of the high-risk youth with whom I worked in Nevada County. In order to establish effectiveness, I was going to need something besides "Well, he is better and no longer having psychotic episodes." I searched the Net and found Dr. Terence Ketter, an associate professor of psychiatry at Stanford University who was an expert on bipolar disorder and brain scan imaging. Since I had nothing to lose and possibly much to gain, I sent him an email on the September 18, 2000.

Proposal for a single subject trial

Sir,

This is admittedly a long shot, but if I don't ask I will never know. I have an adult son who is currently at Live Oaks Hospital in Sacramento. He is diagnosed as bipolar. I am interested in a better way to help him.

On the fourth of October Dr. Bonnie Kaplan, a psychologist from the University of Calgary will be making a poster presentation on the nutritional treatment of 10 bipolar patients at a Conference of the Canadian Psychiatry Association. She will report that 10 patients became symptom free following administration of the supplements. Alberta has funded $500,000 for a double blind placebo controlled study treating bipolar illness with the supplements. These supplements are also proving to be effective in the treatment of fibromyalgia, ADHD, Asperger's disorder, even some cases of schizophrenia. The theory is that on a biological basis these illnesses simply represent different ways the body tries to deal with inadequate nutrition or genetically impaired inadequate metabolic processes. If you front-load the system with the necessary ingredients, then the brain can establish its own homeostasis. For an academic this will sound quite unsophisticated. Being a mental health professional myself I can certainly understand this perception.

I doubt if any brain scans were involved in this preliminary study. Would you be interested in a single trial involving re-

placement of traditional medications with the supplements and documenting progress with brain scans? Given my son's recent history, he would probably require an inpatient stay during the transition process. He is currently taking Zyprexa, Wellbutrin, Depakote, and lithium. The goal of the treatment would be to transition away from these drugs as the supplements restore brain homeostasis.

If this approach were effective, it would result in some significant brain scan changes. Given the polarity of his current thinking with primitive magical black and white aspects, I would expect that his frontal cortex has significantly shut down. My son is a college graduate but he is functioning at a very regressed level now.

I can send you more information on the approach if you are interested. Thanks.

Dave Moyer, Lt Col, USAF, Ret.

Three More Chances

Figuring it would be easy to ignore one message, the next day I tried again. I hoped to engage Dr. Ketter by pointing out possible similarities between his own research and what I was learning about a nutritional approach to bipolar disorder.

September 19, 2000

Sir,
I read with interest your article entitled "Decreased dorsolateral prefrontal N-acetyl aspartate in bipolar disorder." I am an Alaska licensed clinical social worker. I don't know much about biology or chemistry. My previous inquiry to you was based on some very impressive case studies I have read and the fact that a governmental agency in Alberta was willing to pay $500,000 for a double blind placebo controlled study on the effect of the supplements on bipolar disorder. It was not based on any detailed understanding of the science of the supplements.

After learning from your paper that the ratios of N-acetyl aspartate, myoinosital, and choline to creatine-phosphocreatine were high in normals and low in bipolar patients I decided to check the supplements to see if they address that. If inositol and myoinosital are related, then two of the three substances are in the supplements. Among other things, they contain choline and inositol. Clearly, this is not proof of any efficacy, but I found it interesting that the supplements supply substances that you have found to be lacking in bipolar patients. I'm sure it is much more complicated than that, but I wanted to share the general concept with you. If there were any validity in these necessarily sketchy deliberations, it would suggest that your research findings might be consistent with the supplement approach. If you are interested in looking at the biochemistry of this further, here are some sites that may have meaning to you.

Is it possible that inadequate nutrition or genetically inadequate metabolic pathways result in various central nervous system disorders of which bipolar is one? If my son were to improve on the supplements as measured by brain scan, I would think this idea would be interesting to pursue. If you are unable or too busy to pursue this, do you know of anyone else who might be interested? Thanks for considering this proposal.

Dave Moyer, LCSW, BCD
Internet Sites:
http://www.genome.ad.jp/kegg/pathway/map/map00380.html
http://www.expasy.ch/cgi-bin/show_image?H2&down

After two days I had not received a response. I wasn't surprised. I figured he probably had some email filtering device and by now my messages were off his radar screen. I had nothing to lose by continuing to try, so I sent one more.

The Internet and email are wonderful inventions. I could easily access the research from a top scientist from Stanford University, then I could send him a message about it, asking for an opportunity to give my son the exact nutrients that his research showed were low in bipolar patients. I could offer him the opportunity to measure whether the supplementation helped Chris's brain to function better. After all, without treatment implications, of what benefit was academic research?

My chances of getting through the system by phone were negligible. I wouldn't have had the courage or stamina to try, but with email, if he were interested, it was easy. So what if Dr. Ketter or his staff members thought he was getting a crackpot message from a bipolar father of his bipolar son? The worst that could happen is that he would say no or not respond. Two days later I sent the following.

September 21, 2000

Sir,

On the other hand, an article on a failed single trial of a bipolar patient on a nutritional supplement would provide much needed public education for people like myself, who are not happy with the status quo. We are desperate for new solutions because we are worried about our children facing a life of minimal functioning, of which parkinsonian symptoms are but one example. The patients on the ward my son is now on justify such concerns. The developer of this supplement was such a person. After his bipolar wife died by suicide his family consisted of 10 children, three of whom were diagnosed bipolar. These children were reportedly restored to health by the supplements they developed over a several year period, the conceptual foundation of which was a well-established veterinary treatment for ear and tail biting syndrome. I didn't believe it at first either. But then they were treating ulcers in animals with antibiotics long before the medical community ostracized an Australian doctor for having the nerve to suggest that H. Pylori was the cause of human stomach ulcers which could be effectively treated with antibiotics. One of the developer's sons later became psychotic. The supplements restored his mental health too.

If the trial were a dramatic success, or even a partial success with improved function on minimal medications (One of the ten did remain on small amounts of psychotropic medications), then this research would support the public interest also.

If you are too busy to look into this and you know someone or some institution with the time or the interest, I would be most grateful. I would appreciate a referral to any facility where there might be interest in either warning an unsuspecting public of unproven medical "scams" or examining

154

a disruptive technology that may establish biological commonalties among many of the DSM-IV diagnoses. If this approach were effective across a spectrum of illnesses then DSM-IV disorders would have to be viewed in an entirely new light. To my knowledge, although only 10 cases are to be presented on 4 October, hundreds have been treated successfully. However, I do not believe any of these trials involved brain scans to corroborate the clinical picture.

Dave Moyer, Lt Col, USAF, Ret, LCSW, BCD, ACSW

My last, best, and final offer

What more could I do? I had already used up all my titles. Oh well, what the heck. I decided to try one more time. I must admit that my entreaties were becoming increasingly similar to those of one Ray W. Moyer, the self appointed guardian of the morals of the Oregon and California school systems, the man who, like his fellow bipolar and/or cyclothymic mentor, Winston Churchill, would "nevah, nevah, nevah" give up. And here I was, leading the charge for the bipolar "cure." The line between persistence and monomania, between creativity and madness, was admittedly a thin one.

September 22, 2000

Sir,
Here is a follow up to my previous note. These are comments by Dr. Julian Whitaker on the use of anteoplastines which have been used to treat brain tumors for 20 years now and for which the FDA has finally authorized 72 Phase II trials. Five of these trials have reported astonishing results that have not yet received the attention they deserve from the medical and academic communities.

"True cultural advancement is never smooth. It is always bumpy. This is because true advancement requires that an accepted paradigm be replaced with a discovery that more accurately defines reality. The accepted paradigm is always fiercely defended and the resistance to the discovery always incorporates the financial, political and legal institutions of the culture. For instance, the germ theory of disease depended on Louis Pasteur's successful treatment of Louis Meister, a 7 year old who had contracted rabies. If the child died, Pas-

155

teur would have been executed, and that advance- ment would ment would have been postponed for an indefinite period. The discovery that the earth is round took centuries to replace the accepted paradigm of a flat earth."

I don't thinks the risks of a new paradigm of treatment for bipolar illness are as severe as those faced by Pasteur.

Thanks but no thanks

Finally I received a response.

Data: September 23, 2000
Dear Mr. Moyer,

Regarding your request to Dr. Ketter, I do not believe our clinic has the capacity to carry out a single subject trial. Because such a trial would be very expensive, you may wish to approach the supplement manufacturer first to explore whether they are interested in funding research on the compound. Alternatively, a larger pharmaceutical house might be interested in the compound based on your preliminary findings and could pursue the necessary research and development.

Best wishes,
Connie Watkins, Assistant to Dr. Ketter

I had received a response! If I had not traveled down this path I would never have known. Through my persistence I had learned a valuable lesson. Money talked louder than the potential promise of nutritional supplements. The single most important criterion for a single subject research trial was how much money one had.

The only criterion I would now have for our own low budget single subject research would be how well Chris did off the medications and on the supplements. If he did not become hypomanic, manic, or depressed, that would be good enough for us.

We had even been willing and, I thought, able to pay for the hospitalization and the brain scans. Could they have been that expensive? Oh well, we had enough to worry about. I would see about getting data to support a new approach for my high-risk kids from Nevada County later.

After a couple emails to Dr. Kaplan and Tony I realized that brain scans of Truehope clients would not happen for some time. For one thing, the "compound" was not proprietary. For another, the resources of a nutritional company could not compare with those of a Merck or a Lilly.

Computer programmers are familiar with a protocol referred to as "computer busy handshaking." Whenever computers "meet" one another they size each other up and decide on the kind of relationship, if any, they will have. They can pour out their secrets, cut off the relationship, or enjoy a predefined limited and safe relationship. If they do not do a careful and thorough "handshake," one computer could steal secrets from another, or, worse, infect it with a virus. My sending the emails was like "computer busy handshaking." A person who was manic would keep on putting out his hand, irrespective of the response. I knew that no one at Stanford wanted to shake mine so I withdrew it. I had been persistent. It had only been a modicum of mania - this time.

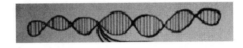

Part III - Perhaps Not

Each patient carries his own doctor inside him. We are at our best when the doctor who resides within each patient has the chance to go to work.

Albert Schweitzer, M.D.

15 - Switches, Widgets, and Brain Cells

So far our decisions had been driven by despair, faith, intuition, hope, and a very positive gut feeling about Tony and Barbara Stephan. Now it was time to find out if the data supported our decisions. I needed a rudimentary understanding of what was broken before I could determine if we were on the proper path to fixing it.

Symptoms and causes

If I wanted my mechanic to repair my car's racing engine, he first would need to find out what was wrong with it. The diagnosis would not be "racing engine." That only described symptoms. Perhaps the throttle was stuck. Perhaps the smog control or the fuel/air mixture was set incorrectly. The mechanic would be no closer to solving the problem if he diagnosed subsets of symptoms such as racing level I or II, level I meaning that the engine routinely goes too fast and level II meaning that the engine goes slowly with occasional bursts of unwanted speed. One would think it strange if the mechanic were to get paid solely for making these diagnoses. Suppose he offered the following diagnosis: Car Racing, Level I. Suppose he didn't fix my car, but got the "diagnosis" right. He would likely not be in business for very long; that is, unless he had a monopoly and customers had no other choices.

What if the mechanic were to tell me that my car had a "functional" problem, a set of symptoms without any known physical cause, but he could fix it by putting something in the gas tank that slowed down the engine. The mechanic who worked in this way would lose out to any mechanic who actually got under the hood to figure out what was wrong and then did his or her best to fix it.

The fact that Chris met the criteria for one of the subtypes of bipolar disorder called Bipolar I Disorder, told me nothing about what was broken or how to fix it. Even the general category of "bipolar disorder" only described a set of symptoms, not causes. I approached the task of finding these mysterious causes with a great deal of trepidation. Although I knew the difference between Bipolar I, Bipolar II, and cyclothymic personality, I was not trained at "getting under the hood." And there was no way I could master the science to give me the answers I was searching for. However, having made the decision to figure out what was broken, I had no choice but to take a look. My wife and son and I were not happy with our mechanics.

161

Stuck switches

The first piece of research I found pertained to switching mechanisms that become stuck in one position. These switches are designed to facilitate back-and-forth communication between the left and right hemispheres of the brain. The following statement by Professor John D. Pettigrew, Director, Vision Touch and Hearing Research Centre, University of Queensland, Australia, explains an experiment to test for evidence of a biological switching defect in bipolar patients.

> *We propose that bipolar disorder is the result of a genetic propensity for slow interhemispheric switching mechanisms that become "stuck" in one or the other state. Since slow switches are also "sticky" when compared with fast switches, the clinical manifestations of bipolar disorder may be explained by hemispheric activation being "stuck" on the left (mania) or on the right (depression).... The interhemispheric switch rate may provide a trait-dependent biological marker for bipolar disorder.*[1]

That was a complicated and intellectually provocative "big picture" hypothesis. The researchers presented a series of circular "grates," with either vertical or horizontal lines, to either the right eye (left hemisphere) or left eye (right hemisphere). The subjects, euthymic bipolar patients, patients in no current distress, and a control group without bipolar disorder, pushed the appropriate key when they figured out whether or not the lines on the grates were vertical, horizontal, or intermediate. Intermediate meant the subjects couldn't tell the direction of the lines. The task required the subjects' brains to switch perception from one hemisphere to another. The rivalry alternation rate was the speed with which the subjects were able to perceive the shape of the grate and press the corresponding key accordingly. The bipolar patients had a low alternating rate compared to the control group, suggesting that they were slower in perceptually changing their visual perception of the lines.

So one possible cause of bipolar disorder was that the switches between the hemispheres were stuck, or, perhaps "sticky" would be a better word. In any event they didn't work right. My initial "So what?" reaction was tempered as I read on.

When the left frontal cortex is injured by a stroke, the patient is more likely to experience depression. If the right frontal cortex is injured by a stroke, the patient is more likely to experience mania.[2] Stroke patients who denied having their disease usually had right-sided parietal lesions. This is why stroke victims injured in their right hemisphere may believe that their left arm works perfectly well, even though it is totally paralyzed from the stroke. This condition is called anosognosia. The ability to critically assess their situation is compromised. Those who are fully aware of their deficits had injuries on the left side of the brain. They maintained their critical awareness in their right hemisphere.[3] Why would this be? Could it be that impairment of the left hemisphere magnifies characteristics of the right hemisphere and impairment of the right hemisphere magnifies characteristics of the left? If so, what are those characteristics?

The left hemisphere's cognitive style is goal-directed, with a coherent plan of action that denies or smooths over discrepancies, while the right hemisphere's style is that of a "devil's advocate" which monitors and seeks to raise discrepancies. The hemisphere inactivated by a stroke can no longer oppose the cognitive style of the opposite hemisphere.[4] Mania caused by stroke is considered by medical professionals to be secondary mania, that is, mania related to a known medical condition as opposed to the more generic bipolar disorder.

Experiments in which sodium amobarbital was targeted to the right and left brain hemispheres confirmed the above. Inactivation of the left hemisphere with sodium amobarbital created negative moods, up to and including crying.[5] Right-sided injections created laughter and elation.[6]

Transcranial Magnetic Stimulation (TMS) is a new technology being studied at the University of Pennsylvania Medical Center. TMS generates powerful magnetic fields that oscillate at specific frequencies to selected locations, inducing either faster or slower metabolism in those areas. TMS of left prefrontal cortex (left hemisphere) is therapeutic for unipolar depression. The left stimulation increased the activity of the left hemisphere to help it balance the influence of the right. TMS to the right prefrontal cortex was halted by the overseeing ethics committee after some initial depression outcomes.[2] EEG studies support greater relative right hemisphere activation in depression, as do imaging studies.[8] Left prefrontal low metabolism is demonstrated in depression but is not present following remission.[9] Other studies show that left hemisphere activation occurs in mania.[10]

The impaired judgment seen in manic patients is probably related to the fact that they do not have access to all the resources in their brains. While normal volunteers are found to have activation in the front of their brain when solving problems, manic patients showed increased activity in a part of their brains located on the left and reduced activity in a part of their brain located on the right.[11] I didn't know brain anatomy — didn't need to. I could tell right from left.

To summarize, there are two hemispheres to the brain. Known specializations still apply such as the association of the left brain with language processing and the right with creativity. However, these hemispheres also perform global functions having to do with internal/external orientation and expansive/depressed emotionality. For most individuals, activation of the right hemisphere promotes negative emotions while activation to the left promotes positive emotions. There is inadequate counterforce to the opposing hemisphere.

When the left hemisphere is more active than the right, there is an association with confidence, elation, and mania. This can cause problems because the left hemisphere is also the action brain, responsible for translating inner intent into outward behavior. Left hemisphere phrases might include the following: "Just do it." "Ignore discrepancies." "Focus on the trees (details)." The external reality of the real world is not of particular concern to the left hemisphere when the right hemisphere fails to provide the necessary input. Chris's self description of events as described in this book reflects a lack of awareness of the big picture.

The right hemisphere is associated with caution, apprehension, and depression. Without input from the left, this hemisphere would think, but not act. This is a recipe for depression. The right hemisphere is the critical stopping brain. Right brain phrases include the following: "Think before you act." "Be careful." "Focus on the forest (context, big picture)." The right hemisphere is focused on the external world. It perceives the world as it is: a sort of world-centered approach to perception.

A normal person is able to integrate both hemispheres quickly and effortlessly. Not the bipolar patient. It is as if the self–centered, egoistic child (left hemisphere) and the critical-thinking adult (right hemisphere) can't communicate with each other. They either alternate very fast, as in mixed states (features of mania and major depression in the same day), or fast, as in rapid cycling (4 times a year or more), or more slowly over longer periods of time. They can even alternate in a seasonal pattern.

I thought it interesting that the familiar political "right" and "left" categories share some of the same characteristics as the right and left hemispheres. Maybe there was some profound simplicity here, the so-called reactive right and the so-called proactive left representing fundamentally different approaches to solving problems. Even though the brain is far too complex for any kind of simplistic or even definitive understanding of bipolar disorder from only these studies, the studies do provide evidence for each hemisphere playing a role in bipolar disorder.

Pettigrew's work demonstrated that bipolar patients may have right/left brain switching problems. The concept of stuck switches preventing the two hemispheres from talking to one another was not unlike my experience with Chris and my father when they were manic. Maybe the two hemispheres relate to each other in the same way the bipolar patient relates to his world. I thought back to Chris's comment that there was not enough room in his mind for the thoughts of others. When the bipolar patient is manic, there does not appear to be enough room in his left hemisphere for his right hemisphere, let alone a parent, wife, teacher, policeman, judge, or jail guard.

Since I wasn't a biologist, I needed to boil down the research to the most basic level before I could understand it. At the risk of oversimplifying, I decided to start a "Bipolar 101 for Dummies" with the following:

> *If you cool down the left frontal cortex and heat up the right, you get depression. If you heat up the left and cool down the right, you get mania. If the switches between the hemispheres are stuck, you lose the synergistic effects of both perspectives and drill down to one or the other one at a time, alternating either rapidly or slowly, depending on the nature of the stuck switches.*

The above does not do justice to the complexity and variation of the human brain. The left and right hemispheres contain much more than a right and left frontal cortex and a right and left section of the cingulate gyrus as discussed in the chapter notes. There have been other studies suggesting that a simplistic model such as I have articulated here does not explain all the data. For example, there have been two reported cases where patients switched handedness depending on whether they were manic or depressed![12] How to explain that one? It is beyond the scope of this book and my abilities to provide the kind of scholarly review such as one would find in a book like Manic Depressive Illness, by Doctors Goodwin and Jamison. If I were even capable of fully understanding the complexity of the circuitry of 100 billion neurons and 100 trillion synapses, it would require chapters of technical minutiae to explain it. The Bipolar 101 perspective, while clearly not rocket science, would have to work well enough for me. So, if Chris had stuck switches how did they get that way? The stuck switch theory explained some symptoms, but what made the switches stick?

Widgets

I found an article in the October 2000 issue of the *American Journal of Psychiatry*. It stated that there were abnormally high concentrations of a protein called vesicular monoamine transporter protein 2 (VMAT2) in 16 symptom-free male bipolar patients with one or more manic episodes, and usually major depressive episodes. According to the author, Dr. Zubieta, the bipolar patients had too many synaptic terminals containing VMAT2 compared to normal controls. The author stated that this could be a trait-related abnormality found in bipolar patients. These differences existed in only two areas of the brain, the thalamus and the ventral brainstem. The high concentrations presumed an equally high level of not only synaptic terminals, but also neurotransmitters. What was most interesting to me about this research was that the higher the level of VMAT2 in these areas, the poorer the patients performed on cognitive tests. The patients had been stable for more than six months and were presumed to be free of symptoms. Dr. Zubieta explained:

> *This is very unlike almost anything else seen in other pathologies.... As far as we know, no one has seen increases in terminal density in any illness and we are postulating that this may be connected to a person's disposition to develop mania or mania and depression.... These findings are telling us that it is very likely that these patients have alterations in the way their brain is wired to start with, so we can begin thinking about new avenues to either change or regulate the systems that appear to be altered. If we can show that these abnormalities start before symptoms are seen, it may develop into a diagnostic tool to screen people who might be at risk for developing bipolar disorder.*[13]

Many of the technical aspects of the article were hard to understand. A site for a company providing antibodies to various neurotransmitters for research purposes provided more information on VMAT2.

> *The regulated exocytotic release of neurotransmitters in response to neural activity requires storage within intracellular vesicles.... Storage depends upon the active transport into the vesicles. Several distinct transport activities have been identified for monoamines, acetylcholine, glutamate, GABA and glycine.*

Okay, so far, so good. According to Kathy's college text on animal physiology, exocytosis is the process whereby large, complex molecules are secreted from cells.

> *Vesicular monoamine transporters (VMATs) catalyze the transport and storage of monoamines, serotonin, dopamine, norepinephrine, epinephrine, and histamine.*

Let's see.... Catalyze means to facilitate. In other words, the VMATs served as facilitators for the transport and storage of neurotransmitters. Hey,

I can understand this after all.

> *The driving force utilized by the VMAT is the H+ electro-*
> *chemical gradient generated by a vacuolar ATP-dependent*
> *H+ pump (V-ATPase) located on vesicular plasma mem-*
> *brane.*

> *VMAT2, previously termed SVAT (synaptic vesicle amine*
> *transporter), is primarily found in monoaminergic cell bod-*
> *ies of the central nervous system and also in stomach but not*
> *in adrenals. Tetrabenazine and psychostimulants such as*
> *methamphetamine inhibit VMAT2 much more potently than*
> *VMAT1. Thus the VMATs show considerable differences in*
> *physiological and pharmacological properties....* [14]

Now I was totally — well, almost totally — lost. This was more than I could digest. I found out that a vacuole is a membrane bound cavity, but I could just see myself looking through a powerful microscope into each cellular factory and seeing a vacuolar ATP-dependent H+ pump along the factory wall pumping H+ to the H+ electrochemical gradient — or something like that. This was a foreign language for me. I didn't know much — I didn't know anything about vacuolar ATP-dependent H+ pumps, but I knew a little about how systems worked. So I decided to utilize a systems perspective to combine what I could understand from the article as well as others I had read regarding VMAT2 and neurotransmitters. After reviewing a number of sources and textbooks it was back to "Bipolar 101 for Dummies" again.

> *For the purposes of simplicity, neurotransmitters are defined*
> *as widgets. They are molecules that transmit impulses from*
> *neuron to neuron. For now, let's just say that widgets are*
> *needed so the brain can function properly.*

> *VMAT2 is a cellular widget-processing factory that facili-*
> *tates transport and storage of these widgets into or out of*
> *little sacs (vesicles) that exist in each neuron. They pour out*
> *widgets as needed near the edge of their neuron's axon, the*
> *synapse, an area that connects two interacting nerve cells.*
> *If the Internet were a brain and a computer a neuron, then*
> *the axon and the synapse would be the phone line in and the*
> *modem. So these little VMAT2s supply widgets, which are*
> *then transported to the synaptic cleft, sort of a great divide*

between neurons. The widgets are also called first messengers because they send messages from neuron to neuron. Second messengers do stuff inside the neuron after the widgets bind with certain receptors, and tell certain G proteins

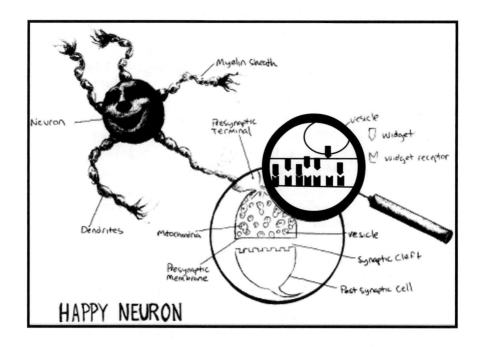

HAPPY NEURON

to do their thing, but more on that later — much later. There are between 80 to 100 different widgets at present, including new subtypes still being discovered.

In the above illustration the widgets leave the vesicles and go to the waiting receptors. If the presynaptic cleft could talk, it might say something like "Message incoming," to which the receptors would respond, "Got it."

Specific widgets are located in specific neural pathways. They do different things throughout the brain. For example, there are serotonin, dopamine, glutamate, and g-aminobutyric acid (GABA) pathways. Serotonin widgets control mood, sleep/wake, feeding, and temperature. Three different kinds of dopamine widgets are involved in muscle tension, emotions, and perceptions, respectively. Glutamate widgets speed up the transmission in the brain while GABA widgets slow down transmission by increasing the inhibition properties of the cells.

If there are too many widgets in a particular neuron, the widget receptors across the synaptic cleft become overactive. Brain functioning is impaired and a person could lose the ability to think clearly. Could even become manic. Too much glutamate can make you over - excited, and kill neurons; too little can make you sedated. Too much GABA can sedate you, and too little can make you excited. Tegretol and Depakote, for example, increase the effectiveness of GABA to prevent seizures and mania. Neurontin, a psychotropic medication and a kind of GABA clone, does the same by mimicking the actions of GABA.

Too much VMAT2 may indicate too much storage of widgets; hence a greater capacity to be released under certain circumstances.

To illustrate one effect of too few widgets, there is a rare, sometimes fatal autoimmune disorder called Stiff Person Syndrome. The syndrome is characterized by constant tension between opposing muscle groups and uncontrollable behavior in response to loud noises. One might think of this as a sort of mania of the cerebellum, if you will. Patients with this syndrome can lose control in response to a loud noise. If you were walking downtown on a sidewalk, heard a loud noise, and then involuntarily crashed into a plate glass window, and you hadn't been drinking, that could be symptomatic of Stiff Person Syndrome (SPS). The condition is, in part, caused by too little GABA. Antibodies interfere with the synthesis of GABA.[15] GABA synapses are the most numerous inhibitory synapses in the brain.

There are noradrenaline widgets that in the brain control arousal, mood, emotion and drive. VMAT2 specifically facilitates the transport and storage of norepinephrine, serotonin, dopamine, and histamine widgets. The details of what VMAT2 does and how it does it are not that important for the level of analysis in this 101 orientation. What is important is that bipolar males have about 30% more widget factories in a part of their brain stem and their thalamus than non-bipolar males and that the higher the number, the more compromised their intellectual functioning. Scientists presume that since they have a higher number of VMAT2s, they

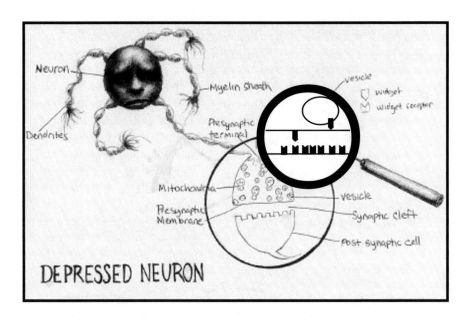

DEPRESSED NEURON

also have a higher number of widgets in their thalamus and brain stem.

In the right amounts, widgets work together to ensure proper brain functioning, but when there are imbalances, functionality deteriorates. The above illustration represents a depressed neuron where, according to the biogenic amine theory, there are insufficient widgets. The message from the presynaptic synaptic cleft might be, "Not much mail today." The illustration at the top of the opposite page represents a manic neuron. Here the message might be "Incoming!" The same symptoms could occur from ingestion of cocaine or antidepressants as well as from a manic episode.

The psychiatrist has many different ways to chemically manipulate the brain. One way is to indirectly increase the number of widgets, such as is done with antidepressants. The psychiatrist can also prescribe lithium to better regulate glutamate and to reduce the responsiveness of receptor widgets caused by too many widget-processing centers storing

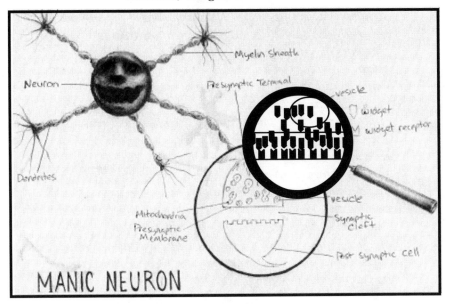

and transporting too many widgets. The psychiatrist can pre-scribe Zyprexa, an anti-widget receptor pill. The patient goes to a pharmacy and buys the pills, then swallows them.

The anti-widgets receptors find their way into the patient's brain, where they seek out receptor widgets in the post syn-aptic axons as illustrated below in the drugged neuron. The molecules from that drug target serotonin, histamine, and

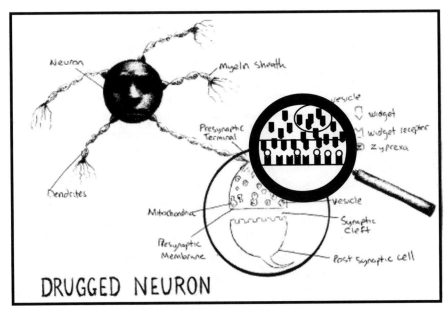

dopamine widget receptors. The substances in the anti-widget pills are said to be antagonistic toward the widget receptors,but actually they have an affinity toward them, so much so that they embrace them so tightly that they became bound together, in effect putting the receptors out of commission. Technically they are called antagonists because they bind to receptors without causing a biochemical response. This lessens the amount of the widget receptors ready to receive all those excessive widgets that VMAT2s specifically store and transport, widgets such as serotonin, histamine and dopamine. The result is that the patient's brain can function better ... sometimes. However, the anti-widget pills also bind with widget receptors that might have been in proper balance before they were antagonized by the anti-widget receptor pills. Also, sometimes the brain grows more receptors (upregulation).

From the standpoint of this backyard mechanic, maybe too many glutamate and too few GABA widgets made Chris's brain race. Maybe the cumulative effect of 2,000 mg of Depakote daily to control his hypomanic behavior facilitated GABA widgets too well, raising cell inhibition thresholds, impairing concentration, and causing depression. Since it is known that medications with a high affinity for histamine receptors promote weight gain, and Zyprexa has such an affinity, maybe the Zyprexa antagonized histamine receptors, causing him to gain 25 pounds during his three-week hospitalization. Did 20 mg of Zyprexa antagonize dopamine receptors, causing his neurons to make more of (upregulate) them, thereby causing his very noticeable muscle tremors (extrapyramidal symptoms) that disappeared when his dose was reduced to 15 mg? Were the intense, almost overpowering sensations of taste, smell, and colors during his manic attacks related to having too many VMAT2s? Were there not enough nutritional supplies to help manage excessive widget processing factories? Did inadequate nutrients impair neuron energy levels, causing sensory overload by firing excessively?

A subset of 40 percent of bipolar patients have generally low levels of GABA widgets, whether they are symptomatic or not.[16] If Stiff Person Syndrome is functionally similar to a "mania" of the cerebellum, and it is caused by too little GABA, then could too little GABA play a role in mania? If too little GABA is a consequence of antibody activity, then could too much antibody activity play a role in mania? If excessive VMAT2 is a trait of many bipolar patients, and if they had a hard-wiring problem, then perhaps, in spite of the side effects, bipolar patients needed a medicine like Zyprexa. Maybe they would need it all their lives in order to limit the excessive widgets available for the storage and transport into the excessive VMAT2s. Maybe

Zyprexa is needed to routinely reduce levels of serotonin, dopamine, and histamine. Again, I had more questions than answers. I called Tony.

"Tony, Chris is doing fine, but I thought I would call you to tell you about an abstract of an article I just read."

"Hi, Dave. Glad to hear he's doing well."

"I found this article in the October issue of the *American Journal of Psychiatry*." I then explained the anatomical differences found in the male bipolar patients, the excessive neurotransmitters, and the corresponding decline in intellectual functioning.

"If excess VMAT2 is related to poor intellectual performance, wouldn't that be a reason for medications to balance the excess neurotransmitters?"

"That is very interesting," Tony said. "I think that might help explain why so many of these people are so creative. Maybe their nutritional demands are greater since they need to manage the excess neurotransmitters they create."

"So you think the brain can do a better job of regulating itself with the proper nutritional foundation than prescription medication?"

"This is what our experience has shown."

"Thanks, Tony. Just wanted to get your take on this."

I shared some of the other highlights of my research, then got off the phone. Tony always had more calls waiting for him.

I had looked at how stuck switches keep the right and left hemispheres of the bipolar brain from talking to each other. I had learned how bipolar patients have imbalances in their widgets (neurotransmitters) affecting the overall functioning of the brain. But what about the cells of the brain, specifically the neurons which make the brain function? They seemed to fire much faster or much slower than normal in bipolar patients. And some didn't seem to fire at all. Were they too hot or too cold, too fast or too slow? What made them misfire? Were some of the cells dead? What happened at the cellular level, and how was that related to the switching problem at the hemispheric level?

Brain cells

While there are any number of environmental and biological insults that can damage brain cells and compromise neuron functioning, I found myself focusing on data suggesting that neurons are killed or impaired by microbes, with far-ranging untoward consequences. Some known viruses associated with bipolar disorder include toxoplasmosis and Borna disease virus, the latter of which appears to be attracted to some specific neural pathways and not others. At the Stanley Foundation at John Hopkins University, researchers are working to discover the role microbes play in bipolar disorder and schizophrenia. The Foundation has been collecting the brains of post-mortem bipolar and schizophrenic patients for a number of years now. They are operating under four central hypotheses:

1. Serious neuropsychiatric diseases are the result of environmental insults occurring in genetically susceptible individuals.
2. Environmental factors include infection and the immune response occurring during the prenatal or postnatal periods or later in life.
3. Genetic factors may include the determinants of the response to infection and the regulation of cytokines and other immune mediators.
4. Different neuropsychiatric diseases such as schizophrenia and bipolar disorder may represent different combinations of these environmental and genetic factors.

In 1996, the Foundation used new electron microscope techniques on post-mortem brain tissue obtained from individuals with schizophrenia and bipolar disorder. They reported that four of five tissue culture samples inoculated with brain tissue obtained from individuals with these disorders displayed alterations in cellular architecture typical of viral infections. How-

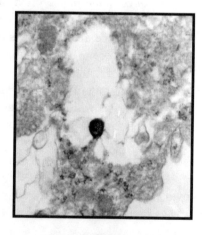

ever, they could not find evidence of an active viral infection, nor could they associate the particular particles with a defined virus. The photo to the right shows evidence of a "virus-like particle." Provided courtesy Dr. Yolken and the Stanley Foundation, it is a thin section of A172 a human glioblastoma cell line, inoculated with brain tissue from an individual with bipolar disorder, showing a virus-like particle budding from the cell membrane. The particle appears to be enveloped, 100-200 mm in size and may be intra- or extracellular. Such particles were not found in any

cells inoculated with brains from normal individuals. The researchers detailed as much as was known of the specific types of viruses and concluded as follows:

> *It is thus likely that the viral particles represent a new human strain of paramyxovirus. Additional studies are currently underway directed at the immunological, biological and molecular characterization of this agent and the further determination of its role in human disease.*[17]

Epidemiological studies have consistently suggested a relationship not only between viruses and bipolar disorder, but also between viruses and schizophrenia. For example, there is a positive relationship between these mental disorders and births in the winter and spring, suggesting an association with viruses. A positive correlation with population density suggests increased viral exposure. Increased antibodies to toxoplasmosis have been found in individuals with both schizophrenia and bipolar illness. Toxoplasmosis, a disease carried by cats, is known to affect human personality traits and to affect neurotransmitters in animal studies.[18]

A more recent study by the Stanley Foundation identified a particular retrovirus unique to schizophrenia. A retrovirus is a particular kind of virus that has in its core RNA rather than DNA and which replicates through a unique process called reverse transcriptase. Dr. Karlsson and others from the Stanley Foundation found evidence of retroviral sequences similar to a virus called HERV-W from 29% of a group of newly diagnosed schizophrenic patients as well as in the post-mortem schizophrenic brains. There were no sequences that could be found in a control group consisting of people without any inflammatory neurological disease.[19]

In addition to evidence of viruses damaging cells, there are microstructural changes in the prefrontal cortex of bipolar patients.[20,21] The mechanisms by which the virus causes cell damage have yet to be elucidated, but it is known that low energy supply to neurons increases excitotoxicity, or the reactivity of the cells, and that such increases promote cell apoptosis, or programmed cell death. Excitotoxins such as aspartate and glutamate can not only cause cell death, but also play a role in seizures and hypoglycemia.[22] The word "apoptosis" is of Greek derivation, and it literally refers to leaves falling from trees. Apoptosis is one of the ways that cells are programmed to die.

At the cellular level, bipolar patients are believed to have compromised activity not only at the level of first messenger activity, but also second messenger activity, so named because it is involved in messaging within the neuron itself. Second messengers are molecules that are inside neurons. They are activated by something called G proteins. G proteins set various cellular switches on the membrane and the nucleus of the neuron. In other words, the G protein/second messenger is a system of communication and monitoring within neurons. It is capable of programming and reprogramming the neurons based on needed changes in the system. No one knows why, but G protein levels in white blood cells are very high during mania and low in depression.[23] Maybe the sensitivity of brain cells is set too high in mania and/or too low in depression for the bipolar patient. One of the reasons lithium ions may be effective at the cellular level is that they help the second messengers to function properly.[24]

There are changes in carbohydrate metabolism at the cellular level in bipolar patients. Insulin sensitivity is definitely increased during mania, and probably decreased during depression. This is clearly seen on PET scans showing the hot spots in the manic brain where the glucose is metabolized much faster. As a matter of fact, bipolar patients have higher rates of diabetes than the general population. Some researchers are suggesting that disturbed carbohydrate metabolism is related to low serotonin.[25] Shoemaker makes the argument that tumor necrosis factor, created by the body in response to viral, chemical, or other toxins, limits the effectiveness of insulin receptors to process glucose. He is speaking of a general population, but if his observations are correct, they would equally apply to bipolar patients whose viral and or other neurotoxin load could compromise their glucose metabolism.

According to the technical VMAT2 discussion quoted earlier, psychostimulants such as methamphetamine (speed) have unique inhibitory effects on VMAT2. If that is the case, does methamphetamine, which is known to make people "high," impair the functionality of first or second messengers through its inhibitory effects on VMAT2? My hunch was that methamphetamine intrudes into the neurons and takes over operations, essentially overwhelming the finely balanced dance of neurotransmitters and receptors that took mother nature millions of years to perfect. Whatever the cause, the result is that some kind of chemical interlopers demand that neurons continually dance the jitterbug until they drop from exhaustion or death.

I had barely scratched the surface, but I had learned enough to know that the old paradigm of "chemical imbalance," was no longer adequate to explain bipolar disorder. While it was still true that too much serotonin, dopamine, and norepinephrine were associated with mania and too little with depression, newer research involving viruses, structural anomalies, first and second messenger systems, and carbohydrate metabolism was elucidating much more complex interdependent systems. There was complex interplay among serotonin, dopamine, noradrenaline, acetylcholine, glutamate, and GABA, as well as an array of second messengers. Even the more professional sounding biogenic amine theory for mania and depression was no longer adequate. And I wasn't even going to try to reduce intracellular calcium ion abnormalities to a Bipolar 101 perspective.

With all this complexity, I again wondered how pharmaceutical companies and/or psychiatrists could know when and where to effectively intervene with such a delicate and complex system as the human brain. As Dr. Marie Asberg stated, "The CNS can be likened unto a net. If you pull any single mesh in the net, the shape of every other mesh will change."[25]

Bipolar 101 for Dummies

It was time to go back to Bipolar 101 for Dummies to try to make sense out of this necessarily superficial and incomplete exploration into bipolar phenomena.

Imagine that there are two teams of mechanics, team A and team B. Each team consists of two mechanics. Both teams are given one hour each to diagnose what is wrong with my car. With team A, both members communicate spontaneously and freely, modifying their perceptions as they test out different hypotheses. One team member is intuitive and quick to act. The other is cautious and questioning. Members of the second team are only allowed to communicate one at a time for a specific period of time, alternating every ten minutes. One of the mechanics has a "know-it-all" attitude. This mechanic springs into action at the first inkling of a solution. The other is a critic who disparages the efforts of the "know-it-all." Which team will be able to diagnose my car first, the team that can flexibly alter their perceptions based on the information they are sharing with each other, or the team locked into rigid communication patterns? The first team benefits because collaborating from different viewpoints leads to synergistic accomplishments. The B team is handicapped by the lack of effective communication between the members as well as their rigid stances. The bipolar brain is like the B team. Each team member (each hemisphere) is unable to improvise his or her learning and communicate it to the other. These hemispheres lack plasticity, the ability to adjust to input. Instead of finding a solution, they don't listen and instead argue with each other.

In other words, programming defects at the cellular level, and concurrent and/or resulting abnormalities at the widget level, result in stuck switches that prevent the two sides of the brain from being on the same team. The bipolar brain can barely get its act together, let alone operate interdependently with brains that are well-coordinated. As the integrity of switches, widgets, and brain cells decreases, the black/white polarity increases.

To illustrate, the following scenarios describe how I might think about writing this book given varying levels of functionality of my switches, widgets, and brain cells. This first scenario presumes they are in good working order, a dubious assumption, perhaps, for a person willing to stop his normal life for two years to research and write a book. The "right" and "left" designation refers to whether the central concept is a left (manic, no discrepancies) or a right (caution, world perspective) hemispheric perspective.

If the supplements help Chris to overcome his bipolar disorder (right), they could help others as well (left). The process of writing can help me to better understand Chris's illness (left). It may help me to help my clients to more effectively

*deal with this illness (right/left). If I called the book "The
Cure for Bipolar Illness," potential readers might presume
that I am manic (right). If I state, as I did originally, that the
supplements are "Too Good To Be True," this would reflect
how most people probably look at the supplementation program and the claims made by it (right). But that would also
convey the message that the claim was too good to be true
and therefore wasn't (right). But if I called it "Too Good To
Be True? Nutrients Quiet the Unquiet Brain," that might
appeal to the right-brained critics and the left-brained optimistic hopefuls (right/left). While I have written papers and
have published several during my career, I have never written an entire book before (right). It would take a lot of work
and research, but I think I could do it (left/right). I could do
a lot more for families with bipolar kids by writing a book
than by trying to help kids in the county system (left). Whether
or not it gets to a publisher and whether or not people buy
the book, writing it could help me (right/left). And, if Chris
can get his switches, widgets and brain cells to operate efficiently, this project will be well worth it, regardless of how
well the public accepts it (left/right).*

In the above perspective, there is frequent shifting between my egocentric view and a more objective world view, between wish-fulfilling expansive claims and real world cautions. There are also words that denote grada-
tions like "probably" and "could." As brain dysfunction worsens, the thinking becomes more primitive and regressive, similar to the thinking of a young
child who can see blacks and whites but not grays. Now consider the same
issues from a hypomanic perspective.

*Big things are about to happen. I found the cure.
I found the truth, and I must tell the world about
it. They will buy the book all over the world. I
will be on Oprah Winfrey, David Letterman.
Thousands will be cured by reading this book.
I will not only transform the entire county mental health system, but the mental health professions of the world as well(left).*

If my switches, widgets, and brain cells become more severely compromised, my thinking becomes more psychotic.

GOD IS REVEALING THE WORDS TO ME AS I WRITE. I DON'T NEED TO SLEEP OR EAT BECAUSE I HAVE TO GET HIS THOUGHTS WRITTEN FOR ALL THE GENERATIONS TO COME. THE TRUTH IS SETTING ME FREE. THE TRUTH IS SETTING CHRIS FREE. <u>THE TRUTH WILL SET THE WORLD FREE!!!!</u> SHARING THE TRUTH IS MORE IMPORTANT THAN ANY EARTHLY NEEDS I USED TO HAVE. GOD IS CALLING ME TO DO IT (LEFT).

Now to shift to a right hemisphere depressed perspective.

I have nothing to offer anyone. I am a failure. I don't know anything. I can't do anything right. People would laugh at me if I tried to write a book about bipolar illness. Nobody would even listen to what I have to say (right).

Assuming a greater degree of impairment, this scenario reflects a psychotic perspective.

God has condemned me. I can smell the sulfur. I am going to hell. Every thought and action I have is bad. I am worthless(right).

When Chris was first hospitalized, he believed the world was going to end in one great apocalyptic finale. His prophecy was correct. His world did come crashing down, never to be the same again. His perception of reality underwent a massive paradigm shift as a consequence of biological processes going on in his brain. His "world" was no longer the world as perceived by others with well-functioning brains. That world is a balance of accurate perceptions of the real world that exists independently of us and the subjective egocentric view of the world that parts of our left hemisphere create for us.

Here is how I saw it. When he was in a manic state, Chris's consciousness was in his left hemisphere, closed off to input that could have helped him maintain a balance with his right hemisphere. When he was depressed, left hemisphere functions were unable to compete with the critical right brain processes that had been held in check when he was manic. Known and unknown physical processes caused this. I wondered why the known biological anomalies like viruses had not been investigated in Chris's case.

If a patient tells his doctor he has pain in the stomach the physician will rule out a number of diagnoses, such as ulcer, acid reflux and tumor. If he tells his doctor he has a cough, diagnoses such as asthma, pneumonia and allergies, among other things, will be ruled out. So why, if he tells his doctor that he has severe mood swings, does his doctor tell him that his diagnosis is severe mood swings, otherwise known as bipolar disorder? Why doesn't the doctor try to find out what is wrong? It seemed so elementary.

Scientists know some of the biological processes involved in bipolar disorder and they are learning more. For now, I would have to be satisfied to view this as a problem of switches, widgets and brain cells. While this problem was highly complex, one approach seemed pretty simple. Provide the body an ample supply of what it needs and then let the brain/body solve the problems for itself rather than trying to guess which widgets, which first or second messengers, which chemical precursors needed tweaking one way or the other in order to ensure proper brain functioning. To me, anyone who claimed to fix the brain with the right kind and amount of widgets and widget receptor antagonists had to be little grandiose, maybe even a bit manic. I wondered if some day we would look back at our current psychiatric practices and compare them to the "snake pit" mentality of a bygone treatment era.

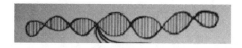

Notes

1. This is how Pettigrew explains his hypothesis.

> *Support for this "sticky" interhemispheric switching hypothesis stems from our recent observation that the rate of perceptual alternation in binocular rivalry is slow in euthymic subjects with bipolar disorder (n=18, median=0.27Hz) compared with normal controls (n=49, median=0.60Hz, p<0.0005). We have presented evidence elsewhere that binocular rivalry is itself an interhemispheric switching phenomenon. The rivalry alternation rate (putative interhemispheric switch rate) is robust in a given individual,*

with a test-retest correlation of >0.8, making it suitable for genetic studies.

Pettigrew, John D., Miller, Steven M., "A 'sticky' interhemispheric switch in switch in bipolar disorder?" 2000.
http://www.uq.edu.au/nuq/jack/procroysoc.html

2. Robinson, R.G., Downhill, J.E., "Lateralization of psychopathology in response to focal brain injury," in Brain asymmetry (eds.), R.J. Davidson & K. Hugdahl, London: MIT Press. 1995, 693-711.

3. McGlynn, S.M., Schacter, D.L., "Unawareness of deficits in neuropsychological syndromes," *J Clin Exp Neuropsych*, 11:143-205, 1989.

4. Ramachandran, V.S., "Phantom Limbs, neglect syndromes and Freudian Psychology," *Int Rev Neurobiology*, 37, 291-333, 1994.

5. Christianson, S.A., Saisa, J., Garvill, J., Silfvenius, H., "Hemisphere inactivation and mood-state changes," *Brain and Cognition,* 23:127-144, 1993.

6. Lee, G.P., Loring, D.W., Meader, K.J., Brooks, B.B., "Hemispheric specialization for emotional expression: a reexamination of results from intracarotid administration of sodium amobarbitol," *Brain and Cognition,* 12: 267-280, 1990.

7. Pascual-Leone, A., Rubio, B., Pallardo, F., Catala, M.D., "Rapid-rate transcranial magnetic stimulation of left dorsolateral prefrontal cortex in drug-resistant depression," *The Lancet* 348:233-237, 1996.

8. Henriques, J. B., Davidson, R. J., "Left frontal hypoactivation in depression," *J Abn Psychol*, 100: 535-545, 1991.

9. Bench, C.J., Frackowiak, R.S., Dolan, R. J., "Changes in regional cerebral blood flow on recovery from depression," *Psych Med,* 25:247-251, 1995.

10. Migliorelli, R., Starkstein, S.E., Teson, A., de Quiros, G., Vazquez, S., Leiguarda, R., Robinson, R.G., "SPECT findings in patients with primary mania," *J of Neuropsychia and Clin Neurosci*, 5: 379-383, 1993.

11. Rubenstein found that when a control group consisting of non-bipolar patients was given problems to solve, the group demonstrated activation in the ventral (towards the belly) prefrontal cortex and the anterior (front) cingulate gyrus, a region going from the front to the back of the brain. On the other hand, manic patients had increased activation in the left dorsal anterior cingulate and decreased activation in the right frontal polar region. The strengths of the relationship correlated with the level of mania. Controls had greater task-related activation in the inferior frontal gyrus than did manic patients. The study showed that manic patients demonstrated abnormal task-related responses in a specific frontal region.
Rubenstein, J., Fletcher, P., Rogers, R., Ho, L., Aigbirhio, F., Paykell, E., Robbins, T., Sahakian B., "Decision-making in mania: a PET study," *Brain*, Vol 124, No. 12, 2550-2563, December 2001.

12. Goodwin, F.K., Jamison, K.R., Manic Depressive Illness, Oxford University Press, New York, 1990, 509.

13. Zubieta, Joh-Kar, "Excessive monoaminergic synaptic terminals associated with bipolar disorder," *Am J Psychiatry,* 157:1619-1628, 2000.

14. Alpha Diagnostic International, Inc., "Vesicular Monoamine Transporters (VMAT) & ... Antibodies," 2000.
http://www.4adi.com/flr/vmat.html

15. Petty, F., Kramer, G.L., Fulton, M., Davis, L., Rush, A.J., (in press), "Stability of plasma GABA at four-year follow-up in patients with primary unipolar depression. *Biological Psychiatry*," UTSW Psychiatrist, Neuroreceptor/Neuroendocrine Research.

16. Levy, L.M., Dalakas, M.C., Floeter, M.K., "The Stiff Person Syndrome: an autoimmune disorder affecting neutotransmisson of gammaaminobutyric acid," *Ann Intern Med*, 131(7): 533-30 Oct 5, 1999.

17. Stanley Foundation, "Report of Research Activities – 1996." http.//www.med.jhu.edu/stanleylab/research/intro.html

18. Yolken, Robert H., and Torrey, Fuller E.K., "Viruses, schizophrenia, and bipolar disorder," *Clinical Microbiology Reviews*, 131-145, Jan 1995.

19. In an article entitled "Retroviral RNA identified in the cerebrospinal fluids and brains in individuals with schizophrenia," Karllson reported finding ten of 35 schizophrenic patients (29%) to have retroviral elements in their cerebral spinal fluid. None were identified among 22 individuals with non-inflammatory neurological disease or 30 with no neurological or psychiatric illness (p<0.001). These sequences were similar to the endogenous (arising within the body) retrovirus known as HERV-W. In addition, five post-mortem schizophrenic brains were found to have retroviral RNA, two of which were consistent with HERV-W while the others had evidence of similarity with HERV-W. This was in contrast to the finding of no retroviral RNA similar to HERV-W among post mortem control brains.
Karlsson, Hakan, "Retroviral RNA identified in schizophrenic patients," *Proc Natl Acad Sci USA*: 98:4634-4639,4293-4294, April 10, 2001.

20. There is a loss of glial cells as well as neurons in bipolar illness. Glial cells comprise much of the brain. Outnumbering neurons ten to one, they support neurons by, among other things, providing energy to the neurons and facilitating the removal of excessive glutamate, an excitatory amino acid. Three types of glial cells are astrocytes, oligodendrocytes, and neuroglia.
Knable, B.B., Torrey, E.F., Webster, M.J., Barko, J.J., "Multivariate analysis of prefrontal cortical data from the Stanley Foundation Neuropathology Consortium," *Brain Research Bulletin*, in press, 2001.

21. Also, in bipolar disorder, there is a decrease in glial fibrilliary acidic protein, a protein found in glial cells, as well as other levels of specific proteins.
Johnston-Wilson, N.L., Sims, C.D., Hofmann, J.P., Anderson, L., Shore, A.D., Torrey, E.F., Yolken, R.H., "Disease-specific alterations in frontal cortex brain proteins in schizophrenia, bipolar disorder, and major depressive disorder," *Mol Psychiatry,* Mar;5(2):142-9, 2000.

22. Henneberry, R.D., Novelli, A., Cox, J.A., Lysko, P.G., "Neurotoxicity at the N-Methyl-D-Aspartate receptor in energy-compromised neurons, an hypothesis for cell death, aging and disease," *Ann NY Academy of Scient,* 568: 225-233, 1989.

23. Avissar, S., Nechamkin, Y., Barki-Harrington, L., Roitman, G., Schreiber, G., "Differential G protein measures in mononuclear leukocytes of patients with bipolar mood disorder are state dependent," *Journal of Affective Disorders*, 43(2), 85-94 April, 1989.

24. Mondimore, Francis Mark, Bipolar Disorder, A Guide For Patients and Families, Baltimore Maryland, John Hopkins University Press, 1999, 92.

25. Goodwin, F.K., Jamison, K.R., Manic Depressive Illness, Oxford University Press, New York, 1990, 445.

26. ibid, 483.

16 - There Has to Be a Better Way

The idea of using vitamin and mineral supplements to alleviate the causes of CNS disorders was not as farfetched as I had originally thought. Not only did I surf the net, but I purchased and read a number of books on the causes and treatment of bipolar and other mental disorders. In spite of the fact that the DSM-IV describes distinctly different mental disorders, I found evidence suggesting that symptoms common to different mental disorders were effectively treated with nutritional supplements. These were scientific studies, not just case studies and testimonials on the Internet. I also found interesting perspectives on food antibodies and heavy metal poisoning that warranted further exploration.

Assuming that nutritional and/or metabolic deficits wreak havoc on the brains of bipolar patients, I wanted to know what else besides anti-widget pills could help. We couldn't talk Chris out of mania or depression, but we could help him get the nutrients he needed to let his body do the job. But first I had to deal with my own epistemological assumptions. Epistemology is the study of truth. How to know what is true? For the manic, that question is easy to answer. Truth is whatever the manic person thinks is true, regardless of any external evidence to the contrary. I thought I could do better. Yet I realized that, in a sense, I had been doing much the same for much of my life. Like all therapists, I had been taught that certain things were "true" and others "false," and I had accepted much of that teaching on the basis of the authority of my teachers and supervisors. Now it was time to become my own teacher, my own supervisor.

This chapter contains a summary of what I learned about nutrition-based treatment approaches for bipolar disorder as well as other CNS disorders. Some studies are in the chapter, while other, more detailed studies are discussed in the chapter notes. A word of caution to the reader is called for here. Some of this material is difficult to understand due to its technical nature. In addition, progression of thoughts will be, to many, awkward and unfamiliar. Many ideas will seem foreign and unfamiliar because they are. In spite of the importance of these ideas today, conventional wisdom, as reflected in, for example, the media, has yet to take note of them. Our culture is influenced by forces beyond our control; therefore, many of you may read this chapter in disbelief. So put on your analytical hat and be prepared to take some unexpected turns as you discover some of the places a nutritional perspective can take us.

Taking the mental out of "mental" illness

People suffering from borderline personality disorder (BPD) not only experience life as a constant emotional roller coaster ride, but they also have to deal with the stigma that they have a disorder of their personality, not a discrete "illness" like bipolar disorder or schizophrenia. While the lay public may not be aware of this, many mental health professionals prefer not to see BPD patients. If the mantras of the bipolar patient change from "Just do it" to "I am worthless" as their moods cycle back and forth over months, the mantra of the borderline patient, "I hate you; don't leave me," can be sounded hourly throughout their chaotic lives: Impulsive behavior, rapid changes of mood, alternating adoration and hatred of others, plus a tendency toward suicide attempts, combine to make BPD patients among the most difficult therapeutic challenges. I had studied this subject a lot ... out of necessity. When a patient put a razor blade to her throat in my office and threatened to cut her carotid artery, I learned fast. As she later explained, it was no big deal. "I only wanted you to hold me."

When I read Masterson's <u>Psychotherapy of the Borderline Adult,</u> I was impressed with his intellectually compelling model of intra- and inter-psychic processes that, without oversimplifying, provided an elegant way to make sense of the self-destructive, unpredictable behavior of many BPD patients. "Intra-psychic" refers to relationships with others, while "inter-psychic" refers to relationships among the component parts of the self. Terms like "abandonment depression," "regression in the service of the ego," "withdrawing object relations unit," and "rewarding object relations unit" all provided an intellectually satisfying framework for understanding borderline behavior — for the therapist.

Such terms defined the "turf" where the work needed to be done. That turf involved intrapsychic symbolic verbal interchange, otherwise known as psychotherapy. The purpose of these symbolic interactions was to enable the patient to mature and grow without the depression caused by fear of abandonment and the regressive behavior accompanying that fear. The therapist facilitated change by empowering patients to "individuate" without fear of abandonment and to give up the regressive behaviors designed to keep abandonment fears at bay. The presumption was that the parent, most likely the mother — who else? — had programmed the BPD patient incorrectly to regress rather than grow.

This thinking reminded me of early work on the "schizophrenogenic" mother whose "double-binding behavior" supposedly played a role in the etiology of that illness in her children. In the 1960s, such notable communication theorists as Satir, Haley, and Bateson from the Palo Alto Group were promoting the double-bind theory of schizophrenia. While a few independent thinkers like Dr. Silvano Ariete found the theory implausible, many mental health professionals were taken in by it. Perhaps it gave them delusions of mastery and control. If we students couldn't master how to properly fit such words as scapegoating, symbiosis, splitting, projective identification, and infantilization into the arcane world of the double-bind theory of schizophrenia, we just had to study harder. I remember the appeal of these concepts, regardless of whether or not they were true. Many therapists bought it hook, line and sinker, unmindful of the fact that if you were a mother and your child was acting crazy, your behavior might be pretty ambivalent too. It was psychobabble then, and it is psychobabble now. But who was to tell the emperor he was wearing no clothes back then? Who will tell him now?

As stated earlier, we therapists need models to give us at least some sense of control in dealing with our patients' dysfunctional thinking and behavior. Psychotherapy helps many therapists to effectively treat borderline patients by providing a coherent model to replace the incoherence and chaos in these patients' lives. When the BPD patient believes he can choose to change, this, I believe is therapeutic, and often the first step toward real growth. I believe Masterson's model has helped a lot of BPD patients. On the other hand, since one of the characteristics of the BPD patient is identity confusion, surely the therapist would have fertile ground for socializing the patient into a BPD identity such as the one articulated by Masterson, creating a kind of self-fulfilling prophecy. Also, this model could not be proven. It was primarily based on an assumption that there were intra-psychic and inter-psychic dynamic processes taking place at some level whereby the behavior of the patient was being shaped to meet psychological needs, no matter how distorted or pathological those needs might appear to be.

The lack of proof had not been a problem to me before. Theories about therapy were like tinker toy sets. We constructed a different kind of set with different kinds of clients. A therapist could take his pick: psycho-education, Gestalt therapy, cognitive therapy, rational emotive therapy, breath work, or whatever "bias" the therapist had. But now my research was forcing me to confront and transcend my own biases. I was surprised to encounter new data about BPD. The information was a wake-up call for me. It is a wake-up call to all of us in the mental health profession.

I came upon an article by a Dr. D. Ebert and his colleagues while doing searches on N-acetyl aspartate (NAA) in the context of bipolar disorder. They found a 19% significant reduction of NAA concentrations in the dorsolateral (back and sides) prefrontal cortex in patients diagnosed as BPD. ($T = 2.554$; $P = 0.01$). This is the first ever study showing evidence of subtle prefrontal structural brain pathology in patients with BPD. The implications are clear. The data supports the hypothesis that disturbed frontal neurotransmission may contribute to the pathogenesis of this disorder.[1]

In other words, it appeared that borderline patients were self-destructive because their brains were broken. They had poor judgment and little control over their impulses not because of either their conscious or unconscious desire to regress in the service of their egos, but because something had gone badly wrong in the neurochemistry of their brains. NAA is a measure of the health of neurons. Low NAA means that either many neurons are functioning marginally or are dead. High NAA means they are functioning correctly and very much alive.

Subtle prefrontal structural brain pathology? Sure sounded physical to me. It was physical. It wasn't "mental" at all. How could I fit that into my seemingly elegant and logical psychodynamic perspectives? I could relate to behavior, thoughts, feelings, and fantasies of the mind. I couldn't relate to subtle prefrontal structural brain pathology. It looked like I might have to make some adjustments to my professional identity. I might have to move away from the "mental" in mental illness. But wait. Maybe as a mental health professional I could still find a way to get around this physical stuff. Yes, their dysfunctional thinking processes must affect their brains. Maybe I could attribute these findings to "stress," just like physicians have done with such disorders as chronic fatigue syndrome, the so-called "Yuppie" disease, and Gulf War Syndrome, a variant of combat fatigue. But then I ran into another problem. The above mentioned results, which were based on actual data rather than abstract theoretical concepts, were not found exclusively in BPD patients.

Gulf War veterans with Gulf War Syndrome also had disturbed frontal neurotransmission, resulting in reduced energy and diminished capacity to plan and organize their lives, as reflected in low NAA levels in parts of their brains. Fleckenstein compared the NAA levels in 25 veterans suffering symptoms of Gulf War Syndrome with the levels of 18 healthy veterans. Using a technique called magnetic resonance spectroscopy, he and his colleagues were able to detect in symptomatic Gulf War veterans a 10 to 25 percent reduction in the amount of NAA in the brain stem region. This suggested a loss of neurons in a critical area controlling movement, memory, and emotion. Many of the afflicted soldiers had worn flea collars that exposed them to small amounts of organophosphate chemicals, or insecticides.[2] Many had also been exposed to as many as 17 different vaccines, including polio, cholera, hepatitis B, influenza, anthrax, plague, rabies, tetanus, and yellow fever. They were also exposed to an experimental anti-nerve gas known as pyridostigmine bromide.[3] There was even the possibility that some were exposed to Saddam Hussein's chemicals and/or biological agents.

So what is the point of all this? "Physical" has a major impact on "mental." Such a concept would seem to be intuitive, were it not for my years of personal and professional socialization into belief systems based on "mind over matter." To successfully complete this odyssey, I might have to ignore my training in "mental" disorders.

Was it possible that exposure to organophosphates or vaccines had played a role in Chris's illness? One thing was clear: I needed to learn more about what role environmental factors played in these illnesses as well as the specific effects of different nutrients on the symptoms of CNS disorders.

Choline

Choline is a part of the B complex, though not formally a vitamin. It is found in liver, kidney, wheat germ, egg yolk, green leafy vegetables, fish, and peanuts. Supplements containing choline were proven to reduce rapid cycling in bipolar patients taking lithium.[4]

The article that was cited earlier by Dr. Terance Ketter and others at Stanford University had the somewhat intimidating title, "Decreased Dorsolateral Prefrontal N-acetyl Aspartate (NAA) in Bipolar Disorder." The authors found that the ratios of NAA, myoinositol (inositol), and choline to something called creatine-phosphocreatine were high in the back and sides of the prefrontal cortex in a control group and low in bipolar patients. The article also pointed out that there was decreased neuronal density or neuron functioning in bipolar patients.[5] If inositol and choline were low in bipolar patients, it seemed logical to me that providing these nutrients might restore the NAA levels to the same level as those not suffering from bipolar illness, as I had suggested to Dr. Ketter.

There was that NAA again, only now linked to low levels of choline and inositol in the brains of bipolar patients. Decreased NAA in the dorsolateral prefrontal cortex in bipolar patients? Sounded familiar. I had read the same thing about BPD and Gulf War Syndrome veterans. They had NAA deficits in parts of their brains, too. Chris's self-mutilating behavior was not unlike what one would see in a case of BPD. Had his frontal neurotransmission been compromised as well? Maybe if the brain received the proper nutrients, NAA levels might increase, and neurons might start functioning correctly. Maybe more NAA was the answer. Where could I get some?

Not knowing what NAA was, I went to Dogpile.com and asked it to fetch me some information on the subject. I learned that NAA is a brain metabolite present in neurons. That is where I learned that NAA levels decrease either when the neurons are functioning poorly or the number of them is low due to cell death. My plans for NAA supplements quickly evaporated. NAA was a by-product of healthy neuronal functioning, not a cause of it.

I looked at a bottle of the Synergy supplements and found that the initial bipolar dose for choline was 400 mg per day.

Inositol

Inositol is a carbohydrate that is found in beans, citrus fruits, nuts, veal, pork, and wheat germ. It is considered a second messenger precursor, a substance the body uses to create second messengers which, as stated earlier, play an important role in programming the responsiveness of neurons. Bipolar patients uptake (absorb) less inositol into their bodies than do non-bipolar individuals.[6] Inositol levels in the brain are lower in depressed patients. Supplemental inositol has proven as effective in treating symptoms of depression, obsessive compulsive disorder, and panic disorder as antidepressants — with no side effects.[7]

An article examined inositol levels in the post-mortem brains of three different groups, including ten suicide victims, eight bipolar patients, and ten normal controls. The inositol levels in the frontal cortex of the suicide victims and the patients with bipolar disorder were significantly less than those of the normal comparison group. No other differences were found in the cerebellum or occipital cortex. The researchers concluded that the results suggested a deficiency of inositol in those with bipolar disorder and in suicide victims.[8]

I looked at a bottle of the E.M. Power supplements from Truehope and found that for bipolar patients, the initial dose of inositol was 132 mg per day. Inositol, like choline, was a nutritional supplement with multiple indications across several DSM-IV diagnoses. To this backyard mechanic, it seemed elementary. These patients either needed more inositol in their system, or they needed a way to more effectively absorb and utilize what they already had. Maybe, to borrow an expression from Dr. Sherry Rogers, they did not have a lithium, Depakote, and Zyprexa deficiency after all.

Lithium

Lithium, considered the gold standard for managing and treating bipolar disorder, is effective in protecting brain cells and may in the future be used to protect against Alzheimer's and other degenerative brain diseases. Lithium even increases NAA levels.[9,10,11] I wondered why it was that if lithium was so effective in protecting brain cells, there was so much evidence that it impaired long-term memory, slowed mental processes, and reduced skill at psychomotor tasks.[12] If it were true that lithium did confer protection to brain cells, it appeared that this required a therapeutic dose, that is, enough lithium to require expert management in order to preclude the risk of lithium toxicity.

Based on my father's history, I knew the major side effects of lithium were hypothyroidism, which he had, weight gain, which he had, and kidney impairment, which he didn't have. During the writing of this book, my father was hospitalized three times for life-threatening esophageal bleeds. According to his doctor, these were secondary to pulmonary hypertension caused by cirrhosis of the liver. I couldn't prove that this condition had resulted from a lifetime of taking drugs to control his bipolar symptoms, but I knew he had never even touched alcohol and had never had hepatitis. I also knew that many of the drugs he took over his life impacted his liver. Therefore, I was not in favor of long-term therapeutic doses of any drug, let alone lithium. Because the drugs had not positively impacted my father's behavior and because of the long-term potential harm, I was more interested in lithium as a nutrient than as a pharmaceutical drug. I found evidence to support such an interest.

Remarkable research from the University of California at San Diego demonstrated an inverse relationship between psychiatric hospital admissions, incarcerations, and the naturally occurring levels of lithium in the drinking water! In other words, the higher the levels of lithium in the water, the lower the admission and incarceration rates. Researchers used data for 27 Texas counties from 1978 to 1987. They established that the rates of suicide, homicide, and rape were significantly higher in counties whose drinking water supplies contained little or no lithium than in counties with water lithium levels ranging from 70-170 micrograms per liter. The differences were statistically significant at the $p=.01$ level. Similarly, there was an association at less than $p=.05$ with the incidence rates of robbery, burglary, and theft. The abstract concludes with the following:

> *Lithium has moderating effects on suicidal and violent criminal behavior at levels that may be encountered in municipal water supplies. Lithium at low dosage levels has a generally beneficial effect on human behavior, which may be associated with the functions of lithium as a nutritionally essential trace element. Subject to confirmation by controlled experiments with high-risk populations, increasing the human lithium intakes by supplementation, or the lithium of drinking water is suggested as a possible means of crime, suicide, and drug-dependency reduction at the individual and community level.*[13]

If a person could obtain some benefit by taking trace amounts of lithium, maybe the larger doses wouldn't be needed after all. Trace amounts might be sufficient to minimize violence and other impulsive behaviors. Perhaps it would even preserve brain cells. Correlation does not necessarily prove causation, but how else could one interpret the data? I doubted that criminals preferred to live in areas where the lithium levels were low. I wondered how many prisons were giving their inmates trace amounts of lithium in their drinking water. When I talked to Tony about this, he said they had tried to include trace amounts in the Truehope supplements, but the FDA had not allowed it.

Magnesium

Before I decided to write this book, I had glanced over the article on lithium in drinking water in Texas and failed to keep the reference. After I decided to write it I tried to find the article again. It was like looking for a needle in a haystack. I tried Dogpile, Pub Med, and even Mama, the mother of all search engines. I tried a number of different Boolean queries such as "Lithium + drinking water + Texas" or "Lithium + psychiatric admissions + water + Texas." Finally, using Dogpile, I hit pay dirt, big time. I happened upon a site by Mr. George Eby entitled, "Rapid Recovery from Severe Depression." In the site was the link to the study in Texas cited above. However, the serendipitous discovery of Mr. Eby's site was like finding a gold mine with rich veins of ore glittering off the various mine shafts. Mr. Eby reported that he was bipolar and that he obtained relief from depression by first taking magnesium glycinate and lithium and, finally, magnesium glycinate alone. He cited evidence that lithium facilitates the utilization of magnesium that is already in the body and suggested that when lithium is not effective, it may be due to the fact that there are inadequate supplies of magnesium to be utilized. He provided exhaustive links: more than 200 on magnesium alone.[14] One of the sites contained an idea that sounded very practical to me, namely, putting hard water with magnesium into juvenile detention facilities to reduce violence. That particular site had an impressive total of 338 references pointing out the salutary effects of magnesium for alcoholism, aggression, arrhythmia, ADD, cerebral palsy, cerebrovascular conditions, diabetes, depression, and a host of other diagnoses.[15]

I looked at a bottle of the Truehope supplements and noted that the starting dose for magnesium amino acid chelate was 1000 mg a day. The word "chelate" simply means that the mineral is bound to an amino acid so that the body can absorb it more readily than would be the case with the pure mineral. All the mineral nutrients in the supplements are chelated. The chelated form of a nutrient is easier for the gut to digest, whereas non-chelated forms found in more inexpensive supplements are not absorbed as well in the body.

One of the links took me to a study in which the cerebrospinal fluid (CSF) of 275 drug-free, recently hospitalized, mostly female psychiatric patients was examined over 6 years. CSF levels of magnesium were found to be significantly lower in those who attempted suicide. Depressed patients who were non-suicidal had comparable magnesium levels to the controls. The study also found that low levels of cerebrospinal fluid 5-hydroxyindoleactic acid (5-HIAA), a serotonin metabolite, were associated with suicide attempts, especially violent ones.[16]

The sites of Mr. Eby and Mr. Mason together contained more than 500 links on the efficacy of magnesium for ameliorating violence, depression, and a host of other conditions. I was fascinated. Even more amazing was the home page of Mr. Eby, the person who developed the site. I was curious as to why the page on magnesium would be part of www.coldcure.com, so I went there only to discover that Mr. George Eby was the person who developed Cold-Eeze®, the closest thing to a cure for the common cold that I had ever experienced. His story was not unlike that of Tony Stephan and David Hardy.

Zinc and the common cold

George Eby, a graduate of the University of Texas with a Master of Science degree in mathematics, worked on the Apollo project for a period of time in Houston, then went back to school, obtaining a Master's Degree in City Planning from Texas A&M University. In 1979, in response to his 3-year-old daughter's leukemia, he came upon a discovery that has changed the way colds are treated. Mr. Eby owns the patent to the formula for the zinc gluconate lozenges.

His daughter, Karen, was suffering not only from leukemia but also the immunosuppressive effects of chemotherapy. Mr. Eby was not trained to treat his daughter. But, like Tony Stephan, he had no choice. He went to the library and extensively researched leukemia. He also researched colds, which had been occurring with more frequency because of his daughter's compromised immune status. Based on his research, Mr. Eby put Karen on supplements, including zinc gluconate pills for her colds, and, as it turns out for her leukemia, but that is another story. Here is the text from the site.

> *About four months after Karen's diagnosis of leukemia, she developed a particularly severe cold. Her throat was swollen and too painful for her to swallow a zinc gluconate (50 mg zinc) tablet. Eby asked Karen to chew the tablet instead. Karen was too exhausted to chew for long, and she soon went to sleep with most of the crushed tablet remaining in her mouth. Several hours later, Karen came into the living room playing with her toys, saying, "I'm all well, Mom!" Karen, still immunosuppressed from chemotherapy, was completely over her cold. Her cold did not return, even though no subsequent treatment was given. The effects of zinc glu-*

conate lozenges on Karen's colds were impossible for Eby to ignore.

The zinc did a lot more than shorten Karen's cold and reduce the severity of her symptoms. It also facilitated a massive proliferation of healthy young blood cells. And for the rest of us who take Cold-Eeze at the first sign of a cold, it reduced the time of the average cold from 11 to 7 days.[17] On this short side trip away from the path I had been on, I rediscovered another truism. Necessity is the mother of invention, especially for parents with nowhere else to turn.

PUFAs and MUFAs

What is a PUFA and a MUFA? The former is polyunsaturated fatty acids and the latter is monounsaturated fatty acids, or, to give an example of each, fish oil and canola oil. Two types of PUFA's include omega-6 fatty acids, made from seeds such as corn and peanut oil, and omega-3 fatty acids, found in cold water fish and flax seed oil. Humans cannot make either omega-6 or omega-3 fatty acids. Why devote a section to fats when they are not in the Synergy supplements? Because I was searching for any nutrients that could be helpful for Chris. In reviewing the substantial research on fats, I learned that increases in the intake of omega-6 relative to omega-3 PUFAs in our culture appears to have had an effect on the incidence and severity of cardiovascular disorders, inflammatory disorders, and depression.[18] I learned that depressed patients had lower levels of PUFAs, lower levels of zinc, higher levels of inflammation, and a compensatory increase in MUFAs.[19,20]

In one study, low levels of serotonin were found to correlate with more lethal suicide attempts[21] and another found a strong relationship between both low PUFAs, low serotonin levels, and impulsive violence, suicide, and depression. Higher PUFA's correlated with higher serotonin levels. The study found that patients taking cholesterol-lowering medications had a higher risk of suicide than those who did not! The medications were lowering their PUFAs.[22] While universal generalizations are risky, given the varieties in the human genome, it seemed to me that Chris would be better off with more omega-3 PUFAs, and less MUFAs and omega-6 PUFAs.

I reviewed Dr. Stoll's ground breaking work at Mclean Hospital, where he tested the ideas of Doctors Hibbeln, Smith, Maes, and others. In a pilot study involving 30 difficult-to-manage bipolar patients, the experimental group took 6,000 mg of fish oil daily, while the control group took a placebo. The patients receiving fish oil had a significantly longer period of remission than the placebo group. They also scored better on tests assessing depressive symptoms as well as other bipolar symptoms. The patients continued taking their bipolar medications during the trial.[23] A deficit of omega-3 fatty acids (PUFAs) contributed to depression and rapid cycling, while a restoration of levels reduced the number of subsequent episodes.

A long list of studies

I purchased a book entitled <u>Nutritional Influences on Mental Illness</u>, by Dr. Melvyn Werback of UCLA. This book contained hundreds of studies on the effects of nutrition on bipolar disorder and other mental disorders. It stopped me in my tracks. Here I had been researching one article after another trying to find out if there was a link between nutrition and mental illness. Werback not only established such a link but did so with numerous well-documented studies. I suspended my analysis of individual research articles on nutrition and relied upon his voluminous work. He had already completed the kind of research I was just starting.

There were 49 research studies supporting the effectiveness of various supplemental nutrients in treating bipolar illness. Some of these included inositol, choline, folic acid, vitamin B12, vitamin C, dietary lithium, magnesium, zinc, fatty acids, and l-phenylalanine.[24] I again checked the Synergy supplements. They contained all of the above, except for the omega-3 fatty acids and lithium. The list of supplements that might help Chris and the high-risk youth I was working with was growing. I wondered why the psychiatrists I worked with did not recommend any of these clinically proven nutrients to my clients or their parents. I assumed they either didn't know about them or they believed the claims to be false.

Food sensitivities

At the end of the chapter entitled "Bipolar Disorder," in Werbach's book, a subheading under a section entitled "Other Related Factors" caught my attention. It stated, "Rule out food sensitivities." The section described a woman with a 10-year history of bipolar illness. Lithium helped somewhat, but she still felt lethargic and depressed. A nutritional evaluation found deficiencies in zinc and magnesium, but supplementation didn't help. She started a diet restricted to fish, vegetables, rice, and meat. Her mood improved significantly, and she returned to work. However, after challenging herself by eating bread, she became depressed for six weeks and had to stop working again. That was when I learned there were tests for food antibodies Immunoglobulin G (IgG) and Immunoglobulin M (IgM) that could determine if patients were sensitive to certain foods. IgG and IgM molecules aid the body in getting rid of pathogens, or substances which the body perceives as foreign. Why was no one looking at these issues with not only Chris but the high-risk kids I was supposed to be helping? They probably had never heard that IgG food sensitivities were related to bipolar disorder or did not believe it.

Having found an abundance of research supporting the utility of specific nutrients for a wide range of symptoms, it was now time, since I had a ready source in my finger tips, to turn my attention to the major CNS disorders and see if specific nutritional regimens helped patients suffering from these disorders.

ADD/ADHD and nutrition

The ADD Nutrition Solution, by Marcia Zimmerman, recommended supplementation including the following: omega-3 fatty acids, omega-6 fatty acids, calcium amino acid chelate, magnesium amino acid chelate, zinc amino acid chelate, potassium amino acid chelate, copper amino acid chelate, manganese amino acid chelate, chromium amino acid chelate, folic acid, biotin, antioxidants, and a B complex consisting of vitamins B1, B2, B3, B5, B6, B12.[25] I examined a bottle of the Truehope supplements and found almost all the same ingredients, except for omega-3 fatty acids and omega-6 fatty acids. The amounts were different, and they weren't exactly the same formulation, but the core supplements were in both. I found additional research confirmed the usefulness of food-elimination diets for ADHD children.[26]

I found studies showing a correlation between zinc deficiency and ADHD and schizophrenia, not to mention growth-impairment, immunocompetence, anorexia, Alzheimer's, and a host of other conditions beyond the purview of this book.[27]

Returning to Nutritional Influences on Mental Illness, I looked up ADHD. I found another study reporting that 73% of an experimental group of children with ADHD responded favorably to a two week multiple-item elimination diet. Excluded foods were dairy, wheat, corn, yeast, soy, citrus, egg, chocolate, peanuts, and artificial colors or preservatives. I reviewed summaries of 37 articles, studies, and case reports on food sensitivities. Thirty-three of those articles supported the relationship between food sensitivities and the symptoms of ADHD. Four did not. I had recently attended an inservice training presentation at Nevada County Behavioral Health where a staff psychiatrist had said there was no evidence linking food sensitivities to ADHD. What was true? What I read, or what I was being told at the inservice meetings? Was ADHD a result of a Ritalin deficiency or could low zinc and low fatty acids play a role?

Studies in Werbach's book not only addressed the low fatty acid/zinc relationship but also substances that lower zinc levels. I had known for years that the Feingold diet included prohibitions against food colorings, among other things, but I didn't know why. Tartrazine (FD&C yellow #5) is a chelator of zinc. That means it binds with and lowers zinc levels in everyone, including ADHD children. Lower zinc levels prevent some children from being able to process what little fatty acids they have in their diet. The caffeine in soft drinks does the same. Incidentally, Werback also reported that phosphorus as found in colas (also processed and canned meats, and instant puddings) caused hospitalized hyper-aggressive children to become even more aggressive within hours of ingestion! I thought of the soft drink vending machines in the schools and wondered if the school boards who authorized their presence were aware of the price some of their vulnerable students paid for ready access to these products. I wondered why I was feeling so tired at work every day that I was purchasing one, sometimes two 12 ounce bottles of Diet Coke to get me through the day. If zinc-chelating beverages could deprive vulnerable students — and the rest of us — of already minimal amounts of zinc which are needed to utilize already minimal levels of fatty acids, and if these same beverages were facilitating aggression in vulnerable youth, why was no one talking about it? Probably because no one believed it or knew about it. I checked the Truehope supplements and found that the starting dose of zinc amino acid chelate was 80 mg a day.

Zinc and depression

Low zinc levels also correlate with what is called treatment resistant depression (TRD). Researcher Dr. M. Maes established that higher zinc levels help reduce inflammation associated with depression.[28] Understanding the relationship between zinc, helper T-cells, suppressor T-cells, and depression changed my understanding of that illness. Maes was not only saying that low zinc is associated with TRD, but also that the ratio of helper T-cells and suppressor T-cells is itself diagnostic of depression.

T-cells are a type of white blood cell called leukocytes derived from the thymus, a small gland in front of the heart. There are different kinds of T-cells, but I was only interested in two. T-cells that fight antigens, those "bad guys" like *Borrelia Burgdorferi*, are called helper T-cells. T-cells that suppress the manufacture of more helper cells are called suppressor T-cells. When the ratio between helper and suppressor is high (high helper, low suppressor), that means the body, or, to be more precise, the peptides, are saying, among other things, "Hey, we need a lot more helper cells over here. More bad guys than we thought." When the ratio of helper to suppressor cells is low (low helper T-cells, high suppressor T-cells), the peptides are saying, "OK, we can relax now. We got the bad guys on the run." Zinc levels were found to be low when the ratio was high, meaning the battle with the bad guys was still raging. To put it another way, a higher ratio of "alarm" cells to "all clear" cells is associated with depression and low zinc. Zinc appears to reduce the immune/inflammation response that contributes to depression.[29,30] So now I was looking beyond neurotransmitters to inflammation and low zinc levels as being a source, or at least a manifestation, of depression. This was a different way to think about depression. I wondered how it fit into the neurotransmitter model, otherwise known as the biogenic amine hypothesis of depression.

Autism and Schizophrenia

If I could find studies showing that diet and nutrition helped patients suffering from severe debilitating illnesses such as schizophrenia and autism, I would have even more confidence that the path we had chosen was a correct one. This was a significant challenge. I knew that some antipsychotic medications targeted excessive dopamine implicated in the dopamine theory of schizophrenia, an old theory which explained some aspects of schizophrenia. I didn't know that gluten contains a neuropeptide that enhanced the very dopamine activity that antipsychotic medications reduce.[31] Gluten is found in wheat, rye, oats, and barley. Would a diet free of these grains preclude the need for anti-widget pills to bind with the dopamine receptors?

To provide some background for the ensuing discussion, it is necessary to define ligands, peptides, and one form of peptides, endorphins. Ligands are molecules such as dopamine or GABA, the "widgets" described in Chapter 15 that bind to receptors. To use a crude analogy, they are the keys specially made to fit in or bind with specially made locks, or receptors. Five percent of the ligands in the body are either steroids or neurotransmitters while the other 95% are peptides. Peptides are strings of amino acids made by the body. Less than 100 chains is a peptide, between 100 and 200 is a polypeptide, and more than 200 is a protein. Peptides bind to receptors to initiate actions in cells, much like a person pressing a button to initiate an action of some kind. In Scotland, a type of peptide was discovered that would bind to opiate receptors. They were called enkephalins. Later, the name was changed to endorpins. Endorphins became popularized when it became known that they produce the runner's high that transforms pain into feelings of well-being. The internally produced endorpins bind with opiate receptors throughout the brain and body. The same receptors, the opiate receptors, can also bind with external opiates such as heroin or morphine. Peptides play a major role in communicating across the endocrine, neurological, gastrointestinal, and the immune system. The very same receptors that exist in the brain can be found on monocytes, immature macrophages. In addition — and this is a revolutionary thought — most of the neuron communication in the brain does not occur at the synapse, but by receptors binding with the particular form-fitted ligands that only they can bind with. As research professor Dr.

Pert Candace in <u>Molecules of Emotions</u> points out, the conventional view of synaptic neuronal circuits is replaced by a much broader confluence of information substances. "The brain is like a bag of hormones." [32] The work described below is consistent with these newer understandings.

There was an orthomolecular psychiatry Web site, edited by Greg Schilhab, that summarized some very interesting research begun by Dr. Robert Cade as early as 1972 at the University of Florida. For example, Schilhab explained that in some patients, cereal proteins are only partly digested, resulting in gluten fragments entering circulation. These fragments happen to be shaped very similarly to endorphins. Because of this similarity, these ligand-like fragments bind to the brain's endorphin receptors just like morphine and heroin, producing similar results. The phenomena is called molecular mimicry. These ligands are agonists in that they bind and produce an effect. Casein proteins in dairy products also have amino acid sequences similar to endorphins that are also capable of binding with these brain receptors. These substances from gluten and casein are called "exorphins" (exogenous endorphins) to describe their pharmacological effects. [33] They are opioids. Their effects are similar to opiates, and they are produced by the incomplete digestion of casein and gluten.

I wondered if this could have something to do with the drugs Chris manufactured in his own body that had such a profound effect that he had "cheeked" the medicines during his first hospitalization in order to maintain the "high."

Next I focused in on two viewpoints regarding autism. One view, proposed by Dr. Hugh Fudenberg, an immunologist, is that vaccinations such as the combined diphtheria, pertussis and tetanus (DPT) decrease the production of liver enzymes, causing undigested protein to circulate in the blood. The body creates antibodies against these proteins (antigens). The resulting antigen-antibody pairs inflict damage such as arthritis, muscle pain, and brain dysfunction. [34] Could that same process have affected Chris? Some of his symptoms mimicked autism, not the least of which were rocking, social unresponsiveness, and being impervious to pain or the threat of pain. This was another path I would have to explore, especially since I was to learn in the near future that Chris's DPT anti-toxoid levels were, according to the New Century Wellness Center, ten times normal!

A similar but different view was proposed by Dr. Robert Cade, who was not only a professor of medicine and physiology at the College of Medicine at the University of Florida, but who also happened to be the inventor of Gatorade. But first some background.

The frequency of schizophrenia is related to wheat consumption. For example, during World War II, when wheat and rye availability dropped, the incidence of new schizophrenic admissions in Finland and Sweden plummeted. In Canada and the United States, where there was no shortage, the number of new admissions increased.[35] The incidence of schizophrenia in Micronesia and New Guinea had been historically very rare, about 2 per 65,000. However, the introduction of cereal grains to the diets there increased the incidence to European levels, about 130 per 65,000. Dohan noted that the coastal communities where wheat was eaten experienced an increase in schizophrenia while the mountain people who subsisted on the taro root did not experience any increase.[36]

To establish if there was more than just a correlation between gluten and the symptoms of schizophrenia, Singh and Kay conducted a 12-week experiment with 14 schizophrenic patients. Their diets were changed from gluten and casein-free, to gluten, then back to the gluten-free diet. Most of the psychopathology measures deteriorated significantly when the gluten was added back to their diets and improved when it was removed. In another study with 102 newly admitted schizophrenic patients, Dohan found that a diet low in gluten and casein reduced hospitalization time compared to a group that ate high amounts of gluten.[37] I wondered how many mental hospitals were putting patients with schizophrenia on casein-and gluten-free diets. Those in charge probably didn't know about it, or, if they did, didn't think the conclusions were true.

My attention was drawn to Dr. Cade when I read a news release from the university about his work. He reported that 95 % of 81 children with autism or schizophrenia had 100 times the normal levels of a milk protein in their blood and urine. His studies were presented at two international meetings in 1999.[38] Milk protein produces morphine-like exorphins that are taken up by areas of the brain where there is clear evidence of cellular malfunctioning. Dr. Cade believes a malfunctioning enzyme in the intestine, one that can't break down the casein in milk, is responsible. According to Dr. Cade, eight of ten of the schizophrenic and autistic children no longer had symptoms of autism or schizophrenia after being put on both a casein and gluten-free diet!

He injected rats with one of the suspect proteins, beta-casomorphin-7, one of the key proteins in milk that coagulate to make cheese. Not only was the protein taken up at 32 different sites in the rat brains, but it also caused some interesting behavioral changes in the rats. Dr. Cade explained what happened in a letter on the Internet:

> *There are a whole number of behaviors that the rat has after beta-casomorphin-7 that are basically the same as one sees in the human with autism or schizophrenia. If we ring a bell beside a rat's cage, it normally looks up to see where the noise is coming from. But the rats after beta-casomorphin-7*

didn't do that — they were completely oblivious to the bell ringing above them. This struck us as interesting because many mothers of autistic children comment that they seem at times to be totally deaf — they talk to their children and they just don't seem to hear them.

He then explained what this data meant:

We now have proof positive that these proteins are getting into the blood and proof positive they're getting into areas of the brain involved with the symptoms of autism and schizophrenia.

We think this process is linked to the production of antibodies in the gut when you eat something you're sensitive to. Both schizophrenics and autistics have a high incidence of [certain] antibodies, and a high incidence of diarrhea, which points to an intestinal disorder. So we think that with autism and schizophrenia, the basic disorder is in the intestine, and these individuals are absorbing beta-casomorphin-7 that they normally should break down in the body as amino acids, rather than peptide chains up to 12 amino acids long.

In other words, these foreign proteins from milk and gluten provoke antibody production in much the same way that microbes provoke antibody production for the defense of the organism.

The letter by Dr. Cade that was displayed on the Internet reported the most current results of his work on diet and schizophrenia and autism. In this letter, he writes about hyperpolypeptiduria. This term refers to a condition in which there are an excessive number of large peptides, or protein fragments, in the blood and urine.

Our studies, which are still in progress, have shown:

I. There is a relationship between diet, hyperpolypeptiduria and schizophrenia and childhood autism.

(a) 95% of patients with schizophrenia or childhood autism have a significant hyperpolypeptiduria.

(b) All of these patients had a greatly increased amount of peptides that have a morphine-like activity and are derived from either casein (milk) or gliadin (wheat).

II. The degree of the polypeptiduria can be decreased by either dialysis, diet, or the two in combination.

(a) As the polypeptiduria decreases, the symptoms of schizophrenia or autism decrease.

(b) If the polypeptiduria can be reduced to normal range, most patients either improve dramatically or become completely normal. A very rigid adherence to a gluten/casein-free diet is required to accomplish this.

(c) When the urine peptides are fractionated, b-casomorphine-7 was found in large amounts in all of the autistic and schizophrenic patients. It was found in small amounts in about half of our normal subjects.

(d) Gliadorphin-7 was found in very large amounts in 84% of schizophrenics and 65% of autistic patients, while it was found in 32% of normals in very small amounts.

III. Both schizophrenic and autistic patients had immunoglobulin abnormalities.

(a) Among autistic children, 30% had high titer IgA antibodies to both gluten and casein. Among schizophrenics, 86% had high titer IgA antibodies to gluten and 67% to casein. In normal individuals less than 10% have IgA antibodies to gluten and casein and these are all low titer.

(b) Among autistic children, 87% had high titer IgG antibodies to gluten and 90% to casein, while among schizophrenic patients 86% had high titer IgG antibodies to gluten and 93% to casein.

(c) The presence of IgG antibodies means that gluten and casein with their morphine-like components get into blood (where they should not be) in large amounts. The presence of IgA antibodies means the intestinal mucosa is sensitive to gluten or casein. This mucosa is the site of the defect. The markedly different incidence of IgA antibodies, comparing autism to schizophrenia, means there are probably two different intestinal abnormalities that allow gluten and casein to enter the blood.[39, 40]

Dr. Cade was making a revolutionary statement. **Autism and schizophrenia, far from being mental disorders, were, in fact, intestinal disorders!** Many patients with schizophrenia and autism suffer from the absorption of exorphins formed in the intestine from the incomplete digestion of gluten and casein.

In private correspondence, Dr. Cade informed me that he found the evidence supporting Dr. Fudenberg's view of a significant role for diminished levels of liver enzymes phosphosulfotransferase and p-450 cytochrome in autism to be weak. Even though Doctors Cade and Fudenberg do not agree on the reason for the digestive problems, they both agree that undigested proteins and antigen-antibody pairs were one of the factors in autism and schizophrenia. Chris didn't have these illnesses. He had bipolar disorder. But maybe the clear differentiation I had in my mind between schizophrenia, autism, and bipolar disorder was not really so clear cut on a biological level. Chris's rocking, his parent deafness, his inability to respond to others appropriately were consistent with behavior I had seen in autistic patients. Once again, how was I to know what was true? I would not connect Dr. Cade's research to bipolar disorder for months.

I read a summary of six prospective double-blind studies in the treatment of schizophrenia. The studies were conducted from observations of 4,000 patients. The regimen consisted of diet, nutritional supplements, and, as needed, psychotropic medications. The diet eliminated processed or prepared foods containing refined sugar and food additives. The patients also underwent elimination diets that removed all food to which the patients were determined to be sensitive. They obtained supplements of B3, B6, and general vitamin formula with additional vitamin C, zinc, and manganese. Acute patients were defined as those suffering their first episode or their second and third episodes with periods of remission between episodes. In a 2-year period, greater than 90% of these patients were symptom-free. Some needed medication occasionally. For chronic patients, about 50% of patients recovered in a ten-year time frame.[40]

My first sojourn into the world of nutrition and mental health had revealed some amazing data. There are measurable physical abnormalities suggesting neuronal death or impairment in the brains of borderline as well as bipolar patients. Organophosphates may be part of the "Gulf War Syndrome," a syndrome not unlike bipolar illness in diminishing the executive planning function of the brain. Food sensitivities can provoke depression. Gluten and casein can provoke symptoms of schizophrenia and autism. Antigen-antibody pairs can promote brain dysfunction. Dietary restrictions and nutritional supplementation restore "mental" health to bipolar patients as well as those suffering from other CNS disorders, including ADHD, schizophrenia, and autism.

This was compelling information. I was learning about a nutritional technology potentially every bit as revolutionary and disruptive to current practices as the impact of computers had been to the typewriter industry. The only difference was that for some reason, this particular technology had yet to hit mainstream America, let alone Nevada County Behavioral Health Services.

Too Good To Be True?

When I taught sociology at the junior college level, one subject I particularly enjoyed teaching was social systems. All social systems, whether a family, school, or even something as large as the justice system, have elements, or, components, in common. The term "component" to describe these elements is impersonal by design, since the student of social systems wants a scientific, objective perspective. Every system has power components, the "bigwigs" who call the shots. There are gate keepers who permit the entrance of "pro" system components, whether ideas, resources, or people, while making sure that "contra" components are expelled or neutralized. In every system, there are system norms, those formal and informal rules that determine how participants are supposed to act in that social system and with components from other social systems. This orientation helped students to understand how social systems operated and to see commonalities shared by even the most diverse of social systems.

Students often had difficulty understanding the concept that power, not usefulness, determines whether or not a change is accepted into a social system. Many students had a difficult time understanding that "he who has the gold makes the rules," that "truth" is what the system power components determine it to be. History abounds with examples. How many years did it take for physicians to believe that hand-washing prevented infections? Suppose that power components in the mental health care system either say that nutrients have no effect on mental illness or go about their work totally unaware of the extensive body of research that exists. In that social system, nutrients will simply have no effect, and any literature stating that they do will be deemed not to exist, regardless of the facts.

I knew that what I had found was true. The information I had found on the effectiveness of interventions based on diet and nutrition was from reliable sources. However, the sociology instructor inside me was not so sure. Social systems such as professional licensing boards, the Joint Commission on Accreditation of Healthcare Organizations, and even the Behavioral Health Services of Nevada County are themselves products of social systems that have no investment in dietary and/or nutritional solutions. These systems decide what is true based not on the facts, but on their own self-interest. There is nothing necessarily personal about it. It's just how systems work — or don't work. If utility were that important, every psychiatric hospital in the county would be giving their depressed patients omega-3 fatty acids and keeping their schizophrenic patients from eating gluten and casein. If utility mattered, the Joint Commission on the Accreditation of Healthcare Organizations would only accredit psychiatric hospitals where schizophrenic patients had a gluten- and casein-free diet. If power mattered, psychotropic drugs would be the primary intervention.

This information was revolutionary and did not fit into existing paradigms of care. It suggested that the current practice of prescribing drugs first

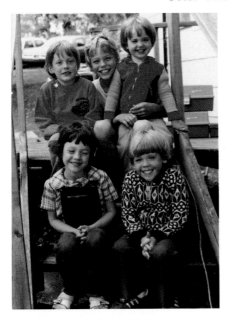

Chris, (bottom right) Kathy, (top
right) and cousins
Washington 1979

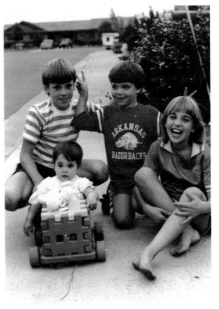

Chris (top left) and Siblings
Atwater, California, 1987

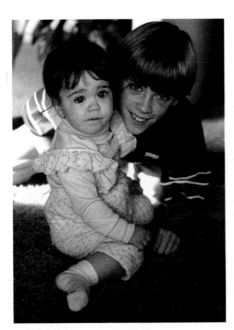

Chris and Elizabeth, 1987

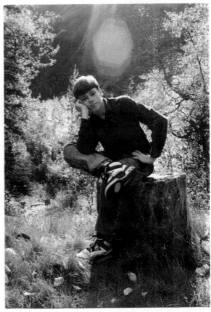

Chris in Alaska, 1991

Fragility of Nature
A Symbolic Representation of the Hemispheres of the Brain

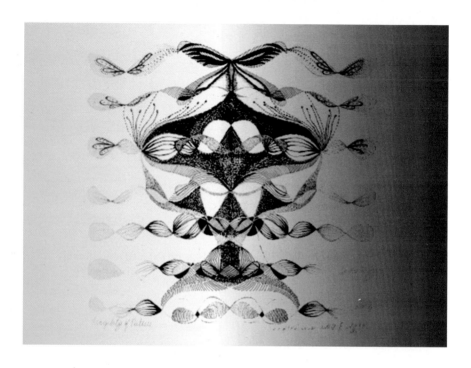

By Judith R. Shamp

The color scheme for this drawing and the cover is based on paintings from the Munch Museet in Oslo, Norway. Munch, who is known for his painting "The Scream," showing a ghostly figure on a bridge, used colors like these in some of his more autobiographical works on display at that museum. The colors represent his energetic, angry, passionate side as well as his helpless, fearful, depressed side. Munch, whose early life included significant family deaths, was hospitalized several times in his life for depression and alcohol abuse.

Brain SPECT

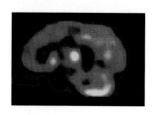

The brain to the left is normal; the one to the right shows multiple perfusion defects in temporal lobe caused by Lyme Disease. (Courtesy Dr. Puneet K. Pakeet Chandak, Harvard University)

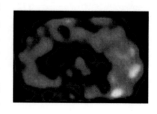

July 31, 2002 SPECT

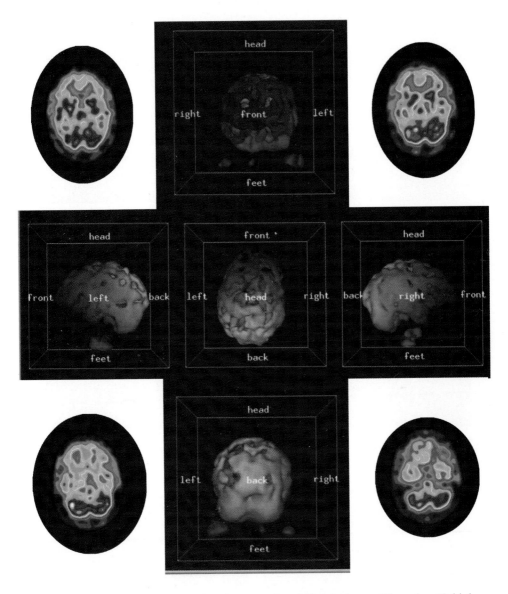

The above SPECT was taken after three months of Chris being on Clozapine, Haldol, Depakote, and Cogentin. He took no Truehope or other supplements. The hypoperfusion, according to the radiologist, is consistent with "Lyme disease, psychiatric illness, or psychotropic medications." A brain that was functioning properly would appear smooth, without the gaps caused by inadequate uptake of the radioisotope. The top of the cross sectional slices is the frontal cortex.

Bad Blood?

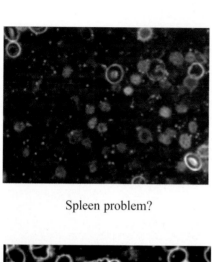

Spleen problem?

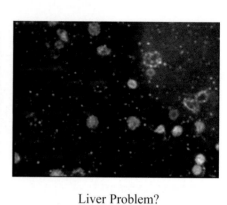

Liver Problem?

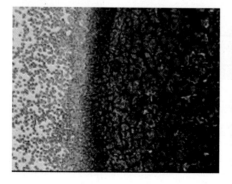

Misshapen cells?

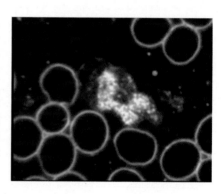

Parasitized Leukocyte?

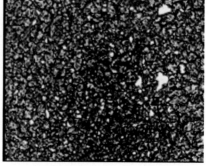

Heavy Metals?

Free Radical Damage?

before understanding biological causes and before attempting, among other things, nutritional solutions, was wrong. The information reported in this chapter supports the central tenet of this book: Nutrients quiet the unquiet brain. Such an idea would be a "contra" to the systems mentioned above.

Maybe these systems are like the bipolar patient after all. Whatever the "system" believe is true, is true. But there is hope. Patients and their families are also part of the system, and their voices have yet to be heard on this matter.

It is all a question of epistomology. How do we know what is true?

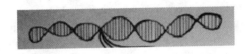

Notes

1. Ebert, D., Van Elst, L.T., Thiel, T., Hesslinger, B., Lieb, K., Bohus, M., Hennig, J., "Subtle prefrontal neuropathology in a pilot magnetic resonance spectroscopy study in patients with borderline personality disorder," *Journal of Neuropsychiatry and Clinical Neurosciences*, 13(4):511-514, 2001.

2. Susman, Ed, "Gulf War Vets Show Brain Problems," United Press International, December 1, 1999.

3. Urnovitz, H.B., Tuite, J.J., Higashida, J.M., Murphy, W.H. "RNAs in the serum of Persian Gulf war veterans have segments homologous to chromosome 22q11.2," *Clinical Diagnostic and Laboratory Immunology*, 6(3):330, 1999.

4. Dr. Andrew Stoll from Harvard University examined choline augmentation of lithium for rapid-cycling bipolar patients. Five of six who were given choline augmentation experienced a substantial reduction in manic symptoms, and four patients had a marked reduction in all mood symptoms during choline therapy. The patients who responded to choline all exhibited a substantial rise in the basal ganglia concentration of choline-containing compounds. Dr. Stoll hypothesized that the action of choline on second messenger systems helped stabilize these patients. The choline was safe to use. Stoll, A.L., Sachs, G.S., Cohen, B.M., Lafer, B., Christensen, J.D., Renshaw, P.F., "Choline in the treatment of rapid-cycling bipolar disorder: clinical and neurochemical findings in lithium-treated patients," *Biol Psychiatry*, 40(5):382-8, September 1, 1996.

5. Winsberg, M.E., Sachs, N., Tate, D.L., Adalsteinsson, E., Spielman D.M., Ketter, T. A., "Deceased dorsolateral prefrontal N-acetyl aspartate in bipolar disorder," *Biol Psychiatry*, 47(6):475-81, March 15, 2000.

6. Banks, R.E., Aitoooon, J.F., Cramb, G., Neylor, G.J., "Incorporation of inositol into the phosphoinositides of lymphoblastoid cell lines establshed from bipolar manic-depressive patients," *Journal of Affective Disorders*, 19(1):1-8, May 1990.

7. Dr. J. Levine, of the Ministry of Health Mental Health Center at Ben Gurion University of the Negev in Beersheva, Israel, reported that inositol in cerebrospinal fluid is lower in depressed patients than a control group. A double-blind controlled trial of 12 grams of inositol daily in 29 depressed patients for four weeks demonstrated sig-

nificant overall benefit compared to placebo on the Hamilton Depression Scale, a scale commonly used to assess the extent to which subjects are depressed. There were no changes noted in hematology, kidney, or liver function. Another study was done with panic disorder with or without agoraphobia, a fear of being outside. The frequency and severity of panic attacks and agoraphobia declined significantly with the inositol compared to placebo. There were minimal side effects. In yet another study, 13 patients with Obsessive Compulsive Disorder (OCD) took 18 grams of inositol while another group took a placebo. The experimental group had significantly reduced obsessive compulsive behavior compared with placebo. These results suggest that inositol has therapeutic effects in the spectrum of illnesses that respond to serotonin selective re-uptake inhibitors, including depression, panic, and OCD. It was not beneficial in schizophrenia, Alzheimer's, ADHD, or autism.

Levine, J., "Controlled trials of inositol in psychiatry," Ministry of Health Mental Health Center, Faculty of Health Sciences, Ben Gurion University of the Negev, Beersheva, Israel, *Eur Neuropsychopharmacol,* 7(2):147-55, May 1997.

8. Shimon H., Agam, G., Belmaker, R.H., Hyde, T.M., Kleinman, J.E., "Reduced frontal cortex inositol levels in post-mortem brain of suicide victims and patients with bipolar disorder," *Am J Psychiatry,* 154(8):1148-50, August 1997.

9. According to the authors, "The study demonstrates for the first time that lithium administration at therapeutic doses increases brain NAA concentration."

Moore, G.J., Bebchuk, J.M., Hasanat, K., Chen, G., Seraji-Bozorgzad, N, Wilds, I.B., Falk, M.W., Koch, S., Glita, D.A., Jolkovsky, L., Manji, H.K., "Lithium increases N-acetyl-aspartate in the human brain: in vivo evidence in support of Bcl-2 neurotropic effects?" *Biological Psychiatry*, 48(1)1-8, July 1, 2000.

10. Another paper demonstrated not only that lithium increased Bcl-2, a known major neuroprotective protein, but also inhibited an enzyme called glycogen synthase kinase 3 beta. This enzyme is known to regulate two substances that play a role in the neurodegeneration found in Alzheimer's disease.

Manji, H.K., Moore, G.J., Chen, G., "Lithium up-regulates the cytoprotective protein Bcl-2 in the CNS in vivo: a role for neurotrophic and neuroprotective effects in manic depressive illness," *Journal of Clinical Psychiatry,* 61 Suppl 9:82-96, 2000.

11. Another study demonstrating the neuroprotective effects of lithium was done at the National Institute of Mental Health. Exposure of selected rat brain cells to glutamate caused rapid increase in two proteins that are known to be proapoptotic, or that facilitate cell death. Long-term treatment with lithium lowered these two proteins while increasing Bcl-2. Once again, the bottom line was that lithium protected brain cells against the effects of excitotoxicity. These authors suggest a possible expanded use of lithium for other degenerative diseases that affect the brain.

Chen, R.W., Chuang, D.M., "Long term lithium treatment suppresses p53 and Bax expression but increases Bcl-2 expression," *Journal of Biological Chemistry*, 274(10):6039-42, March 5, 1999.

12. Goodwin, F.K., Jamison, K.R., Manic Depressive Illness, Oxford University Press, New York, 1990, 707.

13. Schrauzer G.N., Shrestha K.P., "Lithium in drinking water and the incidences of crimes, suicides, and arrests related to drug addictions," *Biol Trace Elem Res,* 25(2):105-13, May 1990.

14. Eby, George, "Rapid Recovery from Severe Depression using Magnesium," 2000.

http://www.coldcure.com/html/dep.html

15. Mason, Paul, "Violence Prevention through Magnesium-Rich Water," 2001. http://www.execpc.com/~cc/prevent.html

16. Banki, C.M., Arato, M., Kilts, C.D., "Aminergic studies and cerebrospinal fluid cations in suicide," *Ann NY Acad Sci,* 487:221-30, 1986.

17. Eby, George, "You mean zinc acetate lozenges can cure my stupid cold?" 2001. http://www.coldcure.com

18. Dr. Ron Smith found a correlation between the increased omega-6/polyunsaturated fatty acid (PUFA) ratio in the Western diet and increased incidence of cardiovascular disorders, inflammatory disorders, and depression. Over time as a culture we have replaced fatty acids from fish, wild game, and plants with omega-6 fatty acids from seeds. I learned from a number of sources that the typical omega-6/omega-3 ration is 20 to one. It should be about one to one.
Smith, Ronald M., "The Macrophage Theory of Depression," *Med-Hypotheses,* 35(4):298-306, August 1991.

19. "The increased incidence rate of major depression since 1913 may be explained by a sharp increase in the rate of omega-6 PUFAs in the diet," wrote Maes and Smith. Maes, M, Smith, R.S., "Fatty acids, cytokines and major depression," *Biol Psychiatry,* 43(5):313-314, 1998.

20. Maes studied PUFAs and MUFAs in 34 inpatients with major depression and 14 normal volunteers. He found that in major depression there is a deficiency of omega-3 PUFAs and a compensatory increase in MUFAs. The results suggest that there is an abnormal metabolism of omega-3 PUFAs in depression and that fatty acid alterations in depression are related to the inflammatory response in that illness, which may persist despite successful antidepressant treatment.
Maes, M., Christophe, A., Delanghe, J., Altamura, C., Neels, H., Meltzer, H., "Lowered omega-3 polyunsaturated fatty acids in serum phospholipids and cholesterol esters of depressed patients," *Psychiatry Res,* 85(3):275-91, March 22, 1999.

21. There is a strong relationship between low serotonergic activity as evidenced by low 5-HIAA, the serotonin metabolite, and a predisposition to more lethal suicide attempts in major depression.
Mann J.J., Malone, K.M., "Cerebrospinal fluid amines and higher-lethality suicide attempts in depressed inpatients," *Biol Psychiatry,* 41(2):162-71, January 15, 1997.

22. This article described how impulsive violence, suicide, and depression are strongly associated with low concentrations of cerebrospinal fluid 5-HIAA and PUFAs. Low levels of 5-HIAA, the serotonin metabolite, are associated with low levels of serotonin. The levels of 5-HIAA and PUFA both correlated with each other. In other words, higher serotonin is associated with higher PUFAs, and lower serotonin is associated with lower PUFAs. The authors point out that increased suicide and trauma had been reported among individuals involved in some cholesterol-lowering trials. They believe this finding may be related to altered concentrations of PUFAs from patients taking cholesterol-lowering drugs. A group of alcoholics was significantly lower in PUFAs than a control group. The author concludes, "Dietary studies are indicated to determine if essential fatty acid supplementation can influence central nervous system serotonin and dopamine metabolism and modify impulsive behaviors related to these neurotransmitters."
Hibbeln, J.R., Linnoila, M., Umhau, J.C., Rawlings, R., George, D.T., Salem, N.,

"Essential fatty acids predict metabolites of serotonin and dopamine in cerebrospinal fluid among healthy control subjects, and early- and late-onset alcoholics," *Biol Psychiatry*, 44(4):235-42, August 15, 1998.

23. Stoll, A.L., Severus, W.E., Freeman, M.P., Rueter, S., Zboyan, H.A., Diamond, E., Cress, K.K., "Omega-3 fatty acids in bipolar disorder: a preliminary double-blind, placebo-controlled trial," *Arch Gen Psychiatry*, 56(5):407-12, May 1999.

24. Werback, Melvyn R., <u>Nutritional Influences on Mental Illness</u>, Third Line Press, Tarzana, California, 1999, 124-142.

25. Zimmerman, Marcia, C.N., <u>The ADD Nutrition Solution</u>, Henry Holt and Company, LLC, New York, N.Y., 1999, 136-165.

26. Laura Stevens, M.S., reports on the common food elimination diet where the foods most commonly suspected in causing brain dysfunction were removed from the diet. According to Stevens, 59 of 78 (76%) hyperactive children improved after eliminating milk, cheese, wheat, corn, chocolate, eggs, and orange juice from their diets. Nineteen of the children were then involved in a placebo-controlled double-blind challenge of the suspected foods. These foods caused significantly more changes in behavior than food given as placebo. A double-blind experiment is one in which an experimental group gets a novel treatment and a control group doesn't, but neither the patients nor the treating doctors know who is getting what. The patients and doctors are effectively "blind" about who does or does not get the novel treatment. Stevens, Laura J., M.S., <u>12 Effective Ways to Help Your ADD/ADHD Child,</u> Avery, a member of Penguin Putnam, New York, 2000, 71-79, 228-229.

27. The purpose of the Zinc-ADHD study was to evaluate the relationships between serum free fatty acids (FFA) and zinc in 33 boys and 15 girls with ADHD and 33 boys and 15 girls with no ADHD. The average serum FFA level in the ADHD group was 0.176 mEq/L and in the control group, 0.562 mEq/L ($p < .001$). The average serum zinc level of the ADHD group was 60.6 micrograms/dl and that of the control group 105.8 micrograms/dl ($p < .001$). A statistically significant correlation was found between zinc and FFA levels in the ADHD group. Both were low. These findings indicate that zinc deficiency may play a role in the etiology of ADHD. Bekaro¨glu, M., Aslan, Y., Gedik, Y., De¨ger, O., Mocan, H., Erduran, E., Karahan, C., "Relationships between serum free fatty acids and zinc, and attention deficit hyperactivity disorder: a research note," *J Child Psychol Psychiatry*, 37(2):225-7, February 1996.

28. Dr. Maes, in an article on zinc and TRD, found that the less zinc, the higher level of treatment resistance to antidepressants and vice versa. Antidepressant treatment had no effect on serum zinc, whereas serum copper was significantly reduced. Maes, M., Vandoolaeghe, E., Neels, H., Demedts, P., Wauters, A., Meltzer, H.Y., Altamura, C., Desnyder, R., "Lower serum zinc in major depression is a sensitive marker of treatment resistance and of the immune/inflammatory response in that illness," *Biol Psychiatry*, 42(5):349-58, September 1, 1997.

29. In another article Dr. Maes states the following:

> There were highly significant correlations between serum zinc and the CD4+/CD8+ T-cell ratio (negative), and total serum protein, serum albumin, and transferrin (all positive). The results suggest that lower serum zinc is a marker of TRD and of the immune/

inflammatory response in depression. It is suggested that treatment resistance may bear a relationship with the immune/inflammatory alterations in major depression.

"CD" refers to clusters of differentiation. The different numbers distinguish different specialized kinds of T-cells.

Maes, M., Vandoolaeghe, E., Ranjan, R., Bosmans, E., Van Gastel, A., Bergmans, R., Desnyder, R., "Increased serum soluble CD8 or suppressor/cytotoxic antigen concentrations in depression: suppressive effects of glucocorticoids," *Biol Psychiatry,* 40(12):1273-81, December 15, 1996.

30. The relationship between CD4+, helper T-cells, and CD8+, suppressor T-Cells, has been shown to predict depression. Maes and others detected a significantly increased CD4+/CD8+ ratio in depressed patients as compared with healthy controls. Higher ratios predict depression with 68% accuracy. Also, low zinc is correlated with a higher number of helper cells, which neutralize antigens, and a lower level of suppressor cells, which tell the body to stop producing so many helpers.

Maes, M., Stevens, W., DeClerck, L., Bridts, C., Peeters, D., Schotte, C., Cosyns, P., "Immune disorders in depression: higher T helper/T suppressor-cytotoxic cell ratio," *Acta Psychiatr Scand,* 86(6):423-31, December 1992.

31. Mycroft, F.J., et al., "MIF-like sequences in milk and wheat proteins," *N Engl J Med,* 307(14):895, September 30, 1982.

32. Pert, Candace, <u>Molecules of Emotion, The Science Behind Mind-Body Medicine</u>, New York, Touchstone, 1999, 24-25.

33. Klee, W., Zioudrou, C., et al., "Exorphins: peptides with opioid activity isolated from wheat gluten, and their possible role in the etiology of schizophrenia," in Uspin, E, Bunney, W.E., Kline, N., (eds.), <u>Endorphins in Mental Health Research,</u> 1977, 209-218.

http://www.orthomed.org/csf/NMH1.96.htm

34. In autism, the mechanism by which the body fails to properly break down certain proteins is hypothesized by Dr. Fudenberg to be a decrease in production of liver enzymes such as phosphosulfotransferase and the cytochrome p450 family. This would not only impair digestion, but also the ability to detoxify the body. DPT immunization in mice results in a decrease of synthesis of both phosphosulfotransferase and cytochrome p450. Intact proteins cross into circulation, and antibodies are formed against them. Antigen-antibody complexes can then enter various organs where the receptors for those antigen-antibody complexes exist. Binding of these antigen-antibody complexes with receptors on the cells causes such symptoms as arthritis in the joints, pain in the muscles and inflammation and cognitive dysfunction in the brain. If Dr. Fudenberg's theory is correct, then I would expect that Chris's high DPT antitoxoid levels, ten times normal according to New Century (Chapter 18), would correlate with low levels of phosphosulfotransferase and p-450 enzymes. In either event, both points of view could justify a Radio Allergo Sorbent Test and a check for hyperpolypeptiduria to help determine if casein and gluten should be removed from the diet.

Fudenberg, H. Hugh, "Typical course of an autistic patient," NeuroImmuno Therapeutic Research Foundation Web site, 2001.

http://www.nitrf.org/autistic.html

35. Dohan, F.C., et al., "Is schizophrenia rare if grain is rare?" *Biological Psychiatry*, 19:385-399, 1984.

36. Dohan, F.C., "Schizophrenia: possible relationship to cereal grains and celiac disease," in Sankarsiva, D. V., (ed.), <u>Schizophrenia: Current Concepts and Research</u>, New York, PDJ Publications, 1969. 539-551.

37. Singh, M.M., Kay, S.R., "Wheat gluten as a pathogenic factor in schizophrenia," *Science*, 191: 401-402, 1976.

38. Ross, Melanie Fridl, "University of Florida researchers cite possible link between autism, schizophrenia and diet," University of Florida Posted March 16, 1999. http://www.health.ufl.edu

39. Cade, R.J., "Exorphins and autism," copy of letter Dr. Cade sent to parents of autistic children, University of Florida Departments of Medicine & Physiology, Health Science Center, Gainsville, Florida 32610-0204.
http://www.paleodiet.com/~paleodiet/autism/cadelet.txt

40. Cade, R., Privette, M., Fregly, M., Rowland, N., Sun, Z., Zele, V., Wagemaker, H., and Edelstein, C., "Autism and schizophrenia: intestinal disorders," *Nutritional Neuroscience*, Vol 3, 57-72, February 12, 1999.

41. Hoffer, A., "Gaining control of schizophrenia," *Am J Natural Med* 5(5):21-2, 1998.

17 - Home Runs and Curve Balls

We thought that we would have difficulty finding a doctor willing to oversee Chris's transition from psychotropic medications to the Synergy supplements, let alone one willing to learn with us. We had no expectation whatsoever of finding a physician who could teach us about biological factors involved in bipolar disorder. As far as we knew, such physicians didn't exist, at least in our area.

A friend of ours who knew of our interest in alternative treatment approaches recommended Dr. Angela Ingendaay, a physician specializing in internal medicine. On October 4 Chris and I drove to Grass Valley to meet with her.

An open-minded doctor

We walked into the converted apartment that was Dr. Ingendaay's office. As we sat in the comfortable waiting room, I leafed through some yoga and health magazines while Chris sat with his eyes closed.

Dr. Ingendaay opened her office door and stepped out. "You must be Chris. Please come on in," she said in a German accent as she welcomed us into her office.

"Hi," Chris said.

I extended my hand. "I'm Dave. We spoke on the phone."

"Yes, of course." She had a strong grip. "Please sit down."

Dr. Ingendaay's office had none of the usual accoutrements of a doctor's office. There was no smell of alcohol, no white coat, no cabinet. There were four comfortable chairs. To my astonishment, I saw a bed in the middle of the room, high up off the floor. The bed had pink sheets. There was a slight, sweet smell of incense. What had I gotten us into now?

"So, Chris, what would you like me to help you with?" asked Dr. Ingendaay.

"I would like to become independent again and move out of my parents' house."

"We'd like that, too," I chimed in. "But there are several issues that need to be resolved first. Here's a summary of Chris's psychiatric history." I handed her a summary that I had written earlier.

"Good, I haven't received the narrative summary yet from Live Oaks."

"I wrote some questions we'd like you to address. Two of them are from reading a book I just recently bought called Nutritional Influences on Mental Illness. It's a compilation of research on the role of nutrition in treating mental disorders. There's a case of a patient diagnosed with bipolar disorder for ten years who was cured when she stopped eating wheat. There's a

213

reference to secondary mania from the presence of IgE antibodies to wheat or rye. We also wanted to check out heavy metal contamination such as lead or mercury."

"We can test for these things, but they may be expensive."

"That's okay. We'll pay for it. Medi-Cal won't cover this, but we don't want to leave any stone unturned. My father is bipolar and had a very rough life. If we can help Chris find some solutions, it will be worth it."

Dr. Ingendaay nodded and turned her attention back to Chris. "So, what medications are you on, Chris, and how much are you taking?"

"I'm taking Wellbutrin, Zyprexa, Depakote, and lithium. Let's see ... I'm on 1,500 mg of Depakote. I don't remember the other amounts."

"They have him on a lot of drugs," I said.

Dr. Ingendaay responded, "Drugs keep you from being curious." I wasn't sure if she was talking about patients or the doctors who prescribed the drugs in the first place. I presumed it was true in both in cases.

I jumped in again. "I work with high-risk kids at County Behavioral Health Services. We give all of them the same treatment — medications — and we don't look for other explanations for their difficulties."

"That is sad, because there are so many different ways to approach a problem."

"Well. That's why we are here. We've already started Chris on the supplement program I told you about."

Dr. Ingendaay asked Chris to give his perspective of his illness. Chris told her about his prophetic visions regarding the end of the world. He reviewed his four previous hospitalizations. He said he wouldn't get manic again, because he realized that his ideas were delusional. He wasn't sure what to believe now. He was afraid to trust his perceptions. He felt depressed.

I commented that Chris saw his difficulties as being spiritual in nature, while I viewed them as biological.

"Maybe you are both right," Dr. Ingendaay said. She talked about how acupuncture has been used for thousands of years to free up energy that is stuck in the body. But she said she was nervous about taking this approach with Chris, because there is often a healing crisis when the energy is freed up. "Maybe we should wait until the current medical crisis is resolved before trying acupuncture. But I may be able to help locally with the knee pain."

She asked Chris about the incident that had led to his most recent hospitalization. He explained in excruciating detail his feelings and behaviors on that day. Some of what he said I had not heard before.

Describing his long walk down Highway 20, he said, "I bit branches off the trees and chewed on them because I wanted to know what it would be like being in hell since I was going there anyway." He explained his belief that his previous writings had condemned him to hell.

"Why did you want to hurt yourself?" she asked.

"I had this image of killing my parents and sister with an electric saw, and I decided that the only way I could prevent myself from doing it would be to kill myself first. I thought of poking out my eyes or castrating myself, but when I saw the broken beer bottle on the road, I decided to use that." He proceeded to give detailed explanation of his desire to die. "I wasn't sure whether I would leave my body looking peaceful so that my parents would know I had gone to heaven, or leave it all mangled up so they would know I had gone to hell."

I listened in pain and not a little surprise. These details were new to me. I wondered if Chris's behavior in biting off the branches of trees was related to the behavior of pigs afflicted with ear and tail biting syndrome, in which, as the name suggests, the pigs bit off the ears and tails of other pigs. As Chris talked, trying to make sense of his behavior, I began to understand more of the psychotic thinking that had held him in its sway the day he'd run amok.

Dr. Ingendaay listened attentively, then spoke. "I've never worked with a person with a mental illness, and I don't know much about this supplement program, but I'm willing to help where I can. I can prescribe smaller amounts as you transition from the drugs."

I wanted to correct her use of the words "mental illness." I would have preferred "central nervous system disorder," but I restrained myself. After all, I had used the words "mental illness" myself. I was grateful that Dr. Ingendaay was even seeing us, and especially that she was so open to alternatives to medication. However, as supportive as she was, her use of the term stuck in my craw. Why call Chris's illness "mental" when it was a brain disorder, one that had been exacerbated by the allopathic care he had received? There were physical anomalies in Chris's brain that caused him to think and act differently from other people.

"I'll order the tests," Dr. Ingendaay said. "We can rule out heavy metals and can test for specific IgE antibodies to common foods. If you send a check with these, it will be faster and cheaper. We can meet again in three weeks."

I gave her the Web site address for Truehope. "Tonight they should post the study presented at the Canadian Psychiatric Association I mentioned earlier. When we see you next time, we'll probably have Chris on a little less medication."

The word is out

That night I checked the Web site. The words jumped out from the screen:

Too Good To Be True?

Successful treatment of bipolar disorder with a nutritional supplement: Ten cases

Presented at the Canadian Psychiatric Association annual meeting
October 4, 2000, Victoria, British Columbia
Bonnie J. Kaplan[1], PhD, J. Steve A. Simpson[1], PhD, MD, Richard
C.Ferre[2],MD, Chris P. Gorman[1], MD, David McMullen[1], MD
[1]Calgary, Alberta, Canada; [2]Salt Lake City, Utah

Recent research on various nutrients has suggested that some mental illness might be ameliorated by supplementation. Much work has focused on essential fatty acids (1), although various minerals are also being studied (especially zinc). We are evaluating a broad-based nutritional supplement that contains primarily trace minerals, plus vitamins and amino acids. Recent work has suggested that crops grown with western farming methods contain fewer of these essential nutrients than they did in years past (2). Although we have been examining the effects of the supplement on a variety of psychiatric symptoms in both children and adults, it appears to be particularly promising for bipolar disorder in adults. We will present an open-case series of 10 male patients aged 20-46 years who thus far have taken the supplement for 1.5 - 6 months. Four were diagnosed with Bipolar I, four with Bipolar II, one with Bipolar Mixed, and one with Bipolar-NOS. In most cases, the supplement has entirely replaced psychoactive medications and the patients have remained well. Side effects (e.g., nausea) have been rare, minor, and transitory. In all cases, the patients have been evaluated periodically with the Hamilton-Depression Scale, the Brief Psychiatric Rating Scale, and the Young Mania Rating Scale. The changes in mean scores for each scale from study entry to the time of the last visit are as follows: Ham-D (20.4 to 8.2), BPRS (37.3 to 9.9), YMRS (16.8 to 6.1), and OQ (75.2 to 48.2). A randomized, placebo-controlled trial of the supplement for Bipolar I has been funded and began in July 2000.

References:

1. Stoll A.L., Severus E, Freeman M.P., Rueter S, Zboyan H.A., Diamond E, Cress K.K., Marangell L.B., "Omega 3 fatty acids in bipolar disorder: A preliminary double-blind, placebo-controlled trial." Archives of General Psychiatry 1999; 56:407-412.

2. Mayer A.B., "Historical changes in the mineral content of fruits and vegetables," British Food Journal 1997; 99:207-211.

The information was now out. That was the good news. But would all this publicity make it more difficult for me to talk to Tony?

A three-way conversation

For three days I tried to call Tony. Chris had been on the supplements and his medications for almost a week, and, although he would not admit it, he appeared to me to be increasingly tired. I wanted to start withdrawing him from the medications before the proverbial ADR hit, but I was concerned that if we started too soon, we would repeat the mistakes of the past. I called Tony's office, his home, even his cell phone, leaving messages each time.

Finally, on Saturday, October 7, Tony returned my call.

"Hi Dave. Sorry I couldn't get back with you sooner, but the phone won't stop ringing around here. We did a spot for Discovery Channel of Canada. I had several interviews for newspapers and TV, and calls have been coming in from everywhere." His voice sounded like he had a cold. "Can you hear me all right?"

"We hear you fine. I appreciate your calling back. You must be pretty busy with all the interest over Dr. Kaplan's presentation. Tony, this is my son, Chris. He's on the other phone."

"Hi, Tony."

"Hi, Chris. Tell me how you're doing."

"Well, I've been taking the supplements for a week. I'm feeling Okay. I don't have the strong thoughts I had when I was in the hospital, but I'm still depressed because I don't know where my life is going."

"Chris, your job now is to sit back and take 120 days to get yourself back together so that you can begin to solve those issues. Do you have waves of sadness that come over you, or is it more like a steady depressed state?"

"More like a constant depression, but not intense like it was."

I joined in. "He tells me he's not having the suicidal or homicidal ideas he had while in the hospital, but he feels trapped, like he doesn't have what it takes to succeed in the world."

"Okay, Chris, those medications you're on are designed to help you not to feel. And they also can be contributing to your confusion and sense of hopelessness. I'd love for you to talk to Jennifer some time. She said we could use her name. Jennifer is a concert pianist with intermittent episodes of mania and depression who was confused, irritable, and unable to work for nine years. She's doing fine now on the supplements and just bought a $40,000 grand piano for her studio. Now, I know what you're thinking, Dave, but no,

217

she did not buy this piano out of her mania, but out of her success as a well-respected piano performer and teacher. Tell me, Chris, are you feeling irritable and hostile now?"

"If I am, I'm able to hide it well."

I broke in again. "From our standpoint, he's doing fine, except for his confusion, memory problems, and lack of energy. He still feels he can't do simple tasks. His highest score on the Truehope questionnaire is the tiredness scale. All the other scores are low."

"That's great. How much medication are you on now, Chris?"

"I'm taking 32 supplement pills and 2 omega fatty acid pills of 1,000 mg each. I don't know how much of the other medications I'm on."

I read from the bottles. "He's taking 1,500 mg of Depakote, 900 mg of lithium, 300 mg of Wellbutrin, and 15 mg of Zyprexa."

"I can't tell you what to do because I'm not a doctor," Tony cautioned, "but if you were my son, I'd start cutting everything by one-third."

"Last time we talked, you said that one-quarter would be a good place to start."

"At Synergy, we're not as conservative as the folks involved in the clinical trials. We've had several years of experience working with the people taking the supplements."

"How fast did you move with your son and daughter?" I asked.

"My son was on lithium, and we stopped that cold turkey."

"I read that sudden withdrawal of lithium can cause seizures."

"We haven't had any problem with that up here. There's a long half-life, so it will stay in your system for up to a week. Now with my daughter, who was on a number of medications, we took her down in thirds, and that took quite a bit longer. The reason I would go with one-third now is that Chris seems to be doing well. He's not irritable, suicidal, or homicidal. He may have more unpleasant side effects down the road if he stays on the supplements and continues with the full dosage of psychiatric medications. It's all up to you."

"Okay, thanks again for getting back to us. We'll start today, if Chris agrees to it."

"I'm willing to do it," he said.

"Call me back in about five days to let me know how things are going. If you need to talk to me sooner, you know my number."

"Thanks Tony. We really appreciate this."

"Bye, Chris. Remember to just kick back and relax. You don't have anything to do except to get your brain working right so you can get your life back together."

"Talk to you later."

I took the box of pills and started figuring which drugs to cut in order to reduce everything by one-third. I was pretty confident at this stage, since

Chris had been stable on much less of the drugs prior to his withdrawal from Zyprexa. "Do you want to start tonight?"

"That's fine with me."

For a week, Chris continued to sleep well and to feel tired throughout the day. See Appendix 2, Psychotropic Drug Withdrawal Log for details.

The diagnostic testing kit arrived from Dr. Ingendaay on October 15. Chris and I went to a local lab, where they took a sample of his blood and sent it off to Great Smokies Diagnostic Laboratories to test for food allergies. While at the lab, I inquired as to whether or not Medi-Cal covered the blood test. The technician said it was covered. I was surprised. If it was covered, then why weren't we having our Medi-Cal-eligible high-risk youth take these tests, or at least the tests for heavy metals and IgE antibodies? The hair analysis, which was not covered, would have to wait for two weeks, as the lab wanted Chris to shampoo regularly with a Johnson and Johnson product before giving them samples. Coincidentally, when we got home I saw a newspaper article about a study done on Beethoven's hair. Musicologists had long speculated as to whether or not the composer's legendary rages had been a consequence of bipolar disorder. In 1997, eight strands of hair taken from his body after his death had been found to have 42 times the lead found in the average of three control samples. While the controls included lead concentrations of .95 to 9.9, Beethovan's hair results ranged from 90 to 250. (Apart from the fact that the differences were significant, the book did not provide further details about the findings.) What was clear was that Beethovan had bipolar-like symptoms, but he had lead poisoning. It most likely killed him.[1]

On October 17, I called Tony again. I told him that Chris's speech was slurred, and he still appeared tired. Tony told us that they had changed the protocol for the double-blind study and were now getting patients off all psychotropic medications within 1 month. I told him that Dr. Ingendaay was nervous about any more medication reductions. I also told him that I was nervous about dropping the Zyprexa too quickly in light of past disasters. Tony said we could do one-quarter or one-third, but that the longer we drew it out, the greater chance of an ADR. We decided to reduce all his medications by another fourth beginning that night.

When feeling better is better

Chris continued to sleep well and to report tiredness upon awakening. Three days after we reduced his medications, he accompanied us to Elizabeth's basketball championship game. Her team won. Afterwards, we went to McDonalds, where Chris quietly sang to himself. Later, in the car, he sang with the girls from Elizabeth's team. We had to ask them to sing more softly. I worried that maybe Chris was enjoying himself too much. Gayle and I were both anxious about the possibility of his becoming hypomanic again.

On October 26, almost three weeks after we'd started reducing Chris's medications, Barbara Stephan called me at work.

"Dave, this is Barb. Tony is out of town, so I thought I'd check in and see if you have any questions."

"I appreciate your calling. Chris is doing very well, almost too well. When he first came home, he seemed very unsure of himself. He didn't feel like he could do simple tasks. Now he's acting more independent. He's doing things he used to say he couldn't do: baking cakes, cutting his pills and putting them in the pill case, doing chores around the house. I know it doesn't sound like much, but he's much more capable then he was just a few weeks ago."

"I know the feelings you're having. Tony had tried magnets, herbs, and when he came up with the supplements, he wanted our son to stop the lithium cold turkey. I went ahead and bought some lithium as an insurance policy, and, you know, that bottle is still unopened today. Our son started getting more energy, and I was afraid he was going to become manic again, but, you know, he never did. My daughter took a lot longer to withdraw from her medications. Now we have had two more of our children diagnosed with bipolar disorder. They are both on the supplements and doing fine."

"Chris has been on half of the discharged dose for about a week and a half now. Do you think we should cut out more?"

"We're finding that a cutback is indicated when they feel excessively tired, or if they have some really good days and then get worse."

"I heard from Tony that in the University of Calgary study, they changed the withdrawal schedule to one month."

"Yes, they're finding that if patients stay on medications too long, they start getting symptoms, and then the doctors want to keep them on medications longer."

"Have you had any cases where withdrawal from the medications has provoked a major depression or a manic psychosis?"

"No, although we have had difficult withdrawals for those who have been on multiple psychotropic drugs for a long time."

When I got home, I told Chris about the phone call. "Barb said that in the double-blind study, they're getting patients off the psychotropic medications in one month. She says normally if you have some really good days followed by a downer, or if you feel tired, then that would be the time to cut again. What do you think?"

"We can cut another third."

"I'll leave it up to you to change the medications in the box."

"Okay."

Two days later, he cut his medication dosage by another third. He remained on 32 pills of the Synergy supplements a day.

The food-sensitivity question

On November 2, Dr. Ingendaay called me at home with the antibody report, then faxed it to me from her office. I looked at the results and got Gayle and Chris together immediately.

"Looks like we've got some good news and bad news here. Chris, you have no IgE antibodies. That's the good news. But out of a possible score ranging from 20 to 240, you have a combined IgE, IgG total of 220. The '220' is all from IgG sensitivities. Look at the foods listed. It says you are sensitive to almost all vegetables, almost all fruits, and all meat except for lamb and oysters. According to this, you should be eating lamb, oyster, bananas, cranberries, peaches, pineapples, sesame seeds, and pears for the rest of your life. You scored a 3+ on almost all vegetables."

"I don't have any allergies."

"This isn't that kind of allergy. It won't give you hives or asthma. Listen to this; it might be very important. According to an article I read, there have been a number of studies showing abnormal immune functioning in patients with psychiatric disorders.[2] I'm not saying this is the case for you, but it is a possibility. IgE antibodies to specific foods provoke immediate symptoms. About 5% of allergies are of this type, but the other 95% are what they call delayed food sensitivities. As I understand it, your body has developed a way to defend against almost all these foods. It has produced IgG antibodies against them. Based on these results, you shouldn't be eating from food groups in which you have 5 or more items with a 3+. According to this chart, you shouldn't eat any vegetables, fruits, and nuts, but you can eat meat and dairy products. Your sensitivity to those foods is still a 1+ or a 2+. I see here that they recommend a rotation diet, but how do you do rotate foods when you're sensitive to almost all of them?"

Chris considered. "If I'm allergic, then what are my symptoms?"

"How about bipolar illness? I can't prove it, but we need to find someone who can make sense of this." I had to go to work, so we left it at that.

After the 20-minute commute, I got out of the car, aimlessly walked to my windowless office enclosed by concrete walls, and closed the door behind me on a clear, crisp, fall morning. My office had once been the kitchen for the Nevada County National Guard Armory, which had recently been converted into the Imaginarium, a place where school kids and the public could marvel at the mysteries of science. It was 9 in the morning, and I was now working half-time, per my agreement with my supervisor. There were six messages waiting on my answering machine. Most were routine, what I called "Tag, you're it." messages. I took notes. Message number 4 clicked on. I heard Barb Stephan's voice.

"Hi Dave. I called to see how Chris is doing." Then she gave her number. I called back on my credit card and told her that Chris was singing around the house and appeared to be doing very well.

"But there is a wrinkle," I added. "When I started my research, I told myself we would leave no stone unturned, so we ordered blood tests for food antibodies and a hair test for heavy metals. We sent his blood to a lab in South Carolina to check it out."

"Just a minute, Dave. I think Tony would like to hear this. He's always interested in new approaches. Tony, Dave is on the line. I'll transfer him to you."

"Hi, Dave."

"Hi, Tony. I was just explaining to Barb that we sent out some blood samples to a lab in South Carolina to see if Chris had any food antibodies. We also sent hair samples to screen for heavy metals. We're still waiting for the hair analysis results, but we just got the antibody report back. It says Chris is sensitive to almost every food imaginable. He almost got the highest score possible on the test. He's sensitive to carrots, celery, citrus fruit, beef, milk, chicken, and turkey. If these foods really are a problem, there is very little he can eat except for oysters, lamb, and pears. Did you ever check for food antibodies with your kids, or do you know of any other bipolar patients for whom this is an issue?"

"No, but I remember one woman who couldn't eat citrus without severe pain and stomach upset. She started on the supplement program and was soon able to eat citrus without any pain. The gut has about 300 enzymes that are required for proper digestion. When she got enough zinc in her system, her digestive problems went away."

"That's interesting. Our doctor suggested we get some pancreatic enzymes. Said it would help his digestion."

"I'm sure that will help, too."

"I don't know the first thing about IgG antibodies, but I've found several articles where high levels were associated with acute psychoses. Zyprexa has an acute antihistamine effect. Histamine increases in response to autoimmune processes. Some of the more common results of the IgG antibodies can include brain fog, moodiness, and perception of heat. Haven't found any direct correlation with bipolar disorder, but some of those symptoms are found in bipolar patients."

I then explained what I had learned about antibodies, GABA, and Stiff Person Syndrome. "If GABA slows the brain down, and if an IgG antibody can reduce the production of GABA, then couldn't the same or similar antibodies play a role in bipolar disorder?"

"I don't know much about this, but it sounds like it would be worth checking out."

"Our problem is finding someone who knows antibodies and can make sense out of these results."

"Good luck with it. Let me know what you find."

"Chris continues to improve. He's down to one-third of his meds."

"Great. In a week, you can take him down to no meds."

"But I thought you said you wanted to go down one-third at a time."

"The longer he stays on the meds, the longer he will not feel like his old self."

"I know you haven't had any bad outcomes, but Chris has gone psychotic three times after getting off his Zyprexa. The last time, he tried to kill himself. How about we go one-half?"

"That would be okay too, but in the study they changed the protocol to one month to be off all meds."

"We're now at about one month and a week. I don't know how many in the study went psychotic three times after discontinuing medications, but I know that Chris did. Also, we don't know how many, if any, have massive antibodies to most foods. I'm not saying it's a cause, but until we know it isn't, I think it's best to be cautious."

"Fair enough. Let me know how it goes."

"By the way, Tony, I've decided to write a book on this. I'm going to call it Too Good To Be True? Nutrients Quiet the Unquiet Mind."

"I'd love to see it when you finish it."

"I'll send you a copy when I finish the draft. See you later, and thanks again for all your help."

There was another message waiting on the answering machine. I pushed the button to listen.

"Dave, this is Mary. I received a complaint today regarding your work with Steven. Someone thought you had made him more agitated. Maybe you shouldn't see him again until we can talk."

High-risk kids

Steven was a third grader diagnosed with ADHD and bipolar disorder. His multiple medicines had not been effective in controlling his behavior. School personnel and I had been telling his psychiatrist for some time that the antidepressants he had prescribed were not working and were, if anything, making Steven even more hyper. I knew that giving antidepressants to bipolar patients could provoke mania. The psychiatrist eventually changed the medications, but instead of stopping the antidepressant, he replaced it with an antipsychotic. I was not happy with this change. It wasn't my role as a social worker to tell a psychiatrist what I'd learned from other psychiatrists: namely, that it was better to change one medication at a time, particularly when that one medication might be part of the problem. In my opinion, he should have waited long enough before starting the other drug to learn the results from discontinuing the first drug. After the change, I had an appointment with Steven at school. He looked drugged. He complained of blurred vision and lay down on the couch while I tried to talk to him. His concentration and schoolwork had improved but, in my judgment, he was overmedicated.

Although privately I was becoming more skeptical about using drugs as the first line of intervention when so many untried alternatives existed, professionally I was doing my job properly, documenting observations and feedback for the psychiatrist and working with Steven to help him adjust better in school. But now I felt unable to keep quiet. I suggested to Steven that he probably had too much medicine. When he returned to class later in the day, he used this as an excuse to get out of doing his schoolwork.

Given his statement and subsequent behavior, it was probably a mistake for me to have told Steven the obvious regarding his medication. But was this just an error in my therapeutic technique, or was I somehow conveying my antipathy toward the very practices I was helping to perpetuate? I had told Tony that if the supplements helped Chris, it would make it more difficult for me to continue working for the county. So far the supplements were helping, and I was having a difficult time. I had been providing Steven's father information about food elimination diets for ADHD children. I was already operating outside my professional boundaries to even suggest he read the research.

My commitments to my clients, my son, and my father had me feeling thinly stretched, but my issues with working for the county were broader than this. I was increasingly questioning our approach to helping high-risk youth. I had written a proposal to provide nutritional respite care where children could be put on a food elimination diet and given appropriate vitamins and minerals. I had shared with the staff information regarding omega-3 fatty acids, only to be cautioned not to share this information with the parents of the bipolar children who needed it. I had expressed my belief that we should be ruling out heavy metal poisoning, food and additive sensitivities, and that we should try vitamin and mineral supplements before considering medications.[3] In eight months of working for Nevada County, I had gotten to know the culture well enough to realize that the leadership was not open to innovation. They denied the need for change. Even if they had tried to change directions, the organizational consequences would have been enormously disruptive. I had made an honest but futile effort to see if I could make a constructive difference.

The good feelings I'd experienced in talking to Barb and Tony were gone now, replaced by a realization that I would not be able to significantly help my clients, the most high-risk school-age children in the county, the very patients who were most in need of innovative treatment options. Maybe my clients were high-risk, not only because of their past difficulties, but also because the tools that counselors like me had at our disposal to help them were so ineffective. When I'd taken this job, I'd told my supervisor up front that if I didn't think I could help my clients, I wouldn't want to stay. Later I'd told her that I often felt as if I were arranging the deck chairs on the Titanic for my clients. One nice thing about being retired was that I could tell the truth to my boss and not have to worry about the consequences. I could always go back to day trading.

After seeing some clients and turning in my documentation, I left early and picked up Chris. We had an engagement in Sacramento.

High and outside

Chris had met Matt during his time in Live Oaks Hospital. Matt was a 35-year-old alcoholic and Valium-addicted bipolar patient with a broad career background. Among other things, he was a computer programer for a Silicon Valley company. We'd first met him on one of our visits when Chris and I were singing while sitting on the hall floor. He later told us that he thought I was a patient. He said he was moved by one of the songs we sang, the same song I had hummed to Chris when he was in his "palace" at Sacred Heart. I liked Matt. He had a lot of spirit. He was the kind of guy who could sell you anything, whether you wanted it or not.

While on the ward, Matt had convinced Chris to come and live with him after they were both discharged. Chris persisted in telling us all the fun things they would do, like riding bikes and going sky diving. He didn't want to come home to his mom and dad. We tried to explain to him that we needed to pull out all stops to get him well. We told him that we didn't think staying with Matt was the answer, and that his judgment was still impaired. It was also true that we did not want our son living with an alcoholic, drug-abusing bipolar patient. After Chris came home, he asked several times if he could go visit Matt. We had other priorities. Matt, who called occasionally to speak with Chris, sent a letter protesting that we were holding Chris back. He invited us to visit him and explained that he was an honorable person with no ulterior motives. We did not suspect ulterior motives, but none of us wanted to drive two hours just so Chris could see a friend he'd met in the hospital. Nor did we want Chris traveling that far on his own, given his difficulty with directions and the fact that he was still on medications.

But this particular weekend, I was attending a human sexuality course at the University of California at Davis extension in order to meet my prerequisites for taking the oral exam for the LCSW in California. Though I was licensed in Alaska, no one else in the family wanted to return there, so I figured I'd better get the California LCSW in case I decided to get a better paying social work job or open a private practice. Chris had called Matt and asked if the two of us could come see him and "crash" at his place over the weekend. Matt had responded in the affirmative. Chris told me that one reason he was eager to visit Matt was to help his friend overcome his drinking problem.

When we arrived at the apartment, the door was open and Matt was inside. The apartment smelled of tobacco and alcohol. Upon seeing Chris, Matt commented on how much better he looked than when he was in the hospital. He noted that Chris's eyes seemed much clearer, more "with it." We talked about the supplement program and how Chris was slowly withdrawing from his medications.

I left and drove to the evening class. After the class, I returned to Matt's apartment, expecting to sleep on his couch. He insisted I sleep in his bed. He said he got up a lot, and it would be better if he slept on the couch. At first, I protested. But after tactfully telling him in as many ways as I could that I didn't want to put him out, I finally accepted his offer graciously and thanked him for his hospitality. It was hard to say no to Matt.

Chris and Matt stayed up late playing video games. The next morning, as I was leaving for that day's class, I noted that Chris was sleeping on the couch and Matt on the floor. After completing the course and having a quick dinner with some of my classmates, I returned once again to the apartment. As before, there was a strong odor of alcohol and tobacco. It was 7:45 p.m. Chris and Matt were playing video games on the TV. I suspected that Chris had been smoking. He claimed he didn't really smoke since he only had a cigarette once in a while, but I was concerned that a powerful drug like nicotine could upset the fragile equilibrium of his brain chemistry. However, this was not the occasion to say anything.

"How was the class?" asked Matt.

"Well, I can't say it was boring because of the subject matter," I said with a smile. "The movies were interesting. I got to learn all about sex toys in a dignified classroom setting."

He laughed. "You could have learned about that in a porn shop."

"Actually, there were some interesting historical perspectives. Did you know that Mr. Graham was down on sex, particularly the solitary kind, and that Mr. Kellogg was down on both solitary and heterosexual sex?"

"So?" said Matt.

"So! I'm talking about Mr. Kellogg as in Corn Flakes and Mr. Graham as in Graham Crackers. Kellogg was even celibate in his marriage. Guess what they came up with to help people curb their carnal desires?"

Both Matt and Chris looked at me silently, with somewhat puzzled expressions.

"I already said it, but the answer is Corn Flakes and Graham Crackers. Hey, I'm serious. Nothing like Corn Flakes and Graham Crackers to kill the old libido! I got it from The New Male Sexuality by a guy named Dr. Bernie Zilbergeld and from the course instructor.[4] Speaking of food, I think I would have rather gone to a class on nutrition and mental illness. I know that sexual behavior is pretty universal, but so is eating, and what do we social workers know about that? So what about you guys? Did you have as interesting a day?"

Chris shrugged. "We wandered around some shops. Matt took me to this great restaurant for dinner. And look at this cool hat he got me!" He showed me a Crocodile Dundee-type leather hat that Matt had purchased for him. It looked expensive.

"Nice hat," I said. "It was very generous of you to get that for him."

Matt took a swallow from a drink. Judging from the odor in the room, I presumed it was alcoholic. I spoke up. "Do I smell alcohol?"

"Yeah. I had a White Russian tonight at dinner and am having my second one now." He showed me a Valium pill that he'd been fingering like rosary beads. "I'm having a hard time not taking this because of the anxiety. That doctor ruined me. He made an addict out of me and ruined my life and my marriage. That is why I decided to sue him. I wasn't addicted to Valium until he started treating me. My malpractice lawsuit against him is starting tomorrow."

"I thought you'd decided not to drink until you got your life back together."

"A few White Russians isn't really drinking."

I grabbed my guitar case and pulled out the guitar. Matt had mentioned that he hoped we could do some jamming during the visit like we'd done in the hospital. Chris and I started singing the song he'd arranged for his senior recital.

> *It's time to slide between cold sheets,*
> *And make them snugly warm,*
> *Time to dream great dreams,*
> *Time to say I love you,*
> *Time to sing I love you with a song.*
>
> *I love you,*
> *Yes I do,*
> *Through the day and night time too,*
> *I'll be here always near, through your days and years.*

Matt's eyes started to well up with tears, as they had on the ward. He talked about how he had never had a good relationship with his father, and how the song moved him. Then he started to enthusiastically talk about the potential he saw in Chris's music.

"Chris's music is pure and clean, not like other artists I've worked with. I'm not usually moved by songs, but his songs move me. I'd like Chris to make a CD of his music. I'll pay for all the expenses. Then I'll travel from Northern to Southern California bugging radio stations until they play it. Chris, your music needs to be on the radio. We can divide any profits by one-third."

"Have you ever done anything like this before?" I asked.

"Sure," he said. "I've produced two CD's. Made some money off both, but neither artist had the talent Chris has."

I spoke up. "That's very generous of you, Matt, but we'd need more music than what Chris has now."

"Yeah," Chris said. "We'd need at least 12 songs for a CD. All I've got now is 'Got to Get a Date' and 'Lullaby.' I'd have to write some more."

I started to get into the act. "Maybe we could modify some of the songs you already wrote." Matt's enthusiasm was contagious, even if the room did smell of alcohol. It was flattering for Chris and me to hear that Chris's music was not only marketable, but that Matt would go all over the state to make sure that his songs were played on the air. I had often told Chris that his songs were much more appealing than the cynical music and rap that filled the airwaves. He had an exceptional ability to write music that touched people.

Here we were getting as intoxicated by Matt's pitch as he probably was on that White Russian. Yet he didn't appear to be under the influence. He didn't appear to be manic. He wasn't talking faster or louder than normal. He acted like a sentimental, aggressive, committed guy who would do anything to get Chris's music on the air.

But the strong odor of alcohol in the room spoke louder than Matt's sales pitch. Reminded me of an Air Force Officer who, according to witnesses looked perfectly sober when he got into his car with a 4.0 blood alcohol level and proceeded to wrap himself around a telephone at 70 miles per hour. I couldn't help wondering whether a high tolerance for alcohol might be masking how drunk Matt really was. I tried to figure out if I was hearing Matt, his alcohol, or his mania. Whatever it was, it felt good. Anyway, hey, I was off duty, and retired.

"Here's a song you could do," I said half-jokingly. "Matt, you might like it. It's about Valium." I sang a song I had written years ago for a Christmas party for the mental health clinic staff at Little Rock AFB. It went to the tune of "Wichita Lineman."

Valium, oh Valium, I can feel your warm waves coming,

So silent, smooth, and numbing,
When I feel glum, I'll take my Valium.

I can feel your presence there before me,
Every morning as I shave my face,
Nice to know there'll always be a friend there,
To reach for and embrace.

Valium, oh Valium, I can feel your warm waves coming,
So silent, smooth, and numbing,
When I feel glum, I'll take my Valium.

I was on a roll. "Here's another one you could do."

They said you must go now, go now to Subic Bay,
Or a mountain will blow, it could blow you away.
Now there's lightning and earthquakes and typhoons, and
more,
For the mountain has blown with a mighty loud roar.
And we're sittin' and shaking and waiting for news.
It must be the time for the Pinatubo Blues.

Chris was joining in with some nice blues sounds. Matt was hitting
the bongo drums.

I got muck in my hair and got mud on my feet.
I got ash in my glasses and grit in my teeth.
I can't drive in my car, just can't see very far.
And the ground 'neath me shakes with so many earthquakes.
There is one thing I got I would sure like to lose.
Ain't it no wonder I got the Pinatubo Blues.

I got the Pinatubo Blues,
I got the Pinatubo Blues,
I got the Pinatubo Blues Blues,
Cause I'm sittin' in front of my radio,
Cain't get no FEN news.

After finishing the fourth verse, Chris and I explained our adventure in
the Philippines. We told Matt how our family had written the song while
rocks from the volcano 15 miles away fell on the roof and the front yard of
the house in which we were staying. We talked about my going down to the
Far East Network (FEN) where they took me up on my offer to record the

song for broadcast. Once the general at Clark Air Base approved it and the power was restored, they played our song on the airwaves as a morale booster. I told Matt how FEN had played it a number of times on the radio, giving me the opportunity to record it for background music for a video I created showing the carnage from the volcano, typhoon and earthquakes.

We were having a great time, a nice break from the ever-present anxiety. We sang some more songs together and discussed Matt's ideas for a CD. While I had some reservations, Matt was able to convince us that his idea was doable. Chris said he would write some new songs. I told Matt I would put some words to the theme from a clarinet solo Chris wrote for his senior recital. While I noted there were more pressing health concerns, I agreed that Chris had what it took to make a quality CD. Matt's enthusiasm was contagious.

I glanced at my watch. It was already 10:15. I mentioned to Chris that we needed to be heading home. We had a family outing planned for early the next day with Ga and Boppie, Gayle's parents, who were visiting us from Seattle.

"Matt invited me to go with him to comedy night," Chris said. "Would it be Okay if I stayed tonight, and then Matt could drop me off at home tomorrow."

"How could he do that? He doesn't have a car."

"He could rent a limo."

"That would be awfully expensive," I said. "Besides, we have been planning this trip for weeks. Let's just go home and stay with the plan."

Matt got up from where he'd been sitting on the floor. "What's the big deal, Chris? I thought you wanted to stay."

The ambience in the room abruptly changed.

"I do. But my dad doesn't want me to, and he would get mad if I stayed."

"Hey, you're 25; you can do what you want!"

Although taken aback, I decided to ignore Matt's remark. "C'mon, Chris, let's go," I said. I wasn't happy that I was being made out to be the bad guy, but I decided to ignore it. I wanted to get Chris out of the apartment in case the situation deteriorated. I didn't have long to wait.

Matt turned on me. "You're trying to control your son. He doesn't need your control."

I started feeling angry as I carried my guitar and clothes out to the car. What was Matt up to? The visit had gone so well, and now here I was getting labeled as the controlling father, no doubt the "manicogenic" father type — the male, mania-inducing equivalent of the schizophrenogenic mother. Was Matt still angling to get Chris to move in with him? What was going on?

He followed us out to the car, drink in one hand, a cigarette in the other. Looking me right in the eye he said, "You know, I really don't like you and never have." He was talking louder now.

"Look," I said, trying to stay calm. "I explained that we have plans for tomorrow."

"I let you stay in my bedroom, and you didn't even thank me. I let you stay with me for the weekend, and you turn around and try to boss Chris around."

That did it. I wasn't the professional social worker now. I wasn't the substance abuse counselor either, though I had worn both hats in the Air Force. I looked Matt in the eye. "If this behavior is anything like what you did to your wife, I can understand why she has a restraining order against you."

Matt stepped to within six inches of me in a threatening manner and yelled, "You stay out of my personal business!"

I thought he was going to hit me. Then and only then did I realize how much drunker Matt was than he appeared. Or, maybe he was manic. I backed away from him and continued loading the car, having decided that further discussion would only cause an escalation. I perfunctorily thanked him for letting us stay with him, and then Chris and I left. What a let down! I had really enjoyed myself until Matt, with Chris's help, turned on me.

On the way home, Chris and I talked about what had happened. He admitted that he had contributed to the turmoil by his comments. We talked about the sudden change in Matt's behavior and whether it was just him, his drinking, or his mania.

After we got home, Matt called and asked to talk to me.

"You know, I'll always be honest with you, and I want you to know that I don't like you one bit. But if I have to go through you to work with Chris, then I'll just have to do that."

"Look, Matt, I have no animosity towards you. You have a lot of good ideas and drive. But I don't like you interfering with our family."

"So if I have to work with you, I will. I want you to know where I stand. Chris has a lot of potential, and I want to help him realize it. You know that I'm in the middle of a divorce settlement with my wife. But I still have money to invest in spite of the $300 an hour my lawyers charge, and I'm prepared to give Chris a $10,000 check right now for the rights to his music. I can come up tonight and deliver it. Like I told you, I will push it, then sell it to a major company like Sony. I can make Chris, you, and me rich."

"That's very generous of you, but right now Chris can't accept that kind of money. He's on Medi-Cal and needs more medical treatment. He wouldn't be eligible for the medical care he needs. Also, you agreed that he didn't have enough music written to fill a CD."

"Do you understand what I'm talking about, man? I'm talking about hundreds of thousands of dollars! I'm talking about big-time CD sales! I'm talking about Chris being on David Letterman. What's a few thousand dollars for medical treatment? Open your eyes, man! Hell, I could give the money to you if you need to hide it."

"What would happen if we took your money and had a major disagreement? I just don't know if I can trust you."

"Hey, this kind of thing is done all the time."

"It doesn't mean we have to do it. Besides, if I were in your shoes, I would be very leery of putting down money on a long shot. You already said you are going through an expensive divorce, suing your doctor, and that you aren't working. Why do you insist that you do this now, with all these other issues going on in your life?"

"Look, I have the money now, and I may not have it in the future."

"That's all the more reason to get through your issues now, then work on a CD when you can really focus on it. It would be the same for Chris. I think it would be great for Chris to write more music and make a CD, but you have to remember that he could have killed himself just two months ago. Our first priority is to get his head right again. Also, I don't know right now if I'm talking to the Matt who is manic or the Matt who is drunk. If you were taking a supplement like Truehope and off the booze and the Valium, you would feel a hell of a lot better than you do now, and I would trust you a hell of a lot more."

"It doesn't fucking matter if I'm manic, alcoholic, or whatever. I can deliver the goods."

"Look, I told you my concerns. I appreciate the confidence you have in Chris, and I agree he is capable of writing and performing some neat stuff. But there is no way I can support taking your money at this time."

Matt stuck to his guns. I cut off the fruitless conversation. Here I was doing more of the same and not even realizing that I was getting more of the same. I should have quit much sooner.

Later, Gayle and I talked with Chris about my conversation with Matt. We suggested that Matt's behavior appeared to be influenced by either his drinking or his hypomanic state, or both. Gayle told Chris that Matt's behavior reminded her of times when he had been similarly insistent and obsessed. While we were talking, the phone rang.

"If that's Matt, tell him Chris isn't here," I said as Gayle reached for the phone. She didn't hear me.

"Chris, it's for you. It's Matt."

We didn't stay to listen but did pick up some snippets of the ensuing conversation.

"Matt, I wouldn't want your ashes if you killed yourself."

And again, later: "When I was manic, I insisted on doing things, and no one could argue with me to change my mind. Sounds like you're feeling like you have to give me the money, but you don't. I'll work with you if we go forward on the CD when the time is right."

Most of the time Chris was listening, as I had been.

After an hour and a half, Chris finally hung up. He informed us that Matt was going to drive in a rented limousine to deliver a $10,000 check to Chris, even though Chris had asked him not to.

"Call him back and tell him he won't be able to come into Lake Wildwood because I won't give permission," I said.

It would have been so easy to take advantage of Matt, given his sudden monomania to get Chris on the airwaves. Yet I had to admit that it would be hard for radio station managers to say no to him ... that is, unless they got so angry that they called the police to escort him from their radio station.

Matt did not bring us the check. What was so surprising about the episode to Gayle and me is that after just two months of being on the supplements, Chris had recognized hypomanic behavior in Matt and shared his own hypomanic experiences with his friend in an effort to help him see reality. Matt had given him the same kind of iconoclastic responses that Chris had once given us, and Chris had held his ground. Chris could easily have swung at Matt's high and outside pitch. He didn't. Maybe we were doing something right. Good eye, Chris.

On November 8, Chris informed me that he was going to discontinue all his meds. We had discussed the pros and cons of this with Tony. I had wanted to keep slowly working down, but Chris decided to proceed on his own, based on the success with the protocol in the double-blind trials. Within two weeks, he was off all medications. He began composing songs again.

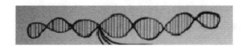

Notes

1. Martin, Russel, Beethoven's Hair, Random House Inc., New York, N.Y. 2000, 234-235.

2. Dietrick, D.E., Schedlowski, M., Bode, L., Ludwig, H., Emrich, H.M., "A viropsycho-immunological disease-model of a subtype affective disorder," *Pharmacopsychiatry*, 31(3):77-82, May 1998.

3. I wrote the proposal after I learned from a county public health employee that the levels of lead in infants in Nevada County were about twice that found in comparable cities in California. I had also learned that the mercury levels in fish in some nearby streams and lakes were unacceptable for human consumption. The mercury was from

gold mining practices in the past as well as current practices. I had been in gold mining stores where I could have bought liquid mercury in order to capture the gold dust in gold pans or sluice boxes. When I found out that money was going to be made available for foster care services for my clients, it seemed only logical to me these children should be screened for heavy metals and then given an opportunity to improve their diet and nutritional intake before they were given drugs.

4. Zilbergeld, Bernie, <u>The New Male Sexuality</u>, Bantam Books, New York, NY, 1992, 71.

18 - Visit to a Parallel Universe

By November 21, 2000, Vice President Al Gore was seeking to divine the will of Florida voters by manually recounting ballots in the most heavily Democratic counties while Governor George W. Bush was challenging the legality of manual hand counts which had the potential to cost him one of the closest elections in American history. All over the country, pundits and citizens alike were wondering, when would enough be enough?

I was asking the same question, blissfully unaware of just how far Chris and I had yet to travel. Chris had been off all psychotropic medications for a week. He had been free of hypomanic, manic or depressive behavior since his discharge. But for me there were still too many unanswered questions. Not expecting to find mainstream doctors able or willing to engage on these topics, I saw no choice but to look elsewhere.

Dr. Bonnie Kaplan refers to the field of alternative medicine as a "parallel universe" to mainstream medicine. This "parallel universe" includes both true paradigm pioneers and charlatans. A fair appraisal of claims demands an open mind and a willingness to research the nontraditional, but mainstream medicine has always had a difficult time distinguishing between the pioneer and the charlatan and tends to see the former as just another instance of the latter. The "gate keepers" of mainstream medicine prefer not to admit the possibility that some alternative medicine approaches might prove to be reliable, safe, and effective.

I was about to enter that parallel universe.

Scouting the terrain

Colleagues at work had warned me that once I started down this path, there could be no telling where I might end up. They were right. For one thing, there was the question of what role, if any, the IgG antibodies played in Chris's illness. Since receiving these test results, I had read a study in which 21 bipolar children were matched for age, race, sex, and socioeconomic status with a control group. The bipolar group had significantly more headaches, allergies, and food sensitivities than did the control group.[1] I also found an article suggesting that allergies can cause depression in some by accentuating cholinergic-adrenergic activity imbalances in the central nervous system.[2]

I called an alternative medicine doctor whose name I had been given, thinking he might refer me to someone who could shed more light on the relation between IgG antibodies and bipolar disorder. He was very helpful over the phone. He provided several references and strongly recommended that I look into the issue of blood pH levels, explaining that a small change in

235

blood pH can lead to a 40% reduction in the ability of the blood to carry oxygen. That sounded important to me, since people with bipolar disorder and major depression have areas of the brain where there is diminished blood flow and low metabolism. The doctor suggested I buy a book called Biobalance, by a Dr. Rudolf Wiley, and referred me to several physicians in Nevada who could help make sense of the "Food-Mood" question. It seemed that many alternative medicine practitioners had moved to Nevada, where the regulatory climate was more favorable to their practices. I asked him if he had heard of the New Century Wellness Center in Reno, and he replied that they had saved a lot of lives and were very competent, though expensive. I made an appointment there for Chris.

I bought and read Dr. Wiley's book. His theory was that persons with acidic blood in their veins were more psychologically vulnerable than those whose blood was slightly alkaline. He stated that the venous pH is the only valid measure of acid/alkaline imbalance, and that the highest and lowest blood pH levels he had ever seen, 7.56 and 7.32, belonged to two individuals who were in mental institutions. He reported that they were both discharged when they achieved the correct biobalance, with a venous pH of approximately 7.46.[3] I did some additional research and learned that the body will do what it can to maintain a critical and narrow pH balance in the blood, even though that may cause other problems.[4]

Dr. Wiley was critical of psychotherapy, which, to be kind, he saw as next to useless. To me, he came across as a crusader more interested in his anti-psychotherapy agenda than in explicating his biobalancing theory. I suspected that he was still hurting from self-inflicted wounds incurred when he'd tried to convince his colleagues at a state hospital of his ideas. I hoped I had not dismissed some good science buried in his book because of his apparent loathing of psychotherapists and the strident nature of his writing. However, his ideas had opened up a new area for exploration that I assumed I could check out with the doctor at New Century.

To complicate matters further, Dr. Ingendaay called and told me that Chris's hair sample had come back with significant levels of mercury and antimony, both heavy metals. I hoped it wasn't enough to make him "mad as a hatter," an expression dating back to 19th century England, where exposure to mercury compounds widely used in the hat-making industry had caused workers to display psychotic symptoms. Perhaps the words "mercurial temperament," derived from the ancient Greek theory of bodily humors, contained a measure of profound simplicity.

Dr. Ingendaay said that she could get us started on a protocol to lower Chris's mercury and antimony levels. Then she drew my attention to Chris's low sulphur values, which, she said, might indicate an amino acid problem. She told me that her contact at the lab had suggested that Chris might need a urine amino acid profile, but that as long as he was taking the supplements, the results would be invalid. Unfortunately, I could not talk to the lab directly, and it seemed as if Dr. Ingendaay wasn't that familiar with the subject. So now we had high levels of IgG antibodies, significant levels of mercury and antimony, and low levels of some sulphur compound ... with Chris having a history of olfactory hallucinations involving the smell of sulphur during his psychotic episodes. How was I to make sense of all this? I didn't think it was a good idea to take him off the supplements just to get a urine amino acid test. And as for the mercury and antimony, I couldn't tell if the results had any clinical significance, because they were just above permissible limits.

On November 29, 2000, Chris accompanied my father and me as we drove to the Reno VA hospital for an appointment. While there, I visited New Century to see if I could change Chris's appointment date, and to scout it out. I was greeted by a large man who resembled a bouncer.

"Can I help you?" he said.

"Yes, I'm here to change an appointment."

"Please proceed to the reception area."

The reception center was two stories high. On the ceiling were two very large round skylights which admitted enough light to give the room a bright, airy feeling even though the sun was obscured by overcast skys. To my right was a large aquarium as tall as it was wide, filled with bright blue, orange, and black fish. Identified by identical purple shirts, staff members bustled about, clearly busy at various tasks. A sign on the second floor referred to New Century Wellness International Research. Upstairs I could see doctors' offices with large picture windows. I felt as if I'd stepped into a spy thriller. I spoke with a clerk and, when asked for my name to reschedule the appointment, restrained myself with some difficulty from replying, "Bond — James Bond."

Back in the parking lot, I noticed a couple walking toward their car.

"Excuse me," I said. "Do you folks have any kind of feel for this place? I've just made an appointment for my son, but I've heard some contradictory reports."

The man spoke. "When we first started coming here, we saw a 20-year-old woman in a wheelchair who had been sent home to die. She had liver cancer. Last time we saw her, her color had improved a lot and she was looking much better."

"Are they helping you?" The man looked very thin.

"Ever heard of scleroderma?"

"Yeah. Matter of fact, I read a case history in their brochure of some patient who had it. She had very high IgG antibodies, just like my son has. I read that her doctor told her there was nothing he could do for her. She came here, and it sounds like she was cured."

"Well, my doctor told me the same thing. He said I have four months to live. My scleroderma moved a lot faster than that lady's did. New Century found I tested positive for Lyme disease, cytomegalovirus, and Epstein-Barr virus. We have the cytomegalovirus under control and are working on the rest now. I'm already feeling a lot better. If you ask me are they helping, I would have to say 'yes.' If you ask me how they're helping, I'm afraid I would have to plead ignorant. When they talk to you, sometimes it sounds like witchcraft. We're trained to understand Western medicine, so when they start talking to us about blockages of energy and electrical circuits in the body, it's a little hard to follow. All I know is that I'm feeling a lot better."

"That's great! Which doctor do you see?"

"Dr. Tang."

"She's the doctor my son is scheduled to see. We're trying to find out if high IgG antibodies to foods could be playing a role in his bipolar disorder."

"She founded the center 18 years ago. Now she's thinking about going into research full time. She has a new drug that helps folks with food antibodies."

"Glad to hear we'll be seeing the founder. Why don't more people know about this place?"

"They don't want the publicity. The AMA has tried to shut them down. They had some test equipment that the police took away because it wasn't approved. The local doctors don't like them taking their patients. Actually, most of their patients are from out of state. We came from Colorado."

"Glad to hear that they're helping you. I can see how they could be considered controversial."

"They try to keep a low profile."

"That reminds me of a doctor named Burzynski in Houston, Texas. He's had phenomenal success treating kids with brain tumors that were 100 percent terminal. A few years ago, the FDA tried to shut him down and put him in jail. He won the suit and now is involved in 73 different FDA-approved trials for all different kinds of cancer."

"We knew someone who went there for a tumor. I don't know about Dr. Burzynski, but New Century has been a godsend for us."

"Thanks for sharing your impressions. I hope things continue to go well for you. Maybe in a few weeks we'll see each other again."

"Good luck with your son."

In anticipation of our appointment at New Century, I wrote a detailed letter to Dr. Tang reviewing Chris's history and our experience with the supplements. Then I wrote a list of specific questions based on what I had learned so far. I asked about the hair analysis results, benefits of fish oil, low sulphur scores, and potential amino acid profile problems. I asked about heavy metals, IgG findings, potential autoimmune problems, food sensitivities, exorphans and their effects on neurotransmitters, benefits of lithium, need for pancreatic digestive enzymes, eating habits, hemoglobin pH, and Synergy supplements for bipolar patients. I didn't want to miss anything.

The vaccination/virus theory

On Wednesday, November 29, Chris and I walked into the cavernous reception area of New Century. Chris filled out a long health history, then underwent a short initial screening interview. From there we went to a room with a microscope and a large video monitor. In walked Dr. Tang, followed by a male colleague, Dr. Oico, and a technician named Terri.

We introduced ourselves and discussed our reasons for being there. I told Dr. Tang about the Synergy supplements and how I believed that taking them was preventing Chris from having further psychotic episodes. Then I reviewed some of the key questions for which I was seeking answers.

She listened attentively, then spoke. "Chris, we need to get your body right so you can go on and live your life. The supplements may be helpful now, but what happens when you become allergic to the vitamins?"

"Allergic to the vitamins?" I responded. "I don't understand."

"Over time, the supplements will not be as useful. I can test him now to see if he's allergic to them."

Time for a credibility check. "Have you had much experience with bipolar patients? How many have you been able to help, and how do you help them?"

"We've seen quite a few. Usually the disorder is a result of the toxic results of DPT or other childhood vaccinations. We can check to see if Chris has high DPT antitoxoid levels. When children grow up, they have their juvenile immune system to protect them, but when they reach about 20, their adult immune system takes over. That's often when you see initial diagnoses of schizophrenia and bipolar illness. The toxic results from early vaccinations begin to have an effect."

"I always wondered why the majority of psychotic breaks occur in the early 20s," I said, trying to maintain a positive ambience. "So how does DPT cause bipolar illness?"

She gave me an article from the *Journal of the American Medical Association* dated 1994, entitled "Adverse Events Associated with Childhood Vaccines Other than Pertussis and Rubella." She showed me a chart of conclusions based on the evidence bearing on causality and stated this as evidence for her theory. I was impressed, but didn't then have time to read the details of the article.[5] Later, when I did read the article, I found it sobering regarding causal relationships between vaccinations and anaphylaxis, death from measles, and death by polio, but there was no specific implication of vaccines in the etiology of bipolar illness.

"The government doesn't want any more claims over adverse effects of vaccinations, so they don't put a lot of resources into it," she said.

"Well, I don't know anything about DPT or MMR, but I believe that Chris would be psychotic if he weren't on the supplements. Just two months ago he was on lithium, Depakote, Wellbutrin, and Zyprexa."

"Doctors usually prescribe medication, then have to treat the results with other medications, but then they don't know if they're treating the illness or the medications prescribed to treat the illness. They treat the symptoms, not the causes. We want to treat the causes."

Now that was something I could agree with. I didn't say anything, but her comment led me to feel we were in the right place. Dr. Tang motioned for the medical technician to prepare for the blood exam.

"Chris, we need a small sample of blood. This will feel like a small prick." The technician stuck his finger and prepared the slide. The video monitor came on.

The dark field microscope: sicker'n a dog

"This is a dark field microscope," Dr. Tang said. "It magnifies the blood 1,000 times."

On the screen were clumps of mostly round cells with white matter flickering between them. There were several large white cells among the others.

Dr. Tang explained what we were seeing. "These large white cells are the lymphocytes. They are involved in the body's defense."

"What are those little things flickering around?" I asked.

"That is waste that the liver hasn't removed yet."

"Is it a problem?"

"For some patients it looks like snow. Now, see the white circles inside some cells? They indicate that the spleen is not doing its job. And these with the dark cells have not been properly cleaned by the liver." I was so curious to know more, I failed to notice that she hadn't answered my question.

"My gosh! What is that thing?" I was looking at a wormlike creature writhing back and forth in the spaces between the cells.

"That is probably a spirochete. Chris might have Lyme disease. We're lucky to be able to see it. Usually, you can't see them in the bloodstream. Lyme disease is now a reportable illness, and it is the third-largest epidemic in this country. It can cause bipolar illness and also cancer. It can cause lesions in the brain such as those found in MS or bipolar illness. See those lines?" She pointed toward some straight, crystal-like images that didn't look like they belonged.

"Yeah."

"Those are called cluster fibrin, and they accumulate from toxic substances such as heavy metals. For example, one can get cadmium into their blood stream from smoking. Now, see these cells with the faint halo around them? These are T-cells that have been knocked out by a virus. We need to find out what kind of virus it is."

Chris spoke up. "I didn't sleep at all last night, Dr. Tang. I either have a bad cold or the flu. I think it's the flu, because my joints are aching. Could that be causing it?"

"You could have a type of herpes virus like Epstein-Barr, cytomegalovirus, herpes simplex, varicella-zoster, or HBLV. We'll see what tests are needed and get back to you in a few minutes, then tomorrow you can see Terri, the technician, who will give your initial feedback." Again, I failed to note that she hadn't answered the question.

Dr. Oico showed us a reprint of a brain scan showing a number of white spots.

"See these scans? If an oncologist saw them, he would say those spots were a tumor. If a neurologist saw it, he would say that the lesions were caused by MS. Actually, this brain contains lesions from Lyme disease." The picture was worth a thousand words, or so it seemed to me.

Witchcraft?

We walked to the lab area. Dr. Tang asked about the supplements Chris was taking. As directed in the welcoming letter, I had brought the pills with me. I gave her two I had in my pocket and showed her the bottle.

"These may work in the short term, but in the long term, as I said before, Chris may become allergic to them. I heard there was a lawsuit over pill casings like this." She took the casings apart, poured the powdered contents into Chris's left hand, and then pinched the casing, creating a cracking sound. "If you can click the casings like this, they have formaldehyde in them. We're going to see if Chris is allergic to the contents of the pills or to the container."

The technician put her left hand on Chris's neck and then stuck her right arm straight out. Dr. Tang grabbed the technician's right arm and pushed down hard, while the technician resisted. Dr. Tang appeared to be putting a lot of energy into pushing the arm down, but she couldn't budge it.

"What are you doing?" I was not hiding my incredulity very well.

"We are checking to see if Chris is allergic to the pills. He's not allergic to the contents, but now let's see if he's allergic to the casings." Dr. Tang turned Chris's hand over, and the powder fell to the floor. She then put the empty casings into his hand. The technician touched Chris's neck again and extended her arm. This time, with what appeared to be moderate effort, Dr.

Tang was able to push the arm down.

I thought I was seeing witchcraft right in front of me. "How does this show anything?"

"This is kinesiology. There is a magnetic field that is disturbed when a person is holding a toxic substance. If the magnetic field is broken by the toxic substance, then I can push her arm down. If it's not broken, then I can't. This is a process that we use a lot here. The vitamins are OK, but he's allergic to the pill casings."

"I just never saw that before. I don't see how that process can possibly show toxic substances." My questions were slowing down a fast and efficient process.

"Even if you're not sure that the casings are toxic, do you want Chris to have to use his own hydrochloric acid to digest these casings when he could take the supplements directly? We have some powder he could mix with the supplement material and then dissolve in a liquid to drink directly. That way he could take the supplements without having to digest the casings."

"I'll look into the issue of formaldehyde and the toxicity of the casings." Actually, I wanted to say something more like, "What the hell is going on here? Sounds like you're setting up a situation to peddle your powder." I thought it, but didn't say it. Probably should have.

My uneasiness about New Century was increasing exponentially. During the dark field microscope exam, while I didn't like or fully understand what we were seeing, I believed I was getting a glimpse into an alien world that might shed some light on the mysteries I was seeking to uncover. When we walked out of the office into the lab, my mind was reeling with possibilities. Maybe Chris's liver wasn't processing the waste well enough. Maybe he had clumped blood cells from dehydration, or, even worse, maybe his spleen or his liver wasn't filtering his blood properly. And what about the blood cells that were not perfectly round, and the T-cells with a "halo" that were allegedly moribund from some virus? And what about the cluster fibrin that showed chemical contamination? And the wormlike spirochetes that were suggestive of Lyme disease? Even though correlation did not necessarily mean causation, the suggestion of Lyme disease along with all the other unexplainable findings like his high IgG scores was puzzling. I had come with a long list of questions. Dr. Tang was not answering them. She was adding more.

The staff left to figure out which lab tests they were going to recommend. Chris and I had a few minutes alone.

"This place is a waste of time," he said. "They don't know what they're talking about."

"I admit the kinesiology left me cold. I felt like I was watching a religious ritual. When they put their hands on you, I was expecting some sort of prayer or incantation."

"This trip was a waste."

"Sounds pretty weird to me, but we can check out their claims. I was impressed with the images of the blood. That wormlike thing was pretty scary."

Who can we trust?

The lab technician returned with a list of recommended tests. There was a standard blood panel for $95, a viral panel for $325, a Lyme Disease antibody Western Blot for $155, a chemical sensitivity blood test for $500, a toxic elements urine for $100, a Lyme antigen test for $110, and a vaccination panel for $450. The total was more than $1,700. It was time to put up or shut up. I crossed out the viral panel, figuring that since Chris already had some sort of viral infection, that test could wait. On the vaccination panel, I crossed out all but the DPT test, since, based on Dr. Tang's comments, that seemed to offer the most promise for a bipolar connection. I authorized all the rest. If it cost this much for a diagnosis, I wondered how much it would cost for treatment?

They took Chris's blood and urine. I paid the bill, about $1,400. As we were leaving, I happened to see the man from Colorado with prostate cancer whom I had questioned on my first visit. I shared with him my skepticism about kinesiology. He said that he'd felt the same way at first, but then he'd secretly "doctored" a pill casing with a substance he knew he was allergic to and had the staff test it for him using kinesiology. The staff member's arm dropped, and, from that moment, the man was a believer.

I wasn't entirely satisfied with his answer, so I turned to a young mother who happened to be nearby in the reception area and had overheard our discussion. "What do you think?"

"I used to think the same as you, but then I started doing it with my daughter, and I can now tell if a medication is good for her or not by using the technique."

"How did you learn this?"

"I watched what the staff was doing and practiced it."

"And is the clinic helping your daughter?"

"She has only one kidney, and the doctors wanted to operate again, but with the treatment here, she's doing a lot better, and we haven't had to have the operation."

I turned back to the man with the prostate cancer, who, I remembered, had also been diagnosed with Lyme disease. "So what happens if they find he has Lyme disease? What might they recommend?"

"They use a hyperbaric chamber to force the spirochetes out of the tissue and into the bloodstream, where they are killed by some substance they add. I don't believe it's an antibiotic."

243

"And about how much would that cost?"

"It would depend on how bad the Lyme is. It might take a few months and about $20,000-$30,000."

"Would he have to live here for the treatments?"

"Often they want to treat him every day for a period of time."

"And still there is no assurance of a cure?"

"When the doctors at the Mayo Clinic told me I had two years to live, they were basing it on my cancer only. They didn't diagnose the Lyme disease. I used to run my tractor on my farm and wake up from seizures from the Lyme. About a year ago, I saw another doctor who told me I had four months to live. This treatment has bought me more time."

As we drove back to the hotel, I thought about our experience. On the one hand, it appeared we were on a wild-goose chase, and an expensive one at that. On the other, perhaps the lab results would give us some answers.

The next morning, Terri, the medical technician, showed us the initial blood results. They indicated an abnormally low level of lymphocytes and a high level of segmented neutrophils. Very generally speaking, lymphocytes are white blood cells that recognize and respond to foreign substances in the body and blood, such as viruses and bacteria. Neutrophils, like macrophages, gobble these invaders up. So, Chris had a low white blood cell count. He could have gotten the same from Zyprexa, which is known for causing, among other things, leukopenia, an abnormal decrease in the number of white blood cells.

Terri explained the findings. "This means that Chris is low on killer, helper, and suppressor lymphocytes. His immune system isn't functioning like it should. It looks like Chris is using up his lymphocytes fighting off everything that he's allergic to. We don't know what to recommend yet because all the results aren't in. You might want to have a test done to see if he has toxoplasmosis, and you could also give him an EEG to determine how his brain is functioning. That would be a lot cheaper than a brain scan."

Chris had already tuned out, having convinced himself that the trip was a waste of time and money, and the staff at New Century didn't know what they were talking about. I hadn't totally tuned out, but I was confused.

On our way home, I mulled over additional questions. I thought of Dr. Fudenberg's research on vaccines and antibodies. If Chris's diphtheria antitoxoid levels were higher than they should have been, that would suggest, at least theoretically, the possibility of impairment in the production of phosphosulfotransferase, resulting in inadequate digestion and excessive antigen-antibody complexes. Inadequate digestion could cause a depletion of tryptophan and other widget precursors. The antigen-antibody complexes allegedly could cause cognitive dysfunction. When Dr. Ingendaay said that someone at Great Smokies Diagnostic Laboratories thought a "sulphur amino acid problem" might exist, was that the same as a deficit in the liver enzyme phosphosulfotransferase? Perhaps there was something to this after all. But other things about New Century bothered me.

Why didn't Dr. Tang answer my and Chris's questions? Why didn't she express any curiosity about the supplements? Based on Chris's history of psychoses when coming off the medications and his hypomanic behavior while on the medications, I had no doubt the supplements were working. I also wondered why I'd felt so rushed, why I'd felt that I couldn't share my views when I heard things I didn't agree with or understand. Had I been in a cult or a medical office, or both? Moving from office to office, waiting alone for the next process, was not unlike what I had experienced during the purchase of our last car. After an interminable period of negotiation, the salesman had moved us from room to room while plugging various features no self-respecting car buyer would ever turn down.

There was a social psychologist named Festinger whose work on cognitive dissonance I remembered from college. He pointed out that there is an innate human desire for our beliefs to be consonant, not dissonant. Experimental volunteers who get more money for doing boring tasks say it is boring while those getting a pittance for the same tasks say it is interesting. They resolve the cognitive dissonance of getting paid next to nothing for doing a task that wastes their time by saying the experiment was worthwhile. The well-paid group sees the experiment as it was, a boring waste of time. They didn't need to justify it because they got paid handsomely for doing it. A corollary of Festinger's theory is that those who have a painful experience value the experience more than those whose experiences are less painful. People love what they suffer for.

Here is an example, of which there are many. A cult leader predicts the end of the world. The members sell all they have and show up to meet the messiah, alien, or whomever is going to take them away. The deliverer doesn't show. At this point the believers can decide if they were right or wrong. Cognitive dissonance theory predicts, as does experience, that the believers decide their deliverer has given the world a second chance to come to the "truth." The deliverer's no-show at the appointed time simply "proves" the truth of their ideas. The members begin a public campaign to convert others since the deliverer has given them a second chance to save the world. The cost associated with the disappointment, in this case selling one's wordly goods and finding no "end of the world," forces the cult members to deal with their cognitive dissonance by declaring that the world has been saved from destruction and the believers have a second chance to save the world. Had Dr. Tang's "believers" spent so much money that cognitive dissonance compelled them to alter their belief systems and praise the staff at New Century — for many, their last hope?

I thought about a time 25 years earlier when we were visiting my mother and stepfather in Fresno. My mom told me that her neighbor had cured herself of some serious, often-fatal disease and now was learning about iridology, a method of diagnosing one's health based on a very close examination of the eye. I saw the neighbor socially, and our conversation drifted to her work with this new technique. I didn't tell her that I thought her newly found beliefs were out in left field, but I did share my curiosity and asked if she would read my eyes. She invited me over, sat me down, and placed a huge magnifying mirror in front of my eyeball. While she divined that my adrenals were weak, that I had an infection, and that my heart might need some checking out, I was looking at my own giant eyeball staring back at me. It seemed like a coincidence that I happened to have a touch of ringworm on my arm. She recommended that I get an EKG to make sure my heart was all right. I thanked her, went home, and told my family about the woman and her weird eye mirror. However, I wasn't laughing quite so hard when, shortly thereafter, I began experiencing heart pain while jogging, so much so that I finally obtained an EKG just to be on the safe side. It was normal. After the EKG I had no further heart pain.

At that time, I had deduced that Milton Erickson's Utilization Theory of Hypnosis might provide a way to understand what had happened. I recalled from workshops I had attended that people are put into a state of hypnotic suggestibility when a novel event occurs for which they have no reference point. Even though my conscious mind was skeptical, and I was submitting myself to the procedure strictly out of curiosity, the novelty of the experience, the surreal appearance of the "eye," and the coincidental existence of an "infection" had combined to put me into a state of hypnotic suggestibility. When my neighbor suggested that I have an EKG, I was unconsciously susceptible to the message and had subsequently developed pain upon jogging, a sort of inadvertent post-hypnotic suggestion. Taking the EKG convinced me that I had no problem, and the pain ceased.

Maybe the novel experience of seeing dark field microscope pictures put patients into a state of hypnotic suggestibility. And when they experienced the pain of paying the bill, even more painful because the health insurance industry does not recognize the existence of the parallel universe of alternative medicine, and often does not cover its treatments, their cognitive dissonance compelled them to conclude it was all worth it.

I wasn't paranoid enough to think that the patients were planted there to lure in unbelievers. I wasn't naïve enough to accept the efficacy of witchcraft. So that was the best I could come up with. If we had spent $30,000 to cure Chris of Lyme disease, I expect I would have had no doubt but that the treatment would have been successful. Any evidence to the contrary would have to have been dismissed. Cognitive dissonance would have compelled us to believe in that for which we had financially suffered.

The first thing I did upon returning home was log onto the Internet. I found several sites reporting that there was no scientific basis to kinesiology. And, by the way, the sites also stated that there was no scientific basis to iridology, which it lumped in with such well-known debunked pseudo-sciences as phrenology (diagnosis by skull characteristics). Multiple references were included. Based on the kinesiology as we experienced it at New Century and on my Internet research, I was not impressed. Did that mean the entire New Century operation was flawed, or just that there were areas in which they were overzealous? The doubt caused by the "witchcraft" led Chris and me to be skeptical about the entire operation. While they had opened up new areas for inquiry, they had also raised credibility issues with us. Chris was ready to throw the baby out with the bath water. I wasn't so sure. They might have opened up fruitful areas in spite of themselves. Amidst all the "witchcraft," New Century may have pointed us in some useful directions. At least they were open to new directions, even though I never got my prepared questions answered.

A week later, New Century faxed the lab results. The Western Blot, with 4½ bands, was strongly indicative of Lyme disease. The ELISA/ACT Lymphocyte Response Assay Results showed strong reactions to aldrin, an organochlorine pesticide; endrin, another organochlorine pesticide; and moderate reactions to xylene, a chemical produced from petroleum; carbon tetrachloride, a chemical found in cleaning fluid and pesticides, among other things; and polysorbate 60, a food additive found in pressurized whipping cream. As I understood it, according to the lab results, Chris was sensitive to all these substances which had at one time or another flowed around in his bloodstream.

In <u>Depression, Cured at Last!</u> by Dr. Sherry Rogers, I had read that there are about 500 chemicals that the average person is exposed to in the home, and the same number in the average municipal water supply. I learned that a rat died after spending the night in a jar with a new piece of carpet. I learned that the body uses up nutrients, particularly choline, in the process of detoxifying chemicals, and that nutritional depletion caused by the constant attempts of the body to detoxify can cause depression.[6] What price was Chris's body paying for trying to cleanse itself of these contaminants?

Contrary to the hair analysis results we obtained through Great Smokies Diagnostic Laboratories, New Century did not find any antimony or mercury in Chris's blood. The results stated that Chris' DPT antitoxoid was 10 times what it should have been, lending support to Dr. Tang's hypothesis that antibodies to DPT may have been playing a role in Chris's bipolar illness. The only problem was that I could find no references to DPT antitoxoid on the Internet, and I didn't really know what it was or if it existed. If it did, then

Chris carried too much of whatever substance obliterated DPT microbes.

To summarize, New Century had answered none of my questions. They had simply raised new ones. I could toss out the kinesiology findings, but the rest of the data, obtained from independent laboratories, raised all kinds of troubling unanswered questions.

A nutritionist's perspective

Shortly after this trip, I was invited to attend a lecture by a visiting nutritionist at the home of a friend. All I needed was more information to confuse me! I was beginning to see the psychological advantages of having only one paradigm, whether it worked or not. At least it controlled the anxiety. But this lecture on nutrition had one thing to recommend it. It wouldn't cost 1400 dollars. It was free. I invited Chris, but he said he was tired of hearing me talk about bipolar illness, allergies, heavy metals, and so on. I asked Gayle to join me instead. She wasn't eager either, and for the same reasons. Yet she would need to be involved if we decided to implement any additional nutritional or dietary plan in Chris's treatment.

The speaker was Glenn Foster, a certified nutritionist and representative of a company called GNLD that made and distributed various health products. He had come to talk about his products. I was prepared to sit through a sales pitch in hopes that he might touch on issues more relevant to our situation. As he was introducing himself, he said something that made my heart feel good. He explained how he had become convinced of the efficacy of nutrition in treating mental illness. After his sister was hospitalized with schizophrenia ten years earlier, he had given her quality nutritional supplements. Her schizophrenia symptoms never returned. I glanced at Gayle, and our eyes met. This was where we needed to be.

One product Mr. Foster was promoting was called Tre-en-en, a grain oil that he said supported adrenal functioning. He said that adrenal weakness is associated with allergies and that vital nutrients in wheat and rice have been removed by modern grain processing. The Tre-en-en grain oils restore those same nutrients and reestablish hormone levels. The product was initially developed in response to chronic fatigue among patients at a hospital in California, including some from the Hollywood set in the 1940s and 1950s. The first person to purchase this product when it became available commercially allegedly experienced a remarkable remission of symptoms of rheumatoid arthritis after years of trying other supplements which had done little to improve the situation. Mr. Foster said that the founder of the company had bought the rights to the oil after its developer had failed to commercialize it. The founder believed in it because it had cured his wife of Lupus. Mr. Foster told a dramatic story about another patient he knew who had been cured of

248

rheumatoid arthritis by taking the grain oil along with salmon oil tablets.

He had some very interesting ideas that were new to me. For example, he said that individuals with inadequately functioning adrenal glands frequently have the following symptoms: fatigue; anxiety and irritability; sensitivity to bright light; salt and sugar craving; nose and eye wrinkles; puffy eyes; contact dermatitis; and a pulse of 84 after a meal. He claimed that Tre-en-en helped to reduce allergies and associated symptoms. Then he talked about other physical signs that can be indicative of systemic problems secondary to nutrition and allergies.

The man was a walking health encyclopedia, citing one study after another. High levels of estrogen and insulin were associated with heart disease. Dehydration facilitates deposits of cholesterol. Dandruff can indicate inadequate fatty acids, B, zinc, and selenium. Bumps on the back of the arm can indicate inadequate zinc. Skin tags are diagnostic of subsequent diabetes about 70% of the time. Calluses in the middle of the hands and fat above the waist can indicate diabetes. White under the eyes was diagnostic of adrenal gland exhaustion, which he called the san paku phenomenon. I found his central tenet, that one could make reasonable hypotheses about a person's health just by looking closely at his or her face and body, to be fascinating.

On the way out, I discussed our situation with him. He suggested that the Tre-en-en might help Chris with his food allergies. From his talk, I had learned that allergies were related to adrenal exhaustion. "Adrenal exhaustion" sounded pretty nonspecific to me, one of those terms from the parallel universe that I had heard and derided before. After all, it was my old neighbor who had said I had "weak adrenals" based on my eyeball, of all things. Even so, it was an interesting concept, particularly the san paku angle. When we got home, I went through some old family pictures of Aunt Harriet, both

as young girl and as a bride. I compared them with her sisters. There was white between her iris and her lower eyelid. The white was more pronounced in her wedding picture. I looked at Chris's senior high school picture. Unlike pictures of the rest of us, there was a slightly exposed white under his left

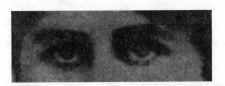

Harriet's Mangram's eyes - san paku?

eye. I told Chris what I had learned. He wasn't interested in either Tre-en-en or san paku. I later bought some Tre-en-en anyway.

Back to the net again

It was time to go back to the Internet to see if I could find data that would corroborate the central role played by the adrenal glands in depression.

In a paper presented at the 27th Anniversary Program of the American Society of Ophthalmologic and Otolaryngologic Allergy in October of 1969 in Chicago, endocrinologist Dr. John Tintera reported that patients had roughly 100,000 times more acute olfactory sensitivity if they had adrenal insufficiency compared to normal subjects.[7] Wow, that could explain Chris's sensitivity to taste and smells!

> *I'm an endocrinologist. In more than twenty years of a busy practice with thousands of patients, I've yet to work with an allergic person whose troubles weren't basically due to his poorly functioning adrenals, or who wasn't relieved of all his allergic woes when his adrenals were put into proper working order. Included among these patients were sufferers from asthma as well as from hay fever, people sensitive to beef protein as well as house dusts or tomatoes or parsnips.[8]*

Incidentally, Dr. Tintera treated all allergies with an injection of an extract of beef adrenals to replenish the adrenal hormones. He did not treat specific allergies because his research demonstrated that the problem was in the adrenal glands.

Also from the Web I learned that san paku is an expression used by adherents of Zen Buddhist Macrobiotics. It is considered a "yin" condition and is considered to be very dangerous. Citing a study without references, the author of the site, Sian Leitch, claimed that as many as 60% of people who died violently were san paku near the time of death.[9]

I found three referenced articles that provided some clues about the connection between adrenal gland functioning and depression. Depressed patients were found to have enlarged adrenal glands.[10] In another study, the average adrenal volume in depressed patients was 38% larger than the volume in a controlled group.[11]

A third article, based on the research of Dr. Ian Goodyer and others from the University of Cambridge in England, reported that specific psychoendocrine factors predicted a subgroup of adolescents who would develop major depression. They assessed the role of cortisol and dehydroepiandrosterone (DHEA) levels in a group of adolescents considered to be at a high risk for depression. They found that 18% of the subjects had an episode of major depression during the study. While stating that the risk may be of genetic and/or earlier psychosocial origin, the authors concluded that psychoendocrine factors were actually involved in triggering the depression. They wrote as follows:

> *Major depression was predicted for both genders by the ad-*

ditive effects of: higher depressive symptoms; personal dis-
appointments and losses only in the month before onset; one
or more daily levels of cortisol at 8 a.m. or DHEA at 8 p.m.
greater than the 80th percentile of the daily mean.... The
findings in this paper suggest a putative causal role for cor-
tisol and DHEA that is not a consequence of highly proxi-
mal recent life events or subclinical depressive symptoms.[11]

Putative is one of those words that experts in medicine use frequently. It essentially means "generally considered or deemed such." Therefore, they generally consider that cortisol and DHEA play a causal role in depression.

So which comes first, the chicken or the egg? Thinking anxious thoughts creates the fight/flight stress response and initiates cortisol release. However, the 82% who did not develop major depression also had a lot to worry about. They were selected for the study based on high risk factors such as losses, family problems, and stressful life events. Even though they had significant worries, they didn't have high levels of cortisol in the morning or DHEA in the evening, and they didn't have major depression. It looked like the stress that mattered had more to do with what was happening inside their bodies than in their environment.

Could inflammatory processes from excessive cortisol or other biological stresses cause an increase in the size of the glands? Once again, I was getting in over my head. I wasn't trying to become a doctor. I just wanted to know how to help keep my son from becoming psychotic again.

By the end of December, my head was swimming with concepts that somehow seemed related to Chris's illness. Adrenal gland anomalies; inflammation; food sensitivities; gluten and casein fragments mimicking endorphins (exorphins); neurotoxins; Lyme disease; heavy metals like mercury and antimony; chemicals; and insecticides ... and somehow I felt I had only scratched the surface. Where was it all going to end? How to separate the wheat from the chaff? Who could we trust? Not only was I getting dizzy, but my family was getting tired of the bipolar theory of the week from me.

It was time for another appointment with Dr. Ingendaay. I prepared by making a notebook of the myriad of lab and research data obtained thus far. When we saw her, she said that she too was overwhelmed by all the data I had accumulated. She recommended that we find a specialist in Lyme disease and make that our first priority. She talked about using colloidal silver (a solution of silver ions in water). Colloidal silver had been used before the advent of antibiotics to fight off bacterial infection, much as mercury had been used in Europe during Beethoven's day. I shared my concerns, having read of some cases where the colloidal silver turned the skin blue permanently. She said that had been a problem but wasn't as much of one now as the concentrations were lower. My research on Lyme disease had been very sobering, suggesting that in its late stages, the disease is often chronic. We discussed whether we could even trust the lab work at New Century given the kinesiology fiasco. She was pleased to see that Chris was on a stable emotional footing but felt she had no more to offer us at that time. When I got home, I started searching for a doctor with Lyme disease credentials.

I contacted Glenn Foster. He said that he did not treat Lyme disease, because that required a physician. However, he could give some recommendations for Chris to strengthen his immune system. I trusted Glenn's integrity. Among other things, besides having a comprehensive grasp of the field of nutrition and helping his sister to overcome the symptoms of schizophrenia, I had learned from listening to one of his tapes that he was an alumni of Westmont College, my alma mater. We made an appointment. He recommended buffered vitamin C, lipoic acid, coenzyme Q10, vitamin E, omega-3 salmon oil, and carotenoid complex, all of which I bought for about $200, enough for one month. He didn't say these supplements would be curative, but he did say that some people get Lyme disease and never have a problem because their immune systems combat it successfully. When I told Glen about our dark field microscope experience, he said that he had read some research suggesting that some who use dark field microscopes do so as a way to get patients to pay for unneeded treatments.

Chris did not want to take the immune-strengthening regimen because he maintained he didn't have Lyme disease. He did not have the classic symptoms such as the initial rash or joint pain. He said he was willing to take it if we came up with a definitive diagnosis. Of interest to me is that the first symptom he reported was being unable to talk to his girlfriend and his friends. He felt "empty." That could have been depression, or it could have been word-finding problems, a symptom of neuro-Lyme disease.

Members of a local Lyme disease support group recommended a Dr. Raphael Stricker in San Francisco, a hematologist who happened to be one of the foremost Lyme disease authorities in California. They told me that the Western Blot ordered by New Century did not examine enough bands, and that the Lyme Urine Antigen Test (LUAT) had not been administered correctly. They said the LUAT was meaningless unless it was administered daily after a period of treatment with antibiotics. One person suggested, and the rest agreed, that IgeneX in Palo Alto was the best place to be tested for Lyme. They also said that all the Lyme patients they knew who had been to New Century had allegedly seen spirochetes on the dark field microscope, an interesting "coincidence" given the supposed rarity of such sightings in the blood. Another member confirmed what Glen Foster had already told me: namely, that there were studies showing that the use of the dark field microscope was associated with excessive unneeded treatments, and that the blood of some patients had been contaminated with pond water in order to convince them of the seriousness of their supposed conditions. My informants were impugning the integrity of dark field microscopy and, by inference, New Century. In the unchartered territory of the parallel universe, the line between a paradigm pioneer and charlatan was hard to find.

Meanwhile, back at the ranch

At work, I continued going through the motions. In December, I happened to meet one of the mental health professionals from Behavioral Health Services during the intermission to "Christmas in Wales" in Nevada City. At work, we had passed in the hall but had never exchanged more than a few words. This time we spoke quite a bit, sharing our impressions of working at Behavioral Health Services. I expressed my frustration over the resistance to new ideas. Having been in charge of mental health clinics in the Air Force, it was frustrating for me to be starting at the bottom, feeling I couldn't do much to improve services for our clients.

I shared my frustration with the documentation process. We had just completed a very time-consuming audit of records to ensure that data put in different places was consistent. I had written software so that all the data was accessible from one database. It wasn't complicated, and it prevented the need to fix problems found in audits. However, I had been informed that a system called Hal, developed by a husband of a former employee, was the system we would be using. Hal didn't integrate the data. On a good day, a day when Hal was working, the user had to remember to input much of the same data on paper products as was inputted into Hal. Therefore, costly audits were needed to fix human errors. I told him of my frustration in trying to get folks to see the advantages of using my system, which I was prepared to make available for free. With my software, all the data was stored in the same database and could be printed to different forms.

He was very verbal in describing what he saw as problems in the organization. "We're just waiting for a lawsuit," he told me. "There will be some bad outcome, and the cards are going to fall."

"What do you mean?" I asked.

"We're not providing the support we should to our clients. They're not being managed properly. We need to be spending more resources to track our high-risk adults."

He also talked about a former staff psychiatrist who had killed himself several months before I started working there. I was amazed that I hadn't heard of it sooner.

"What kind of place is it where it takes me 9 months to learn of an event of that magnitude?" I asked.

I had issues closer to my heart than software but chose not to discuss them. Computers I could talk about. Nutrition? Well, that was a little on the fringe side. I was tempted to talk about my concerns about not properly assessing kids for food sensitivities and heavy metal poisoning before putting them on drugs, but I figured it was probably better if I didn't get started. He was talking about something else anyway, inadequate supervision of high-risk clients. I was surprised by his candor.

Even though I restrained myself, I had been thinking a lot about my increasing frustration. Seeing Chris get better while my clients continued their downward spiral was putting me into an impossible position. My research was suggesting that major innovation was needed. I couldn't help a client without a relationship, and I couldn't establish a relationship when the client was so oppositional that he wouldn't even get out of the car to see me. Neither could I establish a relationship with the client was so distracted that he couldn't focus on any subject long enough to talk to me about it. When I had shared some of the practice implications from my research with the staff, such as Dr. Stoll's work at Harvard using omega-3 fatty acids with bipolar patients, I had gone out on a limb. My supervisor told me that I could be sued if I shared information about nutrition and a parent tried it and had bad results. I said that if I shared research with parents, they would be able to access the research and make their own judgments. Their self-determination would be enhanced.

I knew my chances of moving up the ladder in the organization were poor. I didn't see much of a future with the county, not unless I was willing to ignore what I had been learning and continue doing more of the same. That option assured me a steady paycheck, but it didn't help my high-risk clients.

I enjoyed collaborating with my fellow mental health professionals. When I talked to them alone, they told me of their experiences utilizing alternative approaches for their own health. The diversity was amazing. One took shark cartilage for cancer. One stimulated pressure points for relief of headaches and anxiety. One used breath work. One put his special needs child on nutritional supplements. One stayed on a special low sugar diet. One had mercury removed from her mouth. Few felt comfortable enough to share information outside the scope of care defined by their respective professions. Those that did share their information with clients did so behind closed doors and they made a point not to document their conversation.

If I had shared with county officials the studies in Werback's book demonstrating that phosphorus found in soft drinks and processed foods such as puddings increases aggressiveness in vulnerable children, I would have been criticized for wandering outside my area of expertise. Any attempt to address the proliferation of soft drink machines in the schools would have fallen on deaf ears: schools made too much money from the vending machines to consider removing them. Nor would there be interest in the numerous studies on the behavioral effects of low fatty acids and low zinc. If I had even suggested that deficiencies in zinc, lithium, and magnesium, as well as excesses in phosphorus from soft drinks and processed foods, may play a significant role in violent behavior, my credibility as a professional, such as it was, would have been lost. And if I'd suggested that the juvenile hall provide trace amounts of magnesium and lithium to incarcerated youths lacking these minerals, or that clients be given elimination diets before being treated with medications, or that clients receive the Synergy supplements, I would have been asked, and perhaps none too politely, to leave. There was no way for patients to learn these crucial facts from those who were supposed to be there to help them. The county wanted me to catch alligators. I wanted to drain the swamp.

Near the end of December, I was feeling thinly stretched between making and keeping appointments for Chris and Ray from San Francisco to Reno, working with my clients and their families, and researching this book. I had no more time off for medical appointments. My supervisor wanted me to return to full-time status. I was concerned about neglecting other tasks I had prioritized. In addition to the fact that I was spread so thin, the main issue I was wrestling with was my inability to reconcile what I believed we should be doing for our clients with what we actually were doing to them. We were doing more of the same and getting more of the same. Been there. Done that. It was time for me and the county to part, and so we did.

It had been difficult for me to work in a system that was not open to innovation. My own experiences with Chris and the information I was learning about bipolar illness and ADHD made it more difficult for me to be content with more of the same. My disagreement was not with my fellow mental health professionals. It was with the county system and the systems that had shaped all of us. These systems did what systems do best. They reward the behaviors that support the status quo and extinguish those that don't. We needed to be free to design creative interventions, not to spend so much time and energy addressing internal organizational needs. Of all the clients who needed innovative solutions, the high-risk kids of Nevada County needed them the most. And they weren't getting them. I left at an opportune time.

Murder at mental health

Almost three weeks after I left, an adult patient ran amok at Behavioral Health. He walked into the waiting room and shot and killed a grandmother and a staff member, Laura Wilcox. Laura was a college student who had gone to Nevada Union High School with my son, Thomas. She was one of the valedictorians, a bright and very friendly young woman who had a promising future. The patient severely wounded another staff member with whom

I had worked. He then drove to the local Lyon's restaurant, where he killed a newly hired manager and wounded an employee. He allegedly was unhappy with his mental health care and thought the restaurant was poisoning him. I would have been in the building at that time attending a meeting had I still been working there. The next day, the following article appeared in the *Nevada Union*, our local paper:

> *The Associated Press*
> *Jan 11 2001 5:41a.m.*
> *NEVADA CITY, Calif. (AP) - A man accused of killing three people and wounding two others at a county office and restaurant surrendered peacefully after his brother, a police officer, turned him in.*
>
> *Scott Harlan Thorpe, 40, allegedly walked into the county social services building with a handgun Wednesday and shot three people, two fatally. He then went to a restaurant less than two miles away and killed the manager and wounded a cook, Nevada County Sheriff Keith Royal said.*
>
> *Thorpe was unhappy with the mental-health care he received at the county clinic and believed the restaurant was poisoning him, his brother, Kent Thorpe, told authorities.*
>
> *The Sacramento police officer turned Thorpe in after authorities launched a manhunt. He surrendered following two hours of telephone negotiations.*
>
> *The day's events stunned residents in Nevada City, a town of about 3,000 in a rural area in the Sierra Nevada foothills, about 50 miles north of Sacramento.*
>
> *"It is a dark day for our county," county board Chairwoman Elizabeth Martin said. "I'm here to express our deep grief and horror at this loss to our community and offer our condolences to the families."*[13]

The anxiety of the mental health professional I had spoken with during the intermission of "Christmas in Wales" was based on more than a "gut" feeling. His prediction had been uncannily accurate. He had sensed that a patient was going to do something that would bring discredit to Behavioral Health. He didn't think that his patient would be the one doing it nor did he think that he, along with the county, would be the one sued.

Having served in the Air Force for 28 years, I had seen tragedies of similar magnitude. There was the well-publicized incident in which a patient, Dean Mellberg, killed four and wounded 23 at Fairchild Air Force Base. There were private tragedies of murder and suicide that didn't make the front pages. I knew how easy it was to have hindsight through "Monday morning quarterbacking." Still, I wondered what had caused Scott Thorpe's brain to transform him from a patient into a murderer. Had I still believed that each person created his own world, I would have argued that Scott Thorpe chose to deal with his illness by murder. Seeing my own son overwhelmed with homicidal and suicidal "demons" had shaken the foundation of my "you-are-responsible-for-yourself" philosophy. Now I had a different perspective.

What would have happened if Scott Thorpe had taken trace amounts of lithium or magnesium in his drinking water? Could this tragedy have been averted if he had taken nutritional supplements? Would he have run amok if his brain had received proper nutrition? Would he have kept a better hold on reality if he hadn't been exposed to neuropeptides from gluten and casein? What would have happened if he had undergone kidney dialysis to reduce hyperpolypeptiduria?

I knew nothing about the case except that a schizophrenic patient had killed some people, some of whom I knew. Nonetheless, based on what I was learning, besides whatever other factors predisposed him to this act, maybe, just maybe, Scott Thorpe was right. Maybe the restaurant *was* poisoning him — with gluten and casein. Maybe Scott Thorpe was poisoning himself — with gluten and casein.

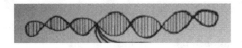

Notes

1. Younes, R.P., Delong, G.R., Neiman, G., Rosner, B., "Manic-depressive illness in children: treatment with lithium carbonate," *Journal of Child Neurology*, 1(4):364-8, October 1986.
2. Marshall, P.S., "Allergy and depression: a neurochemical threshold," *Psychol Bull*, 113(1):23-43, January 1993.
3. Wiley, Rudolf, A., Biobalence, The Acid/Alkaline Solution to the Food-Mood-Health Puzzle, Essential Science Publishing, Hurricane Utah, 1989, 14.
4. Allocca, John A., Clinical Nutrition for the Balanced Body, 2nd edition, Allocca Biotechnology, Inc, Northport, N.Y., 2000, revised 3/29/01, Chapter 18. http://www.allocca.com/1start.htm
5. Stratton, K. R., Howe, C.J., Johnson, R.B., "Adverse Events Associated with Childhood Vaccines Other than Pertussis and Rubella," *JAMA*, 271:1602-1606, 1994.
6. Rogers, Sherry, Depression Cured At Last!, SK Publishing, Sarasota Florida, 1997, 113-119.

7. Henkin, R.I., Gill, J.R., Bartter, F.C., "Study in taste thresholds in normal man - patient with adrenal cortical insufficiency; the role of adrenal cortical steroids and of serum sodium concentration," *Journal of Clinical Investigation,* 42:727-735, 1963.

8. Tintera, John, in "Chronic Fatigue Unmasked 2000: Chapter Two History of CFS." http://www.chronicfatigue.org/Chap%202%202000.html

9. The author includes several qualifications stating that he is only sharing his own ideas. After September 11, I was surprised to see that at least four of the terrorists, including their ringleader, Mohammed Atta, demonstrated very clear indications of san paku in their photos.

Leitch, Sian, "Strange Facts About Krishnamurti," January 1, 21308. http://www.sleitch.nildram.co.uk/kfacts.html

10. Dr. Dumser and others analyzed the weight of adrenal glands in 42 suicide and 37 control cases. The researchers found the following: "Relative combined adrenal weight (weight/body surface) >6 g/m2 may be a morphologic sign of a depressive disorder prior to death if no other disease with a known effect on the adrenals is present. These results are consistent with clinical computed tomographic findings of enlarged adrenals in depressed patients."

Dumser, T., Barocka, A., Schubert, E., "Weight of adrenal glands may be increased in persons who commit suicide," *Am J Forensic Med Pathol,* 19(1):72-6 March 1998.

11. This study looked at adrenal gland volume and both base line and stimulated pituitary and adrenal cortical hormones in 35 unmedicated major depressives and 35 individually matched normal control subjects. The average adrenal volume in the depressives was 38% larger than the adrenal volume of their matched controls. Basal plasma adrenocorticotropic hormone (ACTH) 1-39, a specific kind of ACTH, was significantly lower in depressed patients while basal plasma cortisol was significantly higher in the same group. Overall ACTH was not different between the groups. In addition, there was a positive correlation between adrenal volume and the somatization factor of the Hamilton Depression Scale, which was accounted for by the specific symptoms of somatic symptoms and somatic anxiety.

Rubin, R.T., Phillips, J.J., McCracken, J.T., Sadow, T.F., "Adrenal gland volume in major depression: relationship to basal and stimulated pituitary-adrenal cortical axis function," *Biol Psychiatry,* 40(2):89-97, July 15, 1996.

12. Goodyer, Ian M., et al., "Some adolescents may carry a physiologic risk for major depression," *Br J Psychiatry,* 177:499-504, 2000.

13. The Associated Press, "Calif. Shootings Suspect Arrested," Jan 11, 2001.

19 - Cytokines – Too Much of a Good Thing?

My father, diagnosed and treated in accordance with the prevailing paradigms of mental health care, had been in and out of hospitals and jails throughout his life. The same paradigms had seen my son hospitalized four times for psychotic mania or depression. At different times, both of their brains were so broken that my father said he didn't know who I was, while my son said that he was not only my father, but God. Before I was hired to work at Nevada County Behavioral Health Services, a psychiatrist employed there killed himself. After I left, a patient from the agency killed a co-worker, a grandmother, and a restaurant manager.

Were these unfortunate circumstances and incidents inevitable? Were they bad luck? Or did they point to deficiencies in the way that mental illness is understood and treated? Was I unrealistic to expect better results?

Given that the bipolar puzzle has so many pieces, it should not have been surprising to discover that no one doctor had the big picture. So far, almost every professional we had visited in our odyssey had turned out to have his or her own bias, a bias that usually addressed one or more pieces of the puzzle to the exclusion of all the others. When we saw psychiatrists, Chris had a psychiatric disorder. When we saw an alternative medicine physician, the problem was most likely DPT antitoxins and Lyme disease. What I found most surprising and troubling was that the vast majority of these experts expressed not the slightest curiosity or openness toward differing viewpoints. With the exception of Dr. Ingendaay, they simply ignored facts about Chris's illness that didn't fit their particular paradigm. They were down on what they were not up on, and were either not interested in taking, or did not want to take, the time to get up on what they were down on.

The more professionals I talked to, the more pieces of the puzzle I obtained, but I couldn't fit them together. I seemed to be going in circles. There was no unifying theme. Again and again, I would begin to explore a new path only to end up with more questions than answers. Was my search open-minded or empty-headed? It was no wonder that my family was fed up with my "bipolar theory of the week." Yet now, once more, the Internet was about to lead me to a new path. Would this one be any different?

Call for a new typology

In <u>Psychiatry and the Human Condition</u>, psychiatrist Bruce Charlton argues that there are significant deficiencies in our current understanding of mental illness. In describing the malaise theory of depression, he states, for example, that major depressive disorder should not be considered an affective disorder. Instead, it should be reinterpreted as the behavioral consequences of a unified aversive malaise state called "sickness behavior" that is caused mainly by immunochemicals such as cytokines. According to Dr. Charlton, sickness behavior is a physiological and psychological adaptation to acute infection and inflammatory illness in many species of mammals. The patterns found in sickness behavior include fatigue, psychomotor retardation, impaired cognitive functioning, and loss of motivation for food and sex, or, in other words, many of the same criteria required for a diagnosis of major depression.

Dr. Charlton believes that sickness behavior serves an evolutionary purpose by conserving energy and enhancing immune activity as a sick or infected body mounts, as he writes, a "short-term, all-out attack on an invading microorganism." Depression results from the malaise caused by feeling ill.[1] This malaise occurs when the brain receives feedback from the body, specifically increasing levels of circulating cytokines and similar immune products. Therefore, major depression is not so much a disorder of mood as a response to a disordered physical state. The major emotion is malaise, not sadness. I could relate to that. When I was a teenager, I once felt so miserable during a bout of the flu that I told my parents I could understand how people could feel badly enough to want to kill themselves.

Dr. Charlton views delirium (brain impairment) as a model for understanding psychiatric symptoms. Rather than the "all or nothing" phenomena associated only with the most severe psychoses, he describes delirium as a continuum from mild to severe. Everyday experiences of hypnagogic phenomena and brain fog are located at one end of the same spectrum whose other end is occupied by psychoses. Hypnagogic phenomena occur when a person's brain is impaired in some way, often as a result of sleep deprivation.

I learned first hand about hypnagogic experiences when I worked long hours at the Seattle Mental Health Institute following my graduation from college. Telling myself that I needed to work 60 hours weekly in two jobs to raise money for graduate school, I ignored subtle messages from my brain telling me that there was a price, albeit a small one, to pay. I recall waking up once and seeing a figure moving on a wall; the movements of this figure seemed so full of magical significance that I regretted the end of the apparition when I more fully "came to my senses." Another time, I woke from a brief nap to see strange, disorienting lights. I couldn't put the lights into any meaningful context. It took a moment for my brain to register that I was looking up from a prone position at a chandelier hanging from the ceiling. The scariest experience occurred after I took a nap late at night in my car while on a long trip during my frugal graduate school days. As the sun began to rise, I was stretched out on the front seat, having a nightmare of a car coming at me and being unable to move my hands or feet to avoid the accident; the feeling of doomed helplessness was terrifying. All I could see was the steering wheel and the roof of my car. After I fully awoke, I realized that I had opened my eyes while half-asleep and actually seen my car's steering wheel and roof. These images were then processed into a dream, a hallucination, by my sleep-addled brain. At the time, I didn't know anything about hypnagogic phenomena, and I certainly didn't think of them as a model of psychotic processes. I just figured that these weird happenings were a consequence of my brain not being fully awake. Actually, that's not too bad a definition of hypnagogic experiences . . . or of psychosis, for that matter. If those curious and disorienting mystery moments had expanded to fill my waking consciousness for days, or even weeks, then the staff at Seattle Mental Health Institute might have changed my status from employee to patient.

Dr. Charlton describes such experiences as prototypes of a delirium caused by brain impairment. If I understood the implications of what he was saying, my experiences were not altogether qualitatively dissimilar from what Chris had reported during his second hospitalization. He saw three-dimensional lines through a window converging to a point outside the isolation room where he was confined. He saw himself escaping through the three-dimensional space created by those lines. The only difference between his disorientating experiences and mine was that his persisted. He didn't "wake up" until his medicines took effect. I woke up after a few disorientating seconds.

Dr. Charlton addresses mania by hypothesizing that the production of some endogenous, internally manufactured antifatigue analgesic substance (or taking a drug with the same properties) can switch temperamentally hyperactive people into hypomanic behavior. He suggests that mania occurs when one or more of these substances allows the patient to continue hyperactivity without experiencing the negative feedback of fatigue or pain. Mania can be caused by endogenous opiates such as the endorphins, an example of which is beta-endorphin, made from hormones in the pituitary gland. Beta-endorphin is chemically related to the stress hormone adrenocorticotrophichormone (ACTH), a peptide hormone also produced by the pituitary gland. Dr. Charlton suggests that increased cortisol, which rises in response to stress, may play a role in mania. He also states that exogenous opiates that mimic the actions of endorphins can provoke mania.

This reminded me of a hypothesis of Dr. Abraham Hoffer, the pioneering orthomolecular psychiatrist, that adrenochrome, an oxidative byproduct of noradrenaline, caused schizophrenic symptoms. There is even a street term, "pink adrenochrome," a naturally oxidized adrenal product that some have used in order to get "high."

Dr. Charlton proposes an entirely new classification system of psychiatric illnesses based upon biologically valid psychological variables applied to diseases and to drug effects. He explains:

> *The reason is to pave the way for a new system of classifica-*
> *tion of psychiatric illness, a new nosology based upon bio-*
> *logically valid psychological variables applied both to dis-*
> *eases and to drug effects. And the reason for this is quite*
> *simple — it is to unstick psychiatry from its current concep-*
> *tual stasis and force the subject to emerge from the intellec-*
> *tual ghetto it has occupied for several decades.*
>
> *Whilst occupying this Kraeplinian prison, psychiatry has*
> *learned virtually nothing from biology, and has made no*
> *substantive contribution to the rest of science at all. It is a*
> *pitiful record of misplaced activity, the failure of which has*
> *been blurred, but not obscured, by vast efforts at public re-*
> *lations and hype. We should have no regrets in leaving all*
> *this behind, breaking down the walls, and refreshing the sub-*
> *ject of psychiatry by contact with the scientific disciplines*
> *outside the ghetto. There is a great deal of ground to make*
> *up.*[2]

Microbes and mental illness

I came upon an article by Dr. Robert Bransfield at the Lyme Alliance Web site entitled "Microbes and Mental Illness." The views expressed therein are consistent with, if less strident than, those of Dr. Charlton. Dr. Bransfield addresses the need for psychiatrists to better appreciate the role of microbes, and specifically Lyme disease, in neuropsychiatric illness. Here are some sections from that article:

> *Microbes are the greatest predators of man. As medical tech-*
> *nology improves, there is increasing recognition that infec-*
> *tious disease contributes not only to acute, but also chronic*
> *relapsing illness and mental illness. The evidence to sup-*
> *port this is a combination of insights from theoretical biol-*
> *ogy (particularly Darwinian medicine), research, and di-*
> *rect clinical observations.... With infectious disease, there is*
> *an imbalance between the threat posed by microbes and host*
> *defenses. This imbalance is affected by environmental fac-*
> *tors (including exposure to pathogens) and a number of host*
> *factors such as genetics and/or increased vulnerability as a*
> *result of a state of chronic stress. Although the stress re-*

sponse is adaptive in a short time frame to allocate resources during a crisis, if the stress response is persistent, rather than cyclic, it further increases vulnerability to disease....

Some injury in infectious disease is a result of toxic products or direct cell injury, but a significant amount of injury is a result of host defenses gone awry in response to the infection. Neural injury may occur by a variety of mechanisms, which include vasculitis, direct cell injury, toxins, inflammation, cytokines, autoimmune mechanisms, incorporation of parasite DNA into host DNA, and excitotoxicity. This injury leads to a vicious cycle of disease, resulting in dysfunction of associative and/or modulating centers of the brain. Injury to associative centers more commonly causes cognitive symptoms, while injury to modulating centers more commonly causes emotional and allocation of attention disorders.

Psychiatric syndromes caused by infectious disease most commonly include depression, OCD, panic disorder, social phobias, variants of ADD, episodic impulsive hostility, bipolar disorders, eating disorders, dementia, various cognitive impairments, psychosis, and a few cases of dissociative episodes.

In clinical experience, the link between infectious disease and psychopathology has been an issue with Lyme disease, syphilis, babesiosis, ehrlichiosis, mycoplasma pneumonia, toxoplasmosis; stealth virus, Borna virus, AIDS, CMV; herpes, strep and other unknown infectious agents. In the collective database of patients demonstrating psychiatric symptoms in response to infectious disease, the majority of the cases has been infected by ticks.... When they bite humans, they pose a risk of injecting an infectious cocktail of pathogens into the host.

Patients with psychiatric symptoms from tick-borne diseases are most commonly infected by Borrelia burgdorferi,(Bb) the causative agent of Lyme disease and quite often other coinfections-infections. There is an increasing recognition that many chronic relapsing infections are complex interactive infections in which microbes interact with each other in a manner that contributes to the disease process. The mod-

els most commonly discussed are coinfections associated with HIV and tick-borne coinfections. For example, coinfections associated with Lyme disease may be acquired at the same time, before or after the Bb infection. Interactive infections, however, is a more accurate term than coinfections, since these infections invariably cause an interaction that changes the disease process....

In summary, the complexities of these issues teach us humility. To better understand the clinical syndrome associated with these infections, internists need to recognize the significance of mental symptoms in chronic interactive infections and psychiatrists need to better appreciate the role of microbes in causing mental illness.[3]

The implications of what Doctors Charlton and Bransfield were saying were far-reaching. They could have led me down a dozen different paths. I wondered what relevance cytokines had for me as I continued my increasingly circuitous odyssey in search of the increasingly evasive bipolar "Holy Grail." I had to learn about cytokines before I could either answer that question, or, as had so often been the case, come up with a new set of questions. For now, the "bipolar theory of the week" would remain focused on cytokines.

Cytokines

What exactly is a cytokine? If cytokines create sickness behavior according to Dr. Charlton's theory, how should that lead to a radically different classification system? Whatever they are, cytokines have become increasingly important in the field of clinical psychiatry. I found a recent review by Drs. Kronfol and Remick in the *American Journal of Psychiatry* of the last 15 years of articles on developments in cytokine biology relative to clinical psychiatry. The authors conclude there is growing evidence that cytokines play significant roles over and above that of immune activation and regulation.

Specific cytokines play a role in signaling the brain to produce neurochemical, neuroendocrine, neuroimmune, and behavioral changes. This signaling may be part of a generalized, comprehensive mechanism to mobilize resources in the face of physical and/or psychological stress and to main-

tain homeostasis. The clinical implications of these findings are far-reaching and include a possible role for cytokines in the pathophysiology of specific psychiatric disorders such as major depression, schizophrenia, and Alzheimer's disease. The effects of cytokines in the central nervous system may provide a possible mechanism for the "sickness behavior" of patients with severe infection or cancer, as well as for the neuropsychiatric adverse effects of treatment with interferons and interleukins.... A better understanding of the role of cytokines in various brain activities will enhance knowledge of specific psychobiological mechanisms in health and disease and provide opportunities for novel treatment interventions.[4]

Here again I was venturing into territory in which I was ill-equipped to travel. I couldn't even read the maps. I visited Cytokines On-line Pathfinder Encyclopaedia (COPE), a Web site by Horst Ubelgauft. There were more than 6,650 pages devoted to cytokine research and related subjects, over 15,000 cited references, and more than 50,000 internal hyperlinks.[5] No, I didn't count them. The site reported this. The site was written in English, but it might as well have been in German. If I could grasp just a few main points, I would be doing well. I visited a number of other sites and decided, for the sake of the nontechnical reader, and for myself, to try to make as much sense out of it as possible in my own words. It was time for "Cytokine 101 for Dummies."

Cytokine 101 for dummies

Cytokines are a highly powerful group of amino acids (peptides) produced by a variety of cell types within the body. They are a group of protein mediators that perform important functions in developing and controlling the cells of the immune system.[6]

Protein mediators? Did that mean an amino acid protein which mediated with other proteins? Did the author mean something like protein negotiator? If so, what were they negotiating about, with whom were they negotiating, and how did they do it? Cytokine 101 was getting ponderous already. Maybe my Air Force background could help. I decided to try a different tack.

Too Good To Be True?

Cytokines are an integral part of the body's defensive system, or, if you will, the body's Department of Defense. Cytokines play a central role in command, control, and communication for defense operations. In an organizational chart, the Leukocyte Force (LF) would be directly under the Department of Defense. Within that force are the Mobilization, Intelligence, Attack, and Engineering commands.

Before any force can go to war, it has to mobilize, or, in other words, assemble the right mix of forces to do battle. Within the Mobilization Command, there is a company of helper T- cells, Company H. These cells recognize the presence of invaders and begin to make cytokines to facilitate the growth and responsiveness of B Cells, macrophages, and more T- cells in order to prepare for war. They convey marching orders to Company B (B cells), Company M (macrophages), and Company S (suppressor T- Cells).

Company B, a unit of the Intelligence Command, springs into action by laying a salvo of antibodies on the enemy so that forces from the Attack Command will be able to identify the target. This is like putting a laser beam on the enemy so that the forces from Attack Command will only destroy the desired target. Company B cells circulate throughout the body, marking any enemy (antigen) that shouldn't be there, or that Intelligence Command believes shouldn't be there. As we know, the term military intelligence is an oxymoron. This is why sometimes these forces can identify an incorrect target, like U.S. forces did when they hit the Chinese Embassy during an attack against Iraq. For example, the current conventional view of multiple sclerosis (MS) is that the attack forces mistakenly target the myelin sheath that protects the nerves; they see the myelin sheath as nonself, and attack accordingly. On the other hand, newer understandings suggest that the attack is actually based on a threat. For example, some Lyme disease patients diagnosed with MS have seen symptoms and brain lesions disappear on intra venous (IV) antibiotics.[7] Also, sometimes there are viruses that sneak in like stealth fighters, without the Intelligence Command knowing about it. But more on that later, too.[8]

Company M is a part of Attack Command. It consists of macrophages. This company participates in Operation Phagocytosis. This is somewhat parallel to Desert Storm. Here macrophages ooze out onto the battlefield, engulfing and destroying the enemy that have been identified by the forces of Company B. Enemy forces have antibody markers on them and are an easy target for Company M.

If the battle goes well, Company S directs a cease-fire to prevent fur-

ther carnage, given that there is a price for the defender as well as the ag-gressor in war. T-suppressor cells slow down the pace of battle and start making plans for peace. When the war is going well, the ratio between T-helper cells and T-suppressor cells is about 1.6 to 1.

In the midst of battle, there are many tactical and strategic decisions to be made. Cytokines determine where the forces should go, how many should go, what forces are specifically needed for the task, and how long they should stay at the front. When there is carnage, as there invariably is in battle, the Engineer Battalions from the Engineer Command do a battlefield assess-ment. The cytokines in this battalion rebuild tissue, create inflammation, re-duce inflammation, and promote wound healing, among other things. These cytokines even have an Apoptosis Unit which programs cells to die, as, for example, in certain situations of inflammation. The cytokines realize that the needs of the many outweigh the needs of the few. For the greater good, some cells have to go. Each individual cytokine can have multiple, often-contra-dictory functions depending on its concentration, the kind of cell it's working on, and the presence of other cytokines and mediators.

Many different cytokines together form a system of communication among all the forces of the Department of Defense. Between the different theaters of operations, there is communication from the leukocytes and or-gans and between the companies themselves. The apparently capricious ac-tions of individual cytokines are usually well-orchestrated from a macro per-spective.

This perspective did not come close to the complexity of cytokine pro-cesses, but it gave me a general understanding.

Cytokine inflammation and health

While cytokines are essential in defending and repairing the body, ex-cessive amounts in response to tissue injury or other stimuli can increase inflammation. Some of the proinflammatory cytokines include tumor necro-sis factor (TNF), interleukin-1 (IL-1), interleukin-1B (IL-1B), and interleukin-6 (IL-6).[9] Cytokines initiate the body's responses to threat and tissue repair. One of the cytokines, Interleukin-2 (IL-2), is a powerful immunostimulatory polypeptide that amplifies the immune response.[10] Autoimmune diseases re-sult from the action of the immune system targeting itself. In my Internet search, I happened to find a company called Epogen that is developing ways to ameliorate some of the devastating effects that the immune system can have on the body. This company is looking for ways to rein in cytokines that have "run amok."

Ongoing treatment with cytokines for patients suffering from melanoma is associated with the development of mood and cognitive changes that are believed to be a result of frontal-subcortical cerebral dysfunction. While intuitively one would expect an association between cancer and depression, the CNS effects of cytokines can be disassociated from the effects of chronic disease, other treatments and medications, and psychological responses to illness. The length of treatment and dose are both important factors in the development of mood disturbance. Reducing the dose or stopping therapy may be necessary in some cases.[11] In addition to general changes in mood and thinking, cytokines can also cause mania.

Oncologists have found that a particular cytokine used in the treatment of melanoma, interferon alpha-2b (IFN), provokes mania in some patients. Researchers at Massachusetts General Hospital reviewed four patients whose treatment of melanoma with IFN resulted in mania. They noted that both mania and mood instability can occur with patients being treated with IFN.[12] Interestingly, researchers call such mania "secondary mania." Secondary mania is not the mania found in bipolar illness. The presumption is that a cytokine-induced mania has different roots than the mania found in an illness called "bipolar disorder." Hmm ...

There is evidence that proinflammatory cytokines are capable of causing inflammation and also damage to different parts of the body even as they seek to defend it.

In the cardiovascular arena, proinflammatory cytokines can negatively affect the heart. They change cardiovascular function by, for example, promoting left ventricular remodeling[14] and inducing contractile dysfunction.[15] Increasing levels of certain proinflammatory cytokines that are there to repair the heart can actually harm it. As TNF production increases in response to heart damage, the resulting inflammation to the heart can contribute to congestive heart failure. Enbrel, which binds to TNF, has proven to be useful in reducing inflammation not only with rheumatoid arthritis, but also in the heart. Vasoreactivity in patients with advanced heart failure was improved by taking Enbrel.[13]

I found an interesting discussion among health professionals on the MMI about the relationship between Lyme disease, C-reactive protein levels in the blood, and inflammation. C-reactive protein is a substance the body releases in response to inflammation. High levels are predictive of heart attacks. The MMI members were writing posts about Lyme patients with C-reactive protein above 15 (normal 1.7) and corresponding TNF levels greater than 300 (normal upper limit is 13). Based on these posts, C-reactive protein levels reflect proinflammatory cytokine proliferation. In this scenario, Lyme disease can stimulate cytokine production, stimulate inflammation of the heart, and raise C-reactive protein levels. If cytokines can do this to the heart, I wondered what they could do to the brain.

An epidemiological study of pregnant women with infections established that the presence of proinflammatory cytokines in response to those infections may be involved in neuronal and white-matter tissue injury to the fetuses.[16] Another study compared the maternal blood of 27 adults with schizophrenia and 54 matched control subjects. The researchers retrieved stored blood samples that had been obtained at the end of the mothers' pregnancies. The offspring of mothers with elevated levels of total IgG and IgM immunoglobulins and antibodies to herpes simplex virus type 2 were found to be at increased risk for schizophrenia and other psychotic illnesses in adulthood (p=.03 and p=.04, respectively). No relationship was found with other infections.[17] To me this suggested that either this particular virus, the herpes simplex virus type 2, or its attendant cytokine profile played a role in the increased schizophrenia risk.

Could proinflammatory cytokines be responsible for the decreased N-acetyl aspartate found in bipolar patients? I did a dogpile.com search on variations of "bipolar disorder + cytokines + NAA" and came up with nothing. However, I found general cytokine information bearing on the question of the deleterious effects of cytokines.

> *The cytokine system is a very potent force in homeostasis when activation of the network is local and cytokines act vicinally [in the vicinity of] in surface-bound or diffusible form. When cytokine production is sustained and/or systemic, there is no doubt that cytokines contribute to the signs, symptoms, and pathology of inflammatory, infectious, autoimmune, and malignant diseases.[18]*

The author was stating that in small, targeted doses, cytokines help the body maintain homeostasis, but systemic overproduction can be devastating.

Do cytokines affect adrenal glands to make them disproportionately large in patients suffering from major depression? I found a study done at the Medical Department of Wolfgang Goethe-University in Frankfurt, Germany to be interesting. They investigated the effects of IL-2 treatment of cancer patients on the activation of the hypothalamus-pituitary-adrenal (HPA) axis. They found that cytokines activate the human HPA axis.[19]

Were the large adrenal glands in depressed patients coming from activation of the HPA axis by IL-2? I wondered why the strongest research seemed to be coming out of England, Taipei, and Germany. Was there some bias in universities in the United States away from this model, or was I just not familiar enough with the literature to know?

Lyme, "mental" illness, and IgG levels

It still seemed logical to assume that if excessive amounts of cytokines could inflame the joints and the heart, they could also inflame the brain. So I tried to find the "smoking gun" another way. Looking once again in dogpile.com for "cytokines + brain + inflammation," I returned full circle to a Lyme disease link. Lyme disease causes brain inflammation by stimulating the production of cytokines: IL-1, specifically. IL-1 is the major immunoregulatory molecule produced by macrophages in response to a variety of environmental insults including chemicals, phagocytosis, bacteria, and bacterial products. When macrophages in mice are stimulated by *Borrelia burgdorferi*, the bacteria found in Lyme disease, the production of IL-1 increases. These results suggest that IL-1 in turn may play a role in many of the clinical manifestations of Lyme disease.[20]

In neurologic Lyme disease, about 15-45% of patients have what are called white-matter hyperintensities. These appear as bright spots on an MRI scan and look similar to the demyelinated areas seen in the white matter of the brains of patients with multiple sclerosis. The irritability, memory loss, spatial disorientation, depression, and mania found in cases of neurologic Lyme disease result from damage to the brain by *Borrelia burgdorferi*. Often, antibiotic treatments improve symptoms and neurological test scores, with the white hyperintensities actually diminishing or disappearing.[21] Incidentally, the incidence of bipolar disorder among MS patients is about twice that of the general population.[22]

A study at Queen Elizabeth Hospital found that subcortical white-matter lesions are associated with poor-outcome bipolar disorder. These lesions were deep subcortical areas marked with dots.[23] I concluded that bipolar disorder and Lyme disease both involved damage to the brain.

Single Photo Emission Contrast Tomography (SPECT) provides additional clues to the effects of Lyme disease. SPECT scans of 19 Lyme disease patients revealed that 74% were abnormal. These scans manifested heterogeneous hypoperfusion (poor circulation) with or without globally decreased perfusion. In other words, blood circulation throughout the entire brain was not as complete as it should have been. The patterns of the Lyme patients could be distinguished from those of patients with a diagnosis of Alzheimer's, but not from those with a diagnosis of lupus, cerebral vasculitis, or chronic fatigue syndrome. Of 14 Lyme patients who had an MRI, only 2 (14.3) percent were abnormal with white-matter hyperintensities. The findings suggest that SPECT may provide a more sensitive perspective than MRI for identifying brain abnormalities in Lyme disease patients.[24] I was learning that Lyme disease and the body's response to it were capable of causing significant measurable physical changes in the brain. Could these changes directly cause "mental" illness?

Cytokines — Too much of a Good Thing?

At the University of Rostock, in Germany, physicians evaluated a 42-year-old woman presenting with schizophreniform disorder. This means that she was psychotic but didn't yet have a sufficient history to support a schizophrenia diagnosis. The woman was infected with Lyme disease. In the course of treating that disease with antibiotics, her psychotic symptoms stopped altogether. According to the scientists, "To our knowledge this is the first reported case with an exclusive psychiatric manifestation of Lyme disease." They concluded that when patients first present with manifestation of psychotic disorder, although neurological symptoms are lacking, Lyme disease should be considered and be excluded by cerebrospinal fluid analysis.[25] In another German journal, the authors describe a case of paranoid-hallucinatory syndrome caused by *Borrelia* encephalitis with no neurological signs but marked psychiatric symptoms. After a week of treatment with the antibiotic Rocephin, the symptoms cleared, though there were still some symptoms suggestive of residual organic brain syndrome.[26]

In the MMI, I found a summary of research submitted by a physician who suggested, based on data from Chinese researchers, that *Borrelia burgdorferi* may be an etiological agent in some cases of schizophrenia.[27] The connection was only with schizophrenia, and it was difficult to verify its authenticity; however, a longitudinal study in Europe came up with strikingly similar percentages of psychiatric patients showing evidence of Lyme disease.

A report in the *American Journal of Psychiatry* compared *Borrelia burgdorferi* infection in 499 subjects matched for age and sex. One group was composed of psychiatric patients (no breakdown given, but it included bipolar and schizophrenia patients), the other of healthy subjects. Both were assessed by enzyme-linked immunosorbent assay over a period of four years from 1995 to 1999. The results were striking. Among the psychiatric patients (166), 33% of them were seropositive in at least one of the four assays while 19% of the control group (94) were seropositive. (The China studies cited earlier were 39% and possibly 9%, respectively.) The authors concluded as follows: "The findings support the hypothesis that there is an association between *Borrelia burgdorferi* infection and psychiatric morbidity."[28] If those results were to be replicated with larger studies, it would suggest that as many as one third of all psychiatric patients are seropositive to Lyme disease! Now that was a smoking gun!

Dr. Brian Fallon of Columbia University reported on three patients whose manifestations of Lyme disease included panic disorder, major depression, and bipolar illness — or, perhaps more accurately, symptoms typically found in these disorders. All were treated successfully with antibiotics. Fallon points out that because of a rapid rise of Lyme disease nationwide, and the need for antibiotic treatment to prevent severe neurologic damage, mental health professionals need to be aware of a psychiatric presentation for the disease.[29]

271

Since these "mental" disorders were actually a result of physical infection in the brain, it would only seem logical that the body would be mobilized to fight that infection. I came upon a study that might help explain Chris's high IgG scores.[30] The study looked at heightened immune responses as manifested in the cerebrospinal fluid IgG index. Chris's high IgG scores came from a food antibody assessment. Was there a relationship between the two?

Cytokines and "mental" illness

Even a slight insult to the immune system is capable of compromising mental acuity. Researchers in Israel induced a slight toxic state by two injections of a mild toxin called *Salmonella abortus equi* endotoxin into 20 experimental volunteer subjects while a control group received an injection of saline solution. Though the experimental group had no noticeable symptoms of illness except for a 0.5 degree increase in rectal temperature, significant positive correlation was found between cytokine secretion and anxiety, depressed mood, and decreased memory performance in the experimental group compared to the control group. The following increased in the experimental group: TNF, sTNF, IL-1 receptor antagonist, IL-6, and cortisol.[31] (The prefix "s" means it is soluble in water.)

Major depression is not only associated with activation of the immune system but is actually caused by it. Monokines, one of the cytokines, are created from macrophages, one of the body's key defensive resources against antigens. Dr. Ron Smith, in an article cited earlier in Chapter 16, "The Macrophage Theory of Depression," reported that monokines given to volunteers produced symptoms consistent with major depression. IL-1 provokes the same hormonal abnormalities associated with depression. He attributed the increased three to one female/male ratio of depression to the ability of estrogen to activate macrophages. If Dr. Smith is correct, Mother Nature appears to have assured the perpetuation of our species by designing females with a stronger capability to fight off illness. But there is a cost: greater vulnerability to depression.

Michael Maes, M.D., Ph.D., of the Clinical Research Centre for Mental Healthcare, Antwerp, Belgium, and Dr. Smith described in a *Biological Psychiatry* editorial how a deficiency in essential fatty acid could lead to depression through effects on immune function and cytokine production. They pointed out evidence that depression is accompanied by, and possibly follows from, an acute phase (AP) response in which there is an increased secretion of eicosanoids such as prostaglandins, and of proinflammatory cytokines.

Cytokines — Too much of a Good Thing?

*Inflammatory cytokines .... given to animals or humans pro-
voke an extensive set of symptoms and signs similar to, if not
identical to, those found in major depression .... Cytokines
may be common mediators of external stressors [that is, psychosocial stressors such as adverse life events] and internal
stressors [that is, organic disorders] that are known to play
a role in the etiology of depression.*[32]

I didn't know what an AP response was, or which AP proteins increased from an AP response. I did some Internet sleuthing and learned that activation of cytokines causes an increase in the AP proteins. This is in response to physiological challenges such as inflammation, infection, disease, trauma, or drugs. So basically, the AP response occurs in response to the body's Department of Defense going from DEFCON 4 to a DEFCON 1. An invasion of *Borrelia burgdorferi* could certainly do that.

In order to find out if there is an AP response to major psychiatric illnesses, Maes identified acute phase reactants with 27 schizophrenic, 23 manic, 29 major depressed, and 21 normal subjects. The results suggest that major depression, schizophrenia, and mania are accompanied by an AP response and that this response may be suppressed by chronic treatment with psychotropic drugs.[33] There is evidence that Haldol blocks infection of B-lymphocytes by Epstein-Barr virus[34] and that other psychotropic medications reduce the blastogenic (increase in) response of cultured T-lymphocytes.[35] Lithium, in therapeutic doses, is associated, probably in a dose-dependent way, with higher leukocyte and granulocyte levels in psychiatric patients.[36] Dr. Smith concludes that the immune system may be a key or a primary factor in the action of antipsychotic drugs.[37] It was no accident that in the mid-1950s, chlorpromazine, marketed as Thorazine, was synthesized from a drug used to deworm horses and cows.

Perhaps combating chronic infections and regulating the immune system, rather than regulating neurotransmitters, is what is needed for conditions now classified as mental illnesses. Perhaps the arsenal in today's psychiatric armamentarium will, in the future, prove to have been be crude forerunners of more targeted and effective interventions.

In an article entitled "Depression, Stress and Immunological Activation: the Role of Cytokines in Depressive Disorders," published in *Life Sciences,* T.J. Connor builds on and supports the work of Maes and Smith. The circulating cytokines implicated include IL1-B, IL-6, and gamma-IFN. Positive acute phase proteins and hyperactivity of the HPA-axis was found in the depressed patients. Immunological activation has been found to induce "stress-like" behavioral and neurochemical changes in laboratory animals. While neurotransmitter dysregulation has been implicated for years in the etiology

273

of depression, the author states here that increased cytokine secretion is implicated as a mechanism whereby stress can induce depression.[38]

Additional evidence for the role of cytokine-mediated inflammation in depression comes out of the Department of Adult Psychiatry, Karol Marcinkowski University of Medical Sciences, in Poznan, Poland. Markers of an immune-inflammatory process were examined in patients with major depression and compared to a control group. Comparison of proinflammatory cytokines demonstrated that plasma concentrations of sIL-2R, IL-6, sIL-6, transferrin receptor, C-reactive protein, and alpha 1-acid protein were significantly higher in patients with major depression than in healthy control subjects. The bottom line was that the cytokines IL-2 and IL-6 were elevated in both inflammation and depression.[39]

In another study, systemic administration of three proinflammatory cytokines, IL-1B, IL-6, and TNF, were found to affect in a dose-dependent way consumption of chocolate milk, possibly demonstrating the anhedonia and anorexia effects of the cytokines. The authors state that these cytokines "influence neuroendocrine activity, promote central neurotransmitter alterations, and induce a constellation of symptoms collectively referred to as sickness behaviors."[40] Anhedonia is just a fancy way to say a person gets no pleasure. Anorexia means loss of appetite, a symptom found in patients diagnosed (labeled) as having anorexia nervosa. In yet another study by Levin and others comparing hospitalized depressed patients with a control group, the depressed group was found to have significantly higher cerebrospinal fluid levels of IL-1beta and IL-6, while TNF levels were comparable.[41]

Researchers at the University of Taipei found that immunity was activated in patients with bipolar disorder during manic episodes. With manic patients there was lymphocyte proliferation in response to sIL-2R and phytohemagglutinin, a toxic agent found in many species of beans, but mostly in red kidney beans. This substance, a lectin, is known for its ability to agglutinate red blood cells, alter cell membrane transport systems, alter cell permeability to proteins, and generally interfere with cellular metabolism. (It probably wouldn't be a good idea for a person to ingest phytohemagglutinin when on the verge of a manic episode for fear of exacerbating an already overactive immune system.) More importantly, bipolar mania was correlated with increasing plasma sIL-2R levels that were not found in a control group. There was also a positive correlation between the changes in manic severity and sIL-2R levels. Bipolar patients in remission and normal control subjects did not differ in any of these measures. Interleukin-6R, although associated with depression, was not associated with mania in this study. The researchers concluded, "Cell-mediated immunity activation in bipolar mania was demonstrated and may be through a specifically state-dependent immune response." [42]

In a study of 10 manic patients and 21 healthy volunteers, Maes found that plasma concentrations of both sIL-2R and sIL-6R were significantly higher in the manic patients than in normal controls.[43]

We know that IL-1 is produced by macrophages which stimulate the production of IL-2 cells through T-cells that respond to some kind of antigen. We know that IL-2 stimulates the production of T cells with specific receptors for IL-2. The bottom line is that the IL-2 receptors on the T cells, IL-2R, are expressed in response to the "bad guys," whatever they may be.

Another study reported that detoxified chronic alcoholics had an increased production of proinflammatory cytokines such as IL-6, TNF-alpha, and granulocyte-macrophage colony stimulating factor.[44]

I read a series of powerful arguments by Dr. Smith in favor of the hypothesis that excessive production of IL-2 and IL-2R by gastrointestinal T-lymphocytes is the cause of schizophrenia, the macrophage-T-lymphocyte theory of schizophrenia. Looks like he, as well as Dr. Cade, thinks that schizophrenia is a disease of the gut, rather than the head. Such a hypothesis pulls together the influences of microorganisms and dietary items such as gluten and casein on the immune system. Dr. Smith cites extensive evidence for this; for example, the fact that experimental administration of IL-2 in normal patients causes auditory and visual hallucinations, delusions, paranoia, fear, disorientation, agitation, fatigue, and apathy, as well as other positive symptoms of schizophrenia. [45]

A marker of immunologic activity that has been identified in both schizophrenia and bipolar disorder is quinolinic acid (QUIN). QUIN is considered a neurotoxic product of immune-activated macrophages and microglia, a part of the glial cells that migrate through nerve tissue and remove waste products by phagocytosis. In other words, QUIN is a byproduct of Pac-Man-like organisms eating the bad guys.

Brain elevations of QUIN are a marker for brain inflammation. In a postmortem study of the brain by the Stanley Foundation, QUIN in the cerebrospinal fluid (CSF) was found to be elevated in schizophrenia and bipolar groups compared to unaffected controls with a significance of $p=0.03$ and $p=0.01$, respectively. The study concluded that increases in cerebellar and CSF QUIN levels are found in a subgroup of patients with psychosis. When they looked at brain pH in the cerebellum and frontal cortex, researchers found a significant inverse relationship between cerebellar QUIN and pH in the schizophrenia group.[46] In other words, the more QUIN, the more acidic the brain. Maybe Dr. Wiley was on to something after all with his bio-balance theory.

My initial search to find a relationship between cytokines and inflammation hadn't gone far enough. QUIN, a byproduct of immune activation (specifically, macrophage activity, generated by cytokines), is a substance that actually causes both brain inflammation and damage. I was correct to hypothesize a relationship between cytokine production and brain inflammation, but the relationship was indirect and mediated by QUIN. Did I say mediated? A little knowledge is a dangerous thing.

Even more interesting was a study by Halperin published in *Neurology* comparing 16 patients with CNS *Borrelia burgdorferi* infection, eight patients with Lyme encephalopathy, and 45 controls. The study found that QUIN was "substantially elevated" in patients with Lyme disease. This elevation may contribute to the cognitive problems experienced by many Lyme patients.[47]

This backyard mechanic couldn't explain the differences between complement component 3, C4, or alpha 1-antitrypsin. I couldn't tell a cytokine from an acute phase protein. I couldn't tell the difference between an IL-2 and an sIL-6. To be honest, I didn't really know much about microglia, or, for that matter, QUIN. But it didn't really matter. What I did know was that there was a positive correlation among cytokines, AP proteins, major depression, mania, and schizophrenia. There was a positive relationship between QUIN and psychosis. Lyme disease raised QUIN levels, in turn most likely affecting neural plasticity. That was all I needed to know for now. Immune activation caused cytokines to proliferate. That some of these cytokines played a role in "mental" illness was, for me, indisputable. I was equally convinced that the presence of elevated cytokines was a direct response to danger to the organism, whether the threat was caused by *Borrelia burgdorferi* or its many relatives, any of a multitude of identified or unidentified microbes, or other destabilizing environmental factors.

Repair factors become risk factors. Cytokines, utilized by the body to repair and heal itself, become risk factors for CNS disorders, much as cholesterol, which repairs damage in blood vessels, can eventually choke off the blood supply to the heart. Biological processes that usually heal the body and fend off destructive substances can, under the right (or, rather, the wrong) circumstances, break widgets, switches, and brain cells, or, to be more succinct, break brains.

My cursory look into Lyme disease and "mental" illness had revealed some interesting exceptions. Exceptions usually do not make the rule, but when those exceptions point to mechanisms that can explain phenomena heretofore conceptualized as "functional," then perhaps there is something in those exceptions that could help to establish a new and better rule. Psychiatrists treat symptoms, not causes. They treat the functional manifestations of the illness. Perhaps the mechanisms found in the so-called secondary manias that result from viruses and Lyme disease, along with a host of other illnesses, will help researchers understand the mania found in so-called "bipolar illness." Maybe then researchers will be able to replace the somewhat circular and unproductive "functional" model with a coherent model based on biologically valid psychological variables applied to diseases and drug effects.

Benefits and implications of reducing cytokines

Directly treating the causative low-grade infection or limiting cytokine proliferation can be effective ways to treat some disorders. An article by Dr. Stricker in the *Lyme Times* reports on several patients whose long-term use of antibiotics has successfully treated rheumatoid arthritis, including one woman who was on antibiotics for 35 years![48] In a study with mice deemed the best scientific paper of the year by the American College of Nutrition, Dr. Java Venkatraman demonstrated that a combination of fish oil and vitamin E reduced the levels of inflammation-inducing cytokines that cause the joint swelling and pain characteristic of rheumatoid arthritis. Compared to corn oil-fed mice, those fed fish oil had lower amounts of the following cytokines: IL-6, IL-10, IL-12, TNF-alpha, PGE2, TXB2 and LTB4. Dr. Venkatraman's study showed that mice genetically selected to develop arthritis had significantly lower levels of proinflammatory cytokines on the fish oil and the vitamin E compared with other diets.[49]

In humans, fish oil containing omega-3 fatty acids significantly reduces symptoms of rheumatoid arthritis.[50] The fatty acids cause a decrease in production of cytokines. Daily supplementation of 6 grams of fish oil was found to result in significant benefits with rheumatoid arthritis.[51] Maes and Smith point out in a previously referenced article that the effectiveness of antidepressants in combating depression may be in the potent antiinflammatory activities of this class of drugs. Could the reduction of cytokines be one of the mechanisms by which fish oil prevents recurrences of mania and depression?

There is an over-the-counter product recently introduced in this country called S-adenosyl-L-methionine (SAMe). SAMe is formed naturally in the body by combining the essential amino acid methionine with adenosyltriphosphate (ATP). A deficiency of methionine, vitamin B12, or folic acid results in a decrease of SAMe. SAMe provides an important methyl donor, a subset of specific molecules, in over 35 metabolic processes, many of which are essential for proper brain functioning. It also protects against two proinflammatory cytokines, TNF and IL-1.[52] SAMe has been used to successfully treat both depression and osteoarthritis.

In a long-term, multicenter open trial at the University of Mainz, Germany, the efficacy and tolerance of SAMe were studied for 24 months in 108 patients with osteoarthritis of the knee, hip, and spine. The experimental group improved during therapy with SAMe after the first weeks of treatment and continued up to the end of the 24th month. The authors noted that SAMe administration also improved the depressive feelings often associated with osteoarthritis. To assume that the "depressive feelings" were associated with osteoarthritis is understandable, since a reduction of the pain would be expected to reduce the depression. However, the authors state that the antidepressive effects were more than just relief from pain.[53]

In another open, multicenter study, 195 patients were given 400 mg of SAMe for 15 days. Depressive symptoms remitted after both 7 and 15 days of treatment, with no serious adverse events reported. Further studies with a double-blind design are needed to confirm this preliminary indication that SAMe is a relatively safe and fast-acting antidepressant.[54] While SAMe is an effective antidepressant, it has also been implicated in provoking symptoms of mania, presumably by providing precursors to certain neurotransmitters already present in excessive amounts in bipolar individuals. SAMe would not be appropriate for Chris, but its multifaceted role in counteracting the effects of cytokines and alleviating inflammation and depression lends support to the immune activation-cytokine-inflammation-depression connection.

As discussed in the notes of Chapter 16, Dr. Smith proposes that fish oil is a prophylaxis against depression while omega-6 fatty acids promote depression. Macrophage activation and cytokine proliferation in response to conditions like infection, tissue damage, respiratory allergies and antigens in food are seen as possible causes of depression. Dr. Smith postulated this in 1991, nine years before Dr. Stoll's seminal experiment demonstrating the successful use of fatty acids in treating bipolar patients. The many positive effects of fish oil are amazing.

A number of studies have shown that omega-3 fatty acids are beneficial to the heart. The strongest evidence to date is from three clinical trials, the most convincing of which is the Gruppo Italiano per lo Studio della Sopravvivenza nell'Infarto miocardico (GISSI)-Prevezione study. This study involved 5654 patients divided into one group that received the usual care and the other that received omega-3 fatty acids. Less than 1000 mg daily of Omega fatty acids daily resulted in a 20% reduction in mortality and a 45% decreased risk for sudden death by heart attack.[55]

Even patients with Crohn's disease benefit from omega-3 fatty acids. In a controlled double-blind study, postsurgical Crohn's patients given 2.3 grams of fatty acids had a 34% rate of severe endoscopic recurrences as opposed to a 62% rate in the control group.[56]

What did all this mean? If Chris did indeed have Lyme disease, it could put a chronic load on his immune system. If QUIN and proinflammatory cytokines such as IL-2 were involved, then the resulting inflammation could cause hypoperfusion in his brain and provoke apoptosis or impaired neuron functioning. This could account for the diminished mental acuity noted by his mother and me, and, indeed, himself. While Chris's cognitive performance had improved on the supplements, as evidenced by increased frustration tolerance, access to general information, and an increasing non-manic confidence, it was still possible that evidence of cognitive difficulties would show up as white-matter hyperintensities on an MRI.

The human immune system is designed to mobilize quickly to reduce any threats and then return to alert status. But Chris's defensive forces were engaged in an ongoing battle against both biological and chemical agents. His body had to dedicate more and more of its resources to the war effort, as an army of cytokines tried to counter multiple threats, depriving the component parts of needed resources. Even the simple act of eating put his defensive system into mobilize-identify-attack mode. Deprivation of needed resources caused his system to begin to operate erratically. Order was replaced by chaos. The cumulative effects of the erratic functioning led to his body being overaggressive (mania) or withdrawn (depressed). This intuitively made sense.

I had found relationships between what I previously thought were totally unrelated phenomena. Chris's documented high IgG levels and his presumed high levels of cytokines were likely related to Lyme disease, DPT and other childhood vaccinations, mercury, antimony, aldrin, endrin, xylene, carbon tetrachloride, polysorbate 60, and possibly unknown viruses in his system. These were all foreign and toxic substances against which his body had mounted a defense. The nature of his particular defense was most likely influenced by a combination of genetic factors and nutritional deficits that had contributed to his three episodes of psychotic mania and one of depression — though the latter was iatrogenic, that is, caused by the treatment itself. He could have neurological Lyme disease, which activated high levels of IL-1, IL-2, and IL-2R, the latter associated with mania. These cytokines could be activating his HPA axis through the action of IL-1. With Lyme disease, there was a target. With chemical and heavy-metal contamination, there was a target. With malnourished brain cells, there was a target. We could fight back. Nutrients would contribute ammunition for that fight.

With bipolar disorder, Chris had symptoms of a "mental" illness. Medication for this illness had robbed him of energy and curiosity and held him hostage. I was forced to conclude that four hospitalizations and approximately $90,000 in medical bills had failed to result in a proper diagnosis or treatment of his illness.

I knew that I had barely scratched the surface of the research on Lyme disease and cytokines and their relationship to bipolar disorder. I knew I had not attended to literally hundreds of other highly significant biological findings unique to bipolar disorder and CNS disorders. The point was not that I had found the answer, but that I had found some pieces to a puzzle that could conceivably be different for every patient heretofore given a cookie-cutter diagnosis of "bipolar disorder." I had found a model which appeared to offer a coherent explanation of behavior that had been a total enigma, behavior that had led previous generations to invoke divine displeasure and that had led our generation to invoke "mental" illness as its cause. It was one small but significant step for our family. I felt as if I were looking through a dark glass at patterns that no longer appeared capricious. Beyond the apparent randomness was order. I had a paradigm, the illusion of control, and a logical treatment approach based on it. What more could a therapist ask for?

We would continue to provide Chris with Synergy supplements and to encourage him to strengthen his immune system with omega-3 fatty acids, buffered C, lipoic acid, coenzyme Q 10, Carotenoid Complex, and extra vitamin E. Hopefully, a healthier immune system would reduce the levels of cytokines and other substances that were impairing the functionality of his brain. If competent medical authority told us that Lyme disease was the enemy, we would attack back. If needed, we would seek out and destroy the mercury and specific chemicals to which his body was reacting.

Maybe we would even have his grandfather checked for Lyme. Ray had been bitten many times by ticks as a boy. For that matter, maybe Aunt Harriet had also struggled with an overactive immune system; perhaps the whiteness of her eyes in her wedding photograph, which I had associated with san paku, provided dramatic evidence that something had been wrong in her brain long before she took the life of her son and herself.

What were the implications of Dr. Charlton's call for a new classification system of psychiatric illnesses based on biologically valid psychological variables applied to disease and drug effects? Perhaps some day my son, or any other father's son, would never again be treated for a "mental" disorder defined by a set of similar symptoms which, in actuality, were nothing more than a manifestation of underlying diverse biological disorders. Rather, at some future time, he could be treated for a brain disease, a biologically based illness with specific and effective biological treatments. What a novel idea.

I was another step closer to understanding some aspects of this complex, multifaceted illness. While awaiting better answers to more and more increasingly focused questions, the foxhole phrase "pass the ammunition" would remain apropos. As long as this battle continued, we would give Chris's body all the ammunition it needed in the form of nutritional supplements, including omega-3 fatty acids. Cytokines were pieces of the puzzle, not the entire picture. Gaining a rudimentary understanding of them was enough for the moment.

In the meantime, it was comforting to know that research on bipolar illness was continuing with much more powerful tools. Already scientists using proteomics, the study of human protein sequences, had surveyed 89 post-mortem brain tissues from people with schizophrenia, major depression, bipolar disorder, and normal controls. They identified eight different proteins showing disease-specific alterations in the frontal cortex. I was glad I did not have to try to understand glial fibrillary acidic protein (GFAP), ubiquinone cytochrome c reductase core protein 1, or dihydropyrimidinaserelated protein 2, substances found to be deficient in the brains afflicted with CNS disorders. I didn't know much about GFAP but was intrigued to learn that it is a vital substance in glial cells. GFAP consists of protein strands in glial cells which help regulate excessive glutamate in neurons to prevent cell death. Glutamate can cause mania. I didn't know much about ubiquinone cytochrome c reductase core protein 1, but I was intrigued to learn that ubiquinone was another word for coenzyme Q10, one of the supplements I had been trying to get Chris to take. Ubiquinone, so-called because it is present — ubiquitous — in all cells, is a substance that facilitates effective metabolic processes at the cellular level, and is used not only for Lyme management but for other illnesses as well. It facilitates the mitochondria in the cells which provide needed energy. I would wait to learn if these differences were in fact caused by genetics, by the defense of each unique body against illnesses, by viruses, or by current treatment practices. Researchers believe that proteomic analysis may identify novel pathogenic mechanisms of psychiatric illnesses. I do too.[57]

I was encouraged to learn that others in the medical establishment had also found problems with current models for health care delivery for the "mentally" ill. Dr. Eric Kandel, who won the 2000 Nobel Prize for Medicine for his work on signal transduction in the nervous system, is the founding director of the Center for Neurobiology and Behavior at Columbia University. Reuter's News Service recently quoted him as follows: "Neurology and psychiatry are really one, and should be treated that way." Dr. Kandel pointed out that psychiatry is in crisis, and molecular genetics and imaging are pushing this beleaguered discipline ever-closer to neurology, where he believes the crisis will be resolved.[58] I found a similar sentiment attributed to Dr. E. Fuller Torrey, executive director of the Stanley Foundation Research Programs, which, among other things, is disbursing 20 million dollars annually for the study of the causes of bipolar disorder and schizophrenia. Dr. Torrey recommended that psychiatry as a profession be abolished and subsumed under neurology, where he believes it belongs.[59]

After reviewing and absorbing as much as I could about cytokines, I wondered if so-called "psychiatric illnesses" were, among other things, simply a collection of cytokine mediated brain disorders for which the definitive biological causes had not yet been found. "Psychiatric" was better than "demon-possessed," but we still had a long way to go.

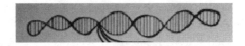

Notes
1. Charlton, Bruce, <u>Psychiatry and the Human Condition,</u> Radcliffe Medical Press:

Oxford, UK, 2000, 75.

2. Ibid., 51-53, 74-78, 105-110, 140.

3. Bransfield, Robert, "Microbes and Mental Illness," Lyme Alliance Spotlight on Lyme, August 1999.
http://www.lymealliance.org/Newsletter/news7/news7.html

4. Kronfol, Z., Remick, D., "Cytokines and the Brain," *Am J Psychiatry* 157(5):683-694, May 2000.

5. Ubelgauft, Horst, "Cytokines Online Pathfinder Encyclopaedia Horst Ibelgauft's Hypertext Information Universe of Cytokines," August 1999.
http://www.copewithcytokines.de/

6. Neta R., Oppenheim J.J., Durum S.K., "The cytokine concept: historical perspectives and current status of the clonal cytokines," in: Stanley, C., (ed.), <u>Lymphokines and the immune response,</u> Boca Raton, Fla.: CRC Press, Boca Raton, Fla., 1990:29-42.

7. Richmond, Ann, "NIH Study participant sees MS reversed by antibiotics," *Lyme Times*, 28: 40-41, Spring, 2000.

8. There is evidence that herpes virus 6, HHV-6, the so-called roseola virus that many of us carry, is not only associated with the brain inflammation of many MS patients, but also increases and decreases based on whether or not the patient is having an MS attack. This would suggest that the body of the MS patient is not so much improperly activating a cytokine defense as it is defending against an attack with resulting inflammation and damage to the myelin sheath.
Regush, Nicholas, <u>The Virus Within — A Coming Epidemic: How Medical Detectives Are Tracking a Terrifying Virus That Hides in Almost All of Us,</u> Penguin Books, New York, New York, 2000, 185-189.

9. Mann, D.L., Young, J.B., "Basic mechanisms in congestive heart failure: recognizing the role of proinflammatory cytokines," *Chest,* 105:897-904, 1994.

10. Sabath, D.E., Prystowsky, M.B., "The molecular basis of interleukin-2 action," in: Stanley C., (ed.), <u>Lymphokines and the immune response,</u> Boca Raton, Fla.,CRC Press, 1990:182-91.

11. Meyers, C.A., "Mood and cognitive disorders in cancer," *Adv Exp Med Biol,* 461:75-8, 1999.

12. Greenberg, D.B., Johasch, E., Gadd, M.A., Ryan, B.F., Everett, F.R., Sober, A.J., Mihm, M.A., Tanabe, K.K., Ott, M., Haluska, F.G., "Adjuvant therapy of melanoma with interferon-alpha-2b is associated with mania and bipolar syndromes," *Cancer,* 89(2):356-62, July 15, 2000.

13. Fichtlscherer S., Rassig, L., Breuer, S., Vasa, M., Dimmeler S., Zeiher, A.M., "Tumor Necrosis Factor antagonism with Etanercept improves systemic endothelial vasoreactivity in patients with advanced heart failure," *Circulation*, 104(25):3023-5, 2001.

14. Pagani, F.D., Baker, L.S., Hsi, C., Knox, M., Fink, M., Visner M., "Left ventricular systolic and diastolic dysfunction after infusion of tumor necrosis factor-alpha in conscious dogs," *J Clin Invest,* 90:389-98, 1992.

15. Finkel, M.S., Oddis, C.V., Jacob, T.D., Watkins, S.C., Hattler, B.G., Simmons, R.L., "Negative inotropic effects of cytokines on the heart mediated by nitric oxide," *Science,* 257:387-9, 1992.

16. Dammann, O., Leviton, A., "Maternal intrauterine infection, cytokines, and brain damage in the preterm newborn," Official Publication of American Pediatric Soci-

ety, Society for Pediatric Research, Volume 42, Number 1, July 1997, Neuroepidemiology Unit, Departments of Neurology, Children's Hospital and Harvard Medical School, Boston, Massachusetts 02115.

17. Stephen, B., Ming, T., Fuller, E., Klebanoff, M., Bernstein, D., Yolken, R., "Maternal infections and subsequent psychosis among offspring," *Arch Gen Psychiatry*, 58:1032-1037, 2001.

18. Slavkovsky, Peter, "1.4.7 Cytokines mediating inflammatory and effector functions," June 27, 1995.
http://nic.savba.sk/logos/books/scientific/node32.html

19. Raab, C., Weidmann, E., Schmidt, A., Bergmann, L., Badenhoop, K., Usadel, K.H., Haak, T., "The effects of interleukin-2 treatment on endothelin and the activation of the hypothalamic-pituitary-adrenal axis," *Clin Endocrinol (Oxf)*, 50(1):37-44, January, 1999.

20. When spirochetes are added to macrophages at a ratio of 10 spirochetes per macrophage, significant quantities of IL-1 are produced. When the ratio is higher, quantities of IL-1 increase proportionately. In addition, IL-1 was found in joint fluids from Lyme disease patients. When IL-1 was injected into the skin on the backs of rabbits, the injection sites became inflamed and warm to the touch after four hours. Lesions similar to those of erythema chronicum migrans, the classic rash caused by a Lyme-infested tick, were seen in some animals after 24 hours. *Borrelia burgdorferi* is a powerful catalyst for IL-1 in Lyme disease patients.
Beck, G., Habicht, G.S., Benach, J.L., Coleman, J.L., Lysik, R.M., O'Brien, R.F., "A role for interleukin-1 in the pathogenesis of Lyme disease," *Zentralbl Bakteriol Mikrobiol Hyg [A]*, 263(1-2):133-6, December 1986.

21. "Lyme Disease Research Studies — Brain Imaging," About.com Lyme Disease January 23, 2001.
http://www.lymedisease.about.com

22. Schiffer, R.B., Babigian, H.M., "Behavioral disorders in multiple sclerosis, temporal epilepsy, and amyotrophic lateral sclerosis: an epidemiological study," *Arch Neurol*, 41:1067-9, 1984.

23. Moore, P.B., Shepherd, D.J., Eccleston, D., Macmillan, I.C., Goswami, U., McAllisteer, V.L., Ferrier, I.N., "Cerebral white matter lesions in bipolar affective disorder: relationship to outcome," *British Journal of Psychiatry,* 178(2):172-176, February 2001.

24. Plutchok, J.J., Tikofsky, R.S., Liegner, K.B., Kochevar, J.M., Fallon, B.A., Van Heertum, R.L., "Tc-99m HMPAO Brain SPECT Imaging in Chronic Lyme Disease," *J Spiro Tick Diseases* 6(3):117-122, 1999.

25. Hess, A., Buchmann, J., Zettl U.K., Henschel, S., Schlaefke, D., Grau, G., Benecke, R., "*Borrelia burgdorferi* central nervous system infection presenting as an organic schizophrenia-like disorder," *Biol Psychiatry*, 45(6):795, March 15, 1999.

26. Barnett, W., Sigmund, D., Roelcke, U., Mundt, C., "Endogenous paranoid-hallucinatory syndrome caused by *Borrelia* encephalitis," *Nervenarzt* 62(7):445-7, July 1991.

27. The original article was written in Chinese by researchers from the Central Hospital of Forestry Industry, Greater Xing-An Mountains, Nei Menggu, China, but I could find no author, journal or even date listed with the abstract in the discussion board submission. I queried the physician. She, too, had been unable to obtain this

information. The researchers reportedly performed a serological survey to detect antibodies against *Borrelia burgdorferi* in 134 cases of schizophrenia and 90 normal control subjects by something called the immunofluorescence assay (IFA). The IFA is an immune test that assesses for Lyme disease by measuring antibodies produced to fight off the disease. The abstract reports as follows: "The results revealed that positive antibody detection was 38.9% in schizophrenics, much higher than in the control group, and spirochetes were isolated from a patient with schizophrenia." The abstract did not reveal the percentage in the control group. In another study from China, this one with the appropriate references, researchers investigated the frequency of Lyme disease in humans and animals in an area considered to be endemic for Lyme disease, the southern foot of the west and middle Arlartai Mountains and forest areas near the mountains in Xinjiang province. Eighteen of 199 (9%) humans were found to be positive for Lyme disease.

Hua ManTang, Lin Tao, Liu ChangLin et al., "Studies on the seroepidemiology of Lyme disease of human and animals in Arlartai area of Xinjiang province." *Zhongguo Meijieshengwuxue ji Kongzhi Zazhi (Chinese Journal of Vector Biology and Control)*, 268-270, 1998.

28. Hajek, T., Pakova, B., Janovska, D., Bahbouh, R., Hajek, P., Libiger, J., Hoschl, C., "Higher prevalence of antibodies to *Borrelia burgdorferi* in psychiatric patients than in healthy subjects," *Am J Psychiatry,* 159:297-301, February 2002.

29. Fallon, B.A., Nields, J.A., Parson, B., Liebowitz, M.R., Klein, D.F., "Psychiatric Manifestations of Lyme Borreliosis," *J Clin Psychiatry,* 54(7):263-8, July 1993.

30. This study was consistent with what members of the local Lyme support group had told me, that Lyme patients suffered from a kind of "hyper-immunity." Their immune systems are always set on high.

Patients with neuroborreliosis demonstrate a blood brain barrier disturbance with 62% showing an elevated albumin ratio and 60% revealing an increased IgG index, indicative of intrathecal IgG synthesis in the cerebral spinal fluid. In addition, 51% of patients exhibited oligoclonal IgG bands and these bands were more likely to be present with a longer time since onset of neurologic symptoms.

Hansen, K., Cruz, M., Link, H., "Oligoclonal *Borrelia burgdorferi*-specific IgG antibodies in cerebrospinal fluid in Lyme neuroborreliosis," *J of Infect Dis,* 161:1194-1202, 1990.

31. Reichenberg, A., Yirmiya, R., Schuld, A., Kraus, T., Haack, M., Morag, A., Pollmächer, T., "Cytokine-Associated Emotional and Cognitive Disturbances in Humans," *Arch Gen Psychiatry, 58:445-452, May 2001.*

32. Maes, M., Vandoolaeghe, E., Neels, H., Demedts, P., Wauters, A., Metzer, H.Y., Altlamura, C., Desnyder, R., "Lower serum zinc in major depression is a sensitive marker of treatment resistance and of the immune/inflammatory response in that illness," *Biol Psychiatry*, 42(5):349-58, September 1, 1997.

33. For the technical reader, they included haptoglobin (Hp), IgG, IgM, fibrinogen (Fb), complement component 3 (C3C), C4, alpha 1-antitrypsin (alpha 1 AT), alpha 1-acid-glycoprotein (alpha 1S) and hemopexin (Hpx). Schizophrenic patients had significantly higher plasma Hp, Fb, C3C, C4, alpha 1S and Hpx than normal controls. Manic subjects showed significantly higher plasma Hp, Fb, alpha 1S and Hpx than

normal volunteers. Depressed subjects had significantly higher plasma Hp, Fb, C3C, C4 and alpha 1S than normal controls. Plasma Hp, Fb, C3C, C4, alpha 1S, and Hpx were significantly higher in schizophrenic, manic and depressed patients who were non-medicated than in those who were treated with antidepressants, antipsychotics or lithium.

Maes, M., Delange, J., Ranjan, R., Meltzer, H.Y., Desnyder, R., Cooremans, W., Scharp'e, S., "Acute phase proteins in schizophrenia, mania and major depression: modulation by psychotropic drugs," *Psychiatry Res*, 66(1):1-11, January 15, 1997.

34. Nemerow, G.R., Cooper, N.R., "Infection of B Lymphocytes by a human herpesvirus, Epstein-Barr Virus, is blocked by calmodulin antagonists," *Proc Natl Acad Sci*, 81:4955, 1984.

35. Baker, G.A., Santalo, R., Blumenstein, J., "Effect of psychotropic agents upon the blastogenic response to human T-lymphocytes," *Biol Psychiatry*, 12:159, 1977.

36. Oyewumi, L.K., McKnight, M., Cernovsky, Z.J., "Lithium dosage and leukocyte counts in psychiatric patients," *Psychiatry Neurosci*, 24(3):215-21, 1991.

37. Smith, R.S., "The immune system is a key factor in the etiology of psychosocial disease," *Medical Hypothesis*, 34:49-57, 1991.

38. Connor, T.J., Leonard, B.E., "Depression, stress and immunological activation: the role of cytokines in depressive disorders," *Life Sci*, 62(7):583-606, 1998.

39. Sluzewska, A., Rybakowski, J., Bosmans, E., Sobieska, M., Berghmans, R., Maes, M., Wiktorowicz, K., "Indicators of immune activation in major depression," *Psychiatry Res*, 64(3):161-7, October 16, 1996.

40. Brebner K., Hayley, S., Zacharko, R., Merali, Z., Anisman, H., "Synergistic effects of interleukin-1beta, interleukin-6, and tumor necrosis factor-alpha: central monoamine, corticosterone and behavioral variations," *Neuropsychopharmacology*, 22(6):566-580, June 2000.

41. Levine, J., Barak, Y., Chengappa, K.N., Rapoport, A., Rebey, M., Barak, V., "Cerebrospinal cytokine levels in patients with acute depression," *Neuropsycholbiology*, 40(4):141-6, November 1999.

42. Tsai, S.Y., Chen, K.P., Yang, Y.Y., Chen, C.C., Lee. J.C., Singh, V.K., Leu, S.J., "Activation of indices of cell-mediated immunity in bipolar mania," *Biol Psychiatry*, 45(8):989-94, April 15, 1999.

43. Maes, M., Bosmans, E., Calabrese, J., Smith, R., Meltzer, H. Y., "Interleukin-2 and Interleukin-6 in schizophrenia and mania: effects of neuroleptics and mood stabilizers," *J Psychiatr Res.*, 29(2), 141-52, Mar-Apr, 1995.

44. Song, C., Lin, A., De Jong, R., Vandoolaeghe, E., Kenis, G., Bosmans, E., Whelan, A., Scharpe, S., Maes, M., "Cytokines in detoxified patients with chronic alcoholism without liver disease: increased monocytic cytokine production," *Biol Psychiatry*, 45(9):1212-6, May 1, 1999.

45. Smith, R.S., "Is schizophrenia caused by excessive production of interleukin-2 and interleukin-2 receptors by gastrointestinal lymphocytes?" *Medical Hypothesis*, 34:225-229, 1991.

46. Bobo, L.D., Yolken, R.H., Torrey, E.F., Paltan-Ortiz, J.D., Herman, M., Briggs, N.C., Velasco, H., Zito, M., Heyes, M.P., "Central nervous system and systemic quinolinic acid in schizohrenia," Stanley Labs Web Site 2001. http://www.stanleylab.org/Document/abstracts/ab98/quinolin.html

47. The researchers summarize their findings as follows: "We conclude that CSF

QUIN is significantly elevated in B burgdorferi infection — dramatically in patients with CNS inflammation, less in encephalopathy. The presence of this known agonist of N-methyl-D-aspartate (NMDA) synaptic function — a receptor involved in learning, memory, and synaptic plasticity — may contribute to the neurologic and cognitive deficits seen in many Lyme disease patients." An agonist is a substance that can interact with receptor molecules and mimic an endogenous signaling molecule.

Halperin, J.J., Heyes, M.P., "Neuroactive kynurenines in Lyme borreliosis," *Neurology*, 42(1):43-50, January 1992.

48. Stricker, Raphael, B., "Antibiotic treatment of rheumatic diseases," *Lyme Times*, 28:40-41, Spring, 2000.

49. Venkatraman J.T., Chu, W.C., "Effects of dietary and omega-6 lipids and vitamin E on serum cytokines, lipid mediators and anti-DNA antibodies in a mouse model for rheumatoid arthritis," *J Am Coll Nutr*, 18(6):602-13, December, 1999.

50. Fung, S.S., Ferrill, M.J., Norton, L.L., "Fish oil therapy in IgA Nephropathy," *Ann Pharm*, 31:112-115, 1997.

51. Geusens, P., Wouters, C., Nijs, J., Jiangy, Dequeker, J., "Long-term effect of fatty acid supplementation in active rheumatoid arthritis," *Arthritis Rheum*, 4:824-829, 1994.

52. Arias-D´iaz J., Vara E., Garcia C., Villa N., Rodriguez J.M., Ortiz P., Balibrea J.L., "S-adenosylmethionine protects hepatocytes against the effects of cytokines," *J Surg Res*, 62(1):79-84, April, 1996.

53. Konig B Institute of General Medicine, University of Mainz, Federal Republic of Germany, "Two-Year Clinical SAMe Trial on Osteoarthritis," *Am J Med*, 83(5A): 89-94, November 20, 1987.

54. Fava, M., Giannelli, A., Rapisarda, V., Patralia, A., Guaraldi, G.P., "Rapidity of onset of the antidepressant effect of parenteral S-adenosyl-L-methionine," *Psychiatry Res*, 28:56(3):295-7, April 1995.

55. Harris, W., Isley, W., "Clinical Trial Evidence for the Cardioprotective Effects of Omega-3 Fatty Acids," *Curr Atheroscler Rep*, 3(2):174-179, 2001.

56. Bang, H.O., Dyerberg, J., Hjoorne, N., "The composition of food consumed by Greenland Eskimos," *Acta Med. Scand*, 200:69-73, 1976.

57. Johnston-Wilson, N.L., Sims, C.D., Hofmann, J.P., Anderson, L., Shore, A.D., Torrey, E.F., Yolken, R.H., "Disease-specific alterations in frontal cortex brain proteins in schizophrenia, bipolar disorder, and major depressive disorder," *Mol Psychiatry*, 5(2):142-9, March, 2000.

58. Reuters Health, "Nobelist predicts marriage of psychiatry, neurology," *JAMA*, 285:601-605, 2001.

59. Mencimer, S., "Brain Storm," *Washington City Paper*, June 16, 1998.

20 - A Progress Report

I had been asking Chris since mid-December 2000 to write an update on how he was doing. In January 2001 he reluctantly agreed to do so. From our viewpoint, he was doing great because he hadn't displayed any hypomanic, manic, or depressed behavior since starting the supplements. He was composing music, playing the piano at nursing homes, attending a class at church, and studying the life and work of Martin Luther and the history of the early Christian church. While Chris was focused on religion and philosophy, I continued to focus on the biology of the brain. I wanted him to have at least some of the same burning drive that I had to understand the workings of his brain, but it was not to be.

Gayle and I were concerned that if Chris didn't develop insight from his past, he would repeat it once he left home and we were no longer around to make certain he took his supplements. Even now we often had to remind him to do so. Our other suggestions, that he follow some kind of sleep discipline and quit smoking, fell on deaf ears. But it wasn't difficult to look on the bright side: He was acting like himself for the first time in four years.

All in his brain

Chris was taking a maintenance dose of 16 supplements a day and was no longer exhibiting any hypomanic behavior. That in itself was a tremendous accomplishment. After a four-year history of hypomania between psychotic hospitalizations, and the recent iatrogenic depression caused by Dr. Lund, Chris was back to "normal." He had begun volunteering to help with household chores. He had lost the 25 pounds he'd gained in the hospital, seemingly without effort. The supplements were definitely making a difference. The so-called positive symptoms of the illness — pressured speech, grandiosity, flight of ideas, the boundary problems — were gone, but negative symptoms such as lack of motivation, disorganization, problems with his memory and directions still remained. He slept from 10 to 12 hours a night.

I suggested he make small goals and organize his time more effectively, using this time at home to develop his portfolio of compositions, for example. He argued with some justification that he had nothing to organize for, since he remained in limbo, waiting for a disability determination, further knee assessments and possibly surgery, an evaluation of his hand, and resolution of the Lyme disease and the chemical and heavy metal issues. I point out that the discipline of writing his compositions and creating a portfolio of his music could be more rewarding both personally and financially than just going with the flow every day.

Chris expressed exasperation toward my "monomania" on the subjects of Lyme disease and his health. Navigating the intricacies of father-son relationships is difficult enough without trying to understand, let alone write a book about, a complex illness like bipolar disorder. Maybe Chris was simply tired of all my talking and writing. Maybe the illness had compromised his insight due to cognitive impairment. Maybe there wasn't enough "room in his brain" for other perspectives. Or maybe he just wanted to be independent; after all, Chris was 25, a young man eager to make his mark on the world yet compelled by circumstances to live at home with his parents. Whatever the reasons, he drifted through each day continuing to deny or minimize a biological role in his illness. Considering that his illness had so negatively affected his life, and almost ended it, I had a hard time understanding his point of view.

We agreed on one thing: that New Century had damaged their credibility with the kinesiology fiasco. Yet I still believed they may have made a major contribution to understanding Chris's illness. Kinesiology aside, I had found much in my research to support their statements about the role of Lyme disease, environmental toxins, and vaccinations in neuropsychiatric disorders. Chris, however, had a different perspective. In my opinion, he continued to operate under the delusion that he and he alone determined his destiny.

All in my mind

My dad asked that I write something about my current progress, although I've told him that there's not much to report. I've delayed quite some time in writing because I do not feel there is much to say. When I have intellectual dilemmas, or when I am mired in deep depression, I find it very easy to write. I write when I have a lot of angst. I write when I have thoughts that need to be sorted out. Lately, I haven't been having a lot of thoughts. I'm just living simply day to day. I wake up in the morning usually between 10:00 and 12:00, I eat breakfast, I watch a little TV or surf the Internet, I spend some time petting the cats and dog, I go to my Yamaha keyboard and plunk out a couple of tunes. Sometimes I go for walks. Sometimes I'll read books, and sometimes I'll play on the Sega Dreamcast. I usually spend about one to two hours a week talking to my good friend, Sandy, who lives in Michigan. Sometimes we play Cribbage or checkers over the Internet, which can be quite fun.

Here in California, living with my parents, I feel as though I'm killing time, waiting for my life to start. In four months, after I receive the final word on my disability status , I would like to move up to the Seattle area. There I may be able to get a position at a security company my best friend, Dan, works for. If not, I can get a position in sales just about anywhere. I'll also be closer to many of my friends who live in the Seattle area, as well as my grandparents and other relatives.

Am I happy with my life right now? Not particularly. Do I have any more thoughts about ending it? Absolutely not. Do I feel the nutritional supplements have given me my life back? To be honest, I can't really tell that they are having an effect. I no longer conjure up images of myself being God, or one of the two witnesses of Revelation, or of being the Antichrist. I no longer dwell on the end of the world and the return of Christ. I no longer feel the burning desire to reach out to the "lost" souls who do not know Christ and who have no desire for truth. But can I say that this can be attributed to the fact that I'm taking a nutritional supplement that is intended to heal the person afflicted with bipolar? I don't think so. During each of my previous three manic attacks, I was given hospital drugs such as Depakote, lithium, and Zyprexa, and, even under heavy dosage, I never faltered in my belief that the coming of Christ was imminent and it was my responsibility to do something drastic to prepare myself and the world for his return. My taking of the supplements did not curb my obsession with God, Christ, Revelations, and the end times. I did. I lost interest. Not in God per se, but in anything that has to do with prophecy or Armageddon. I used to constantly read articles about biblical prophecies, and I always kept an eye out for newspapers with words like "peace treaty," especially when they involved Israel. I searched Revelations meticulously for clues as to how the end would come. I became so wrapped up in end-times theology that it became my reality. I became so entrenched in it that I came to believe that I would be one of God's main players in this final battle between good and evil. From that point on, it escalated ever more, until finally, at the pinnacle of my subjective experience, I was God, creator of the universe and everything in it.

Did bipolar disorder cause this hallucination? In some respects, yes. Bipolar contributed to the loss of boundaries I experienced while in this manic state. However, had I not been so fascinated in the end-times to begin with, the episodes would not have gotten so out of hand. Many people with bipolar have experienced much milder episodes, where perhaps they go on a shopping binge, or they become argumentative and agitated. The imminence of Christ's return and/or the end of the world were the catalysts for all of my manic episodes, and they led me to do outrageous and unthinkable things. The things which held so much fascination for me then are no longer important to me. I don't care about them anymore. But not because I'm apathetic. I don't care about them anymore because I don't believe they are true.

I don't believe that God, by way of his two witnesses, will rain terror down on Earth to all unbelievers, terrorizing them with plagues, boils, insect infestations, and many other destructive things in order to make them repent.

I don't believe fire will come down from heaven and consume all of the unbelievers and Satan as they surround God's camp, sending them to eternal torture in a lake of burning sulphur. These things that were depicted in Revelation seem more suited to the world of dreams and fantasies than to the real world.

Over the past several years, I have learned a lot about what the brain is capable of when it is under tremendous stress. A man who expects the world to end can dream up a number of horrifying images and truly believe they will happen. That was certainly the case with me, although I had always considered myself a very rational person. However, I cannot take full credit for the dreams I had. They were all inspired by a man named John, the author of Revelation, who set the precedent for end-times hallucinations. John was sent to perish on an island called Patmos, alone, because of his faith in a man who claimed to be the Son of God. This man, Jesus, promised his followers that someday he would return and judge the world. With all of the time John had to himself in prison, it is no wonder he dreamed some of the most vivid dreams written about in the Bible. He depicted such gruesome things as locusts with the stings of scorpions sent to torture those who did not have God's mark on their forehead, as well as earthquakes and plagues sent by God to destroy non-believers. His feeling that the end was right around the corner, and Christ would return in full glory, inspired him. These descriptions used to terrify me when I believed that John's words were God-breathed and infallible. Now I realize that John is not that much different than me, and the mental imagery he had is not so different from the mental imagery I had while undergoing a bipolar episode.

Since the main catalyst for my previous manic attacks is no longer something I am concerned about, does that mean I have no more to fear from bipolar? Perhaps. Personally, I'm content to just keep taking the nutritional supplements as if they were actually doing something (and they are, because they are loaded with vitamins and minerals that are healthy for me, regardless of whether or not they are helping with the bipolar) and leave it at that. However, my dad has a different opinion, one with which I wholeheartedly disagree.

Ever since he took me to the New Century Wellness Clinic in Reno, Nevada, and the doctors found a particular type of spirochete (a wormlike organism) they thought to be associated with Lyme disease in my blood, my dad has been obsessed with the disease. He's done enough research to convince himself that there is a link between Lyme disease and bipolar disorder. He thinks Lyme is causing my bipolar disorder, and believes, as the Century Wellness doctors do, that treating the Lyme disease will cure the bipolar. Never mind that a tick hasn't bitten me in 18 years. According to the doctors, Lyme disease can lie dormant for many years before affecting the human *body. I think they could be wrong about what type of spirochete it is, or if it even is a spirochete.*

There are many different types of "wiggly" things swimming around in our blood, and I'm sure they are not all harmful. I was rather surprised at how quickly the doctor came to a tentative Lyme diagnosis after seeing the spirochete. It's interesting to me that Lyme disease is quite rare, and in Arkansas, the only place I've lived where I've been bitten by a tick, fewer than 1,000 cases are reported year to year. Even more interesting is that typical Lyme symptoms include fever, nausea, rashes, and other symptoms that I am not currently experiencing. Statistically, the odds of me contracting an uncommon type of Lyme disease that causes bipolar disorder, and then going nearly two decades before experiencing the effects of that disorder, are quite low. Add to that the fact that Lyme disease is often misdiagnosed, and I become extremely skeptical that I have it.

It doesn't help that the doctors at Century Wellness used a type of hocus-pocus procedure called kinesiology to test if I was allergic to the supplements I was taking. As if it wasn't enough for them to tell me I was allergic to the plastic capsules, they wanted me to mix my supplements with their own special powder. They wanted me to purchase their pills based on their little muscle strength test. Do they take me for a fool? Perhaps. They also wanted me tested for Diptheria, which they claimed could cause the bipolar.[1] Needless to say, I did not have a very positive opinion of Century Wellness as I walked out. They seemed to have their own agenda, and they didn't really take time to listen to our concerns.

They just sent us a list of procedures they think will take care of the Lyme disease, including two straight weeks of intravenous fluids, bottles of nutritional herbs and remedies, shots that I would have to take regularly for an entire year, and several other things. The total cost would be over $20,000. Let's say I agree to the treatment, and this does kill the spirochetes. How do we know I'm cured? Because the spirochetes disappear from my blood? Do my symptoms go away? No, because I never had any symptoms to begin with. Do I feel better physically and mentally? No, because I feel fine physically and mentally right now. So we end up spending thousands of dollars, and I waste an entire year of my life killing a few worms in my blood that have no affect on my life whatsoever. I don't see much point in that. If I was currently experiencing symptoms of bipolar, then I might consider undergoing the treatment. But since there are currently no symptoms, there is really no way of knowing that the treatment is effective. I think it would be an extreme waste of money and time, and I believe it would be destructive for me in my life. I want to get on with my life, not sit at some clinic in Reno waiting for my regular shots. Well, that is about all I have to say at the moment.

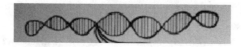

Notes

1. Actually, the test was a diptheria antitoxoid, a measure of the body's defense against the original DPT vaccine. According to the test, Chris's level was ten times higher than it should have been. Dr. Tang did not explain the mechanism by which this caused bipolar disorder, but from my limited research I assumed it had something to do with decreased levels of certain enzymes needed to properly digest proteins, the so-called cytochrome p450 family and phosphosulfotransferase connection. Rats immunized with DPT showed decreased production of these essential enzymes. The cytochrome p450 family is a group of enzymes involved in metabolizing drugs and dietary substances and in synthesizing steroid hormones and other extracellular lipid signalling molecules.

21 - Back to the Mainstream

After all the tests were in, New Century sent us a treatment plan. It consisted of 20 IV treatments at $200 each to treat Lyme disease; coenzyme Q10 to facilitate oxygen utilization at $45 a bottle; a botanical extract for infection at $250 a bottle; chalcedonum drops for the immune system at $75 a bottle; injections of Glyrexal three times a week at $25 a shot; home-care visits for 3 months at $150 a set; and chemical desensitization for aldrin and endrin at $140 a set. This treatment was to target Lyme disease; aldrin, an organochlorine pesticide; endrin, another organochlorine pesticide; xylene, a chemical produced from petroleum; polysorbate 60, a food additive; and carbon tetrachloride, all of which, according to Dr. Tang, were circulating in Chris's bloodstream.

After carefully considering the input from New Century and the Lyme support group members, Chris and I decided to go back to mainstream medicine for a second opinion. Since several patients recommended Dr. Stricker in San Francisco, and since he also took Medi-Cal patients, on January 29, 2001, we went to see him.

Dr. Stricker had the reputation of being one of the foremost Lyme disease specialists in the state. He was not impressed when we told him about the wormlike creatures we had been shown in Chris's blood. He said that it would be very unusual for spirochetes to be visible in the blood. At the same time, he told us that even though New Century had not administered the correct tests, the results of the tests they had administered were highly suggestive of Lyme disease. He reordered the Western Blot and ordered some specialized tests to look at T-cell functioning. He also ordered an MRI to rule out white-matter hyperintensities, which he said usually cleared up after treatment. He told us that if Chris had Lyme disease, he would need at least three months of IV antibiotics.

The most effective treatment for Lyme disease involves the antibiotic Rocephin. In one study, when Rocephin reached a certain level in the host, motile organisms disappeared. Achieving the same level with both penicillin and doxycycline failed to remove the organisms. It was nice to know that Rocephin got all the motile organisms, the ones that squirm around in human tissue, but there could still be a problem. *Borrelia burgdorferi* can morph into cysts and other forms that are impervious to antibiotics. According to Dr. A. Kersten, "Encysted borrelia, granules, and the remaining blebs might be responsible for the ongoing antigenic stimulus leading to complaints of chronic Lyme borreliosis."[1] Rocephin could kill all the motile organisms, but if some morphed into cysts, granules, or blebs, it could not touch them. Even if Chris did have Lyme disease and was treated for it with Ceftriaxone (Rocephin), the *Borrelia burgdorferi* could still survive.

293

The last word on Lyme?

Several days before our next appointment with Dr. Stricker, Ray came to the breakfast table giddy with excitement.

"Last night I had a dream where I went to see a doctor. He found out I had about 200 spirochetes and killed them all. I felt more energetic than I ever had before. Felt 20 years younger."

As he spoke, I could feel the excitement in his voice as he thought about getting rid of parasites that might have robbed him of so much of his life.

"If Chris has it, I'd like to be tested for Lyme, too."

"Great idea," I said. "I'll set it up." Ray had multiple tick bites while growing up in the woods of Mt. Veeder.

On February 20, I drove to San Francisco with Ray and Chris for Chris's scheduled follow-up appointment with Dr. Stricker. The MRI had not been done.[2] The Western Blot results were in.

Dr. Stricker got right to the point. "The Western Blot came back with 6 positive bands for Lyme disease. There's no doubt, Chris. You have Lyme disease."

Chris responded, "When I saw the doctor for my disability assessment, he said that even if I had Lyme, it wouldn't account for the bipolar illness."

"That's not what the 30 or so doctors I talk with in an Internet discussion group are saying," Dr. Stricker replied. "They say they are increasingly amazed at the number of patients whose only manifestation of Lyme disease is neuropsychiatric symptoms."

Dr. Stricker confessed to being surprised by the lab results. He had given Chris an exhaustive T-cell panel he had developed especially for Lyme patients. While there were some minor anomalies, the results were not what he was used to seeing for patients with Lyme disease. The panel included various combinations of T-cell values as well as the relationship of various CD values to one another.

"The blood work doesn't reflect the fact that you have 6 bands positive for Lyme disease. Normally, we get a low CD 57. You got 100 in a range of 60 to 360. Also, the helper/suppressor ratio (CD4+/CD8) appears to be normal. This suggests that your immune system is in good shape, which, again, is surprising considering that you have Lyme disease."

I spoke up. "Could this be because of the supplements he's been taking?"

"It could be. There are two things we can do. Normally I recommend a three month period of IV antibiotics."

Chris gave very clear nonverbal negative feedback.

"Well, since your immune system appears to be functioning so well, we could do a trial of 3 months with antibiotics by mouth. The three months are needed because of the life cycle of the spirochetes."

"Don't they form blebs that are unaffected by antibiotics?" I asked.

Dr. Stricker nodded. "That's another reason why we have to treat for so long. Eventually, they decide to come out again to eat, and that's when the antibiotics get them."

I spoke up again. "According to the guy who developed the supplements, bipolar clients regress when they take antibiotics by mouth."

"They probably have a Herxheimer reaction, where the die-off of bacteria temporarily overwhelms the body's ability to handle the toxins and waste. Then they get the same symptoms associated with the Lyme disease."

"That's not what he says. He says the die-off of essential digestive microorganisms in the gut reduces the digestion of minerals. Without the right precursors for neurotransmitters, the patients crash. Sometimes Truehope customers need antibiotics for various medical disorders. He says if they get them by IV, they don't have a problem. If they give them by mouth, they do. We may be talking about two different things here; that is, unless every bipolar patient has Lyme disease — I'll check with him and see if he can clarify this further."

We discussed whether lithium would be useful as a neuroprotective agent, given that Lyme disease can cause brain damage. I showed Dr. Stricker an article on the neuroprotective aspects of lithium, the one showing the increased NAA resulting from lithium. But Dr. Stricker was not inclined to give Chris lithium as long as his symptoms remained under control. He mentioned that he had used Elavil in small amounts to achieve the same results. He said he didn't give enough for an antidepressant effect.

"My concern is that Chris could become psychotic again," I responded. "Perhaps his levels of IL2-R could became elevated in response to the dead spirochetes."

"You know more about this stuff than the psychiatrists," Dr. Stricker said with a wry smile.

"Well, I've been studying it pretty intensively for about six months now." I felt flattered.

"Yes, the cytokines will become elevated as his body deals with the dead spirochetes. Also, it will be important to eat yogurt and acidophilus to resupply the bacteria in the gut."

"Would you have any objection to our boosting his immune system with lipoic acid, buffered C, Carotenoid Complex, and Co Q10?"

"I know of a doctor on Long Island who has patients taking vitamins and minerals, but there's no formal research on this. Nutrition isn't my area, but I suspect that as long as Chris doesn't get an overdose of any of the vitamins like E or A, they certainly wouldn't hurt. Let's get together again in a month."

"Okay, thanks."

As planned, I brought Ray into the examination room for his appointment. I described his medical and psychiatric history, including his need for a heart pacemaker, his diabetes, and his history of esophageal bleeds. Dr. Stricker said that Lyme disease can cause heart problems because of excessive cytokines. He recommended that we go to the same lab Chris had gone to in order to give a blood sample for the Western Blot. We did.

We had lunch in Chinatown. I asked Chris how he felt about the findings.

He shrugged. "Indifferent."

Later in the meal, he asked his grandfather, "Would you really want to know if you had Lyme disease?"

Ray didn't hesitate. "If I could feel younger by getting rid of it, I'd want to know."

Tony's take

I called Tony to find out what he could tell me about the risks of taking antibiotics by mouth. It took him about a week to call back.

"Sorry it took so long to get back with you, Dave. The pace keeps on picking up. Today, for example, I have 80 calls to make."

Chris got on the extension and explained the situation to Tony. I asked for any data Tony might have concerning how frequently oral antibiotics are a problem for people taking the supplements.

"My son developed a bad infection after he had his wisdom teeth taken out," Tony told us. "The doctor said that if we didn't treat it with antibiotics, the infection could go to his brain. He agreed to bag him and there was no problem. Under no circumstances would I recommend putting antibiotics in the digestive track, especially for three months. It is asking for trouble, Dave. Proteins and carbohydrates can still be digested, but it's not that easy to digest minerals if the gut is constantly bombarded with antibiotics."

Chris spoke up. "Do you get any warning if there's going to be a problem, so you could stop the treatment in time?"

"No. When your brain runs out of serotonin, the change to psychosis is very sudden. You could get away with taking them for about a week, and then you would likely become psychotic again."

"But do you have any numbers as to how many people can get away with it and how many can't?" I asked.

"When we look at our charts and there is a sudden exacerbation of symptoms, it's almost always caused by taking antibiotics by mouth. I argued with one of our clients who had been doing very well on the supplements. He insisted on taking oral antibiotics prescribed for some infection. His wife called about 10 days later. He was suicidal and depressed and blamed me for his depression. I told his wife to take him to the hospital. We see this all the time. People think they are somehow special, and it won't happen to them. But unfortunately, it doesn't matter who you are. There's nothing personal about it; if your neurotransmitters aren't right, your brain won't function properly. It's that simple. If you're taking oral antibiotics now, Chris, I would recommend you stop immediately."

"We wanted to talk to you first before we decided what to do," I told him. "So you don't see this as a Herxheimer reaction, but as simply the gut being unable to digest foods properly?"

"Dave, I don't know much about Lyme disease, but I can tell you that those we've worked with who have gotten better on the supplements cannot risk taking antibiotics by mouth. I would not recommend taking antibiotics by mouth, especially for three months."

"Okay, Tony. Thanks for getting back with us."

We were back to square one. Chris decided not to take the risk, but instead went along with Dr. Stricker's first and best recommendation for IV antibiotics.

The Cure?

We went to San Francisco, where a nurse placed a peripherally inserted central catheter, otherwise known as a PICC line, into Chris's left arm. The PICC ran from his left arm up into his vena cava, where the vessels enlarge just before entering the heart. Then we drove to Option Care, a home care facility in Chico, to start the treatment. Dr. Stricker had ordered that Chris receive IV Rocephin every day for three months. It was up to Option Care to determine how best to deliver it. They gave Chris his first treatment, in which they "pushed" 2 grams (gm) of Rocephin in 20 milliliters (ml) of fluid, a concentration of 100 mg per ml. They taught us how to push the Rocephin, flush it with saline water, and then add heparin to prevent blood clots daily at home. A nurse from Option Care would come weekly to check on progress and to clean the insertion site.

I contacted the Lyme Support Group to reassure myself that we were on the right track. I was shocked to learn from one member that she and her son both had to have their gall bladders removed after the same treatment. The woman believed that being on the daily schedule of Rocephin had caused her gall bladder to fail. She said that she thought a five day on/two day off schedule might give Chris's gall bladder more time to recover between treatments. On the Web, I read an article by Dr. Burrascano, a noted Lyme-literate M.D. (LLMD). He recommended a 5-2 schedule precisely to spare the gall bladder. I called Dr. Stricker and left a message on his answering machine the next day, but he didn't call back. Figuring it was better to be safe than sorry, Chris and I made an executive decision and asked Option Care to switch to a 5-2 schedule until we could talk to Dr. Stricker about it.

I had incorrectly assumed that I could be less hyper-vigilant now that we were back in the world of mainstream medicine. Two weeks after this incident, Chris continued to do well. But just to reassure myself that we were on the right track, I talked with another member of the Lyme group — only to make another shocking discovery.

Jay Fowler was a neuro Lyme patient who had done his homework. He'd had to. After being bitten by a tick and developing the characteristic rash, he'd taken the dead tick with him to his doctor and suggested that he might have Lyme disease. Neither that doctor nor four subsequent doctors had made the correct diagnosis. It wasn't until he found Dr. Stricker that his original suspicions were confirmed. Unfortunately, by that time he had developed chronic Lyme disease.

Jay told me that he did not let his home care agency start him on a "push" because the rate was too fast and the mix was not diluted enough. He told me that according to the Physicians Desk Reference (PDR), Chris should be getting a maximum concentration of 40 mg per milliliter.

I checked the PDR. Jay was right. Upon closer examination, I learned that the 100 mg to 1 ml ratio was the dilution to reconstitute the antibiotic. It was to be followed by additional dilution, presumably in accordance with the PDR. I wondered if this could explain why the woman and her son from the Lyme disease support group had lost their gall bladders. I was painfully reminded that Chris's health, my health, virtually anyone's health could be jeopardized by a trusting, wholehearted delegation of personal responsibility to the professionals, no matter how qualified they seemed to be. Apart from the risk of a lawsuit, the professional does not have to live with the consequences of care. The patient does.

We met with Dr. Stricker again, and he confirmed that the dilution should be 40 mg per ml. I talked to the pharmacist. He agreed to give Chris a large syringe with a pump in order to conform to the PDR protocol. From then on, we properly diluted the mix and had Chris administer it with the larger syringe. Later Dr. Stricker said he was okay with the five on/two off schedule. There were no studies showing one as any better or safer than the other. Although he personally favored a more aggressive approach, we opted to remain conservative.

At that appointment, Dr. Stricker reported the results from Ray's Western Blot. Three of the bands were positive. This was considered an equivocal result. Given his heart problems and his history of bipolar disorder, Dr. Stricker suggested a three-month trial of 100 mg of doxycycline by mouth twice a day. We proceeded with the plan for oral antibiotics given that Ray had not exhibited a manic or depressive psychosis for more than 15 years. However, after a month, due to unrelated ongoing complex medical problems, we decided to discontinue the treatment.

A visit with Dr. Fudenberg

Meanwhile, I continued my research. When I'd started this odyssey, I'd felt like an explorer traveling down a multitude of twisting and intersecting paths. Some of those paths had turned out to be dead ends. Others, like the Lyme disease path, had led to interesting and useful detours. Lately, however, I'd been feeling more as if I was stumbling around in a house of mirrors. As I entered each room, the complexity of the passageways and the mirrors made navigating ever more difficult. Even when I successfully navigated one room, the next was still more complex and disorientating. The scope of my research — and, indeed, this book — had broadened so much that I started looking for professional consultation to help me digest the increasingly technical information I was uncovering.

I began an email relationship with Dr. Hugh Fudenberg, a physician and immunologist whose ideas about nutrition were consistent with the direction my research was taking me. Immunologists work to increase the biological activity of cells that kill viruses, while virologists work on ways to kill viruses directly, bypassing the body's own defenses. Dr. Fudenberg is the head of research at the NeuroImmuno Therapeutics Research Foundation in South Carolina. He has more than 800 publications to his credit, including articles in *Drug Research and the Annual Review of Pharmacology*, *Science*, *Nature*, *New England Journal of Medicine*, *Lancet*, and *Clinical Immunology*. Dr. Fudenberg was the chief editor for *Clinical Immunology* for 20 years. He has successfully treated subsets of Alzheimer's, autism, chronic fatigue syndrome, and A.L.S. with Transfer Factor (TF). TF consists of small protein molecules that passively transfer immunity from one mammal to another by stimulating cell-mediated immunity.

I was pleased when Dr. Fudenberg expressed an interest in my book and agreed to review it. After I sent him a draft, I received an email from him suggesting we meet in San Francisco since he was flying out for the weekend to visit friends.

On April 29, while waiting in the lobby of the Clarion Hotel in South San Francisco, I saw a man who also appeared to be waiting. I introduced myself. It was not Dr. Fudenberg, but a physician friend of his who was also there to visit with him at the same time I was, 7 p.m. I thought that maybe Dr. Fudenberg wanted the three of us to get together. We talked about his work with Dr. Linus Pauling and about my book. He talked about TF, and also some research he had done at Stanford measuring differences in the blood that corresponded to various disease states. By 8:15, the physician could not wait, having other engagements, so he left. I waited until 9:45 when an elderly man slowly walked out of an elevator leaning on a cane. He was wearing dark glasses. I approached somewhat warily and introduced myself, but this time I had the right man; the dark glasses, I learned, were necessitated by an extreme sensitivity to light. We went to the bar since it was too late for dinner. There Dr. Fudenberg and I ate popcorn, drank beer, and talked about an assortment of topics.

Dr. Fudenberg told me that he liked the book and thought the public should be aware of the ideas in it. He said he understood the technical aspects but thought it might be hard for nonprofessionals to follow. I agreed. He said he thought the book needed more emphasis on TF, Borna virus, mercury, and autism, particularly the work of Dr. Reichelt from Oslo.

Dr. Fudenberg also talked about his and another doctor's discovery that sulphur oxidase is low in autistic patients. I asked him if sulfur levels could be high in the blood when sulfur oxidase is low. He said that it could. Then I told him how Chris had reported tasting the salt, the Heparin, and the Rocephin when those substances were pushed through his PICC line. I wondered if, instead of having olfactory hallucinations as had been thought, Chris had actually tasted or smelled sulfur compounds when he became psychotic. Dr. Fudenberg affirmed that this could indeed be the case. In other words, instead of an olfactory hallucination related to temporal lobe seizure-like activity, he could actually be smelling sulfur compounds going through his brain.

We talked about various environmental stressors such as malathion, an insecticide to which our family had been exposed at Clark Air Force Base in the Philippines. We discussed Chris's mercury levels. He asked if Chris had hyperacusis, or acute sensitivity to hearing. I mentioned that he heard crackling sounds when there was a loud noise. He suggested that this could be due to mercury, which can cause pseudo-autism in children, chronic fatigue syndrome in adults, and Alzheimer's in senior adults. It can also impair immune functioning. He said that mercury suppresses the immune system and should be removed. He commented that Chris's high DPT antitoxoid antibodies were a result of his immunizations.

I had researched TF before meeting Dr. Fudenberg, following up on suggestions he had made in emails about the possibility of creating a Lyme-specific TF. However, my Internet searches kept taking me to what were obviously commercial alternative health sites that seemed to lack scientific clout. I told Dr. Fudenberg that I could find nothing on TF at PubMed or Medline, and what this meant to me was that mainstream medicine either hadn't discovered it yet or had repudiated it as a treatment approach. Dr. Fudenberg replied that the "TF" at most Internet sites consisted of bovine colostrum, which, because of the casein in it, could be dangerous. This was not the TF of which he was speaking. I also told him that Dr. Stricker claimed some patients suffered long-term negative symptoms from TF. Dr. Fudenberg responded that while there were short-term complications, he knew of no long-term problems. If there were, it was most likely a result of the TF advertised on the Internet. His own Web site warned against indiscriminate use of TF from colostrum from cows. We shook hands and parted. Dr. Fudenberg headed back to South Carolina. I went back to the Internet.

TF transfers cell-mediated immunity from a donor that is positive for an antigen such as a virus, parasite, or tumor cell to a recipient lacking immunity to that antigen. For example, calves have a better chance of surviving when fed naturally rather than through bottle feeding because of TF. Similarly, humans transfer immunities to their children through breast-feeding. Given that many people test positive for Lyme and have no symptoms, the presumption is that they have an immunity to the disease. Thus, they could donate the substances with the positive immunity against the specific antigen for TF which would then be given to the person lacking such immunity.

Dr. Fudenberg's pioneering work, which he said had been replicated by others, showed that myasthenia gravis and multiple sclerosis are immunological in origin and that they can be reversed with large amounts of TF.[3] Dr. Fudenberg has also used TF successfully in a subset of autistic patients.

He studied 40 infantile autistic patients from 6 to 15 years of age. Twenty-two exhibited what he called classic infantile autism: that is, onset at the age of 12-18 months, often one day to one week after administration of live virus vaccines. Eighteen had onset before 12 months or after 20 months, a group he called "pseudo-autism." In the classic autism group, all had antibodies to myelin basic protein and to neuron axone filament proteins. Of the 22 from this group, 20 responded to TF derived from cells of others in the family. Responders improved as measured on symptom severity score, and 10 became completely normal and were put in regular classes. While there was some regression after termination of treatment, overall functioning remained above base line measures. More than half of all the autistic children had food and or respiratory hypersensitivity due to a deficiency of the enzymes phosphosulfotransferase and cytochrome P-450. Many had marked hypersensitivity to phenols, man-made chemicals used in manufacturing plastics.[4]

While researching TF, I came across a letter by Dr. Fudenberg in the February 17, 1997 issue of *The Scientist*. In that letter, he responded to a previously published article about AIDS that focused primarily on new mainline treatments. Dr. Fudenberg reported effective treatment of AIDS using HIV-specific TF. He claimed that TF reduced viral load better than AZT, causing clinical symptoms to disappear. Two collaborators obtained the same findings, one at the University of Paris and one in Bologna, Italy. Dr. Fudenberg stated in this letter that AIDS patients could get their viral loads significantly lower for about one dollar a day using HIV-specific TF. He went on to state that the AIDS program in the United States was a scandal, listing several references in support of this contention.[5] Dr. Fudenberg was reporting break-throughs to the professional community that probably also sounded "too good to be true." While I was not in a position to assess these claims, I felt a responsibility to report them.

Termination issues

Once we got the initial bugs worked out, Chris's treatment proceeded without a hitch. He continued to function well. He did not experience a Herx. Given that he really had no positive symptoms, we had not expected any dramatic improvements, except that it was our hope that stopping his Lyme disease would stop his bipolar symptoms. After almost three months of IV treatment, our last appointment with Dr. Stricker was on May 24, 2001, ex-actly seven years to the day of my mother's death. (The coincidence felt ironic in that I was doing for Chris what I hadn't been able to do for her: explore new paths toward effective alternative treatments. But more on that later.)

At Chris's request, Dr. Stricker had authorized a new test from IgeneX called the Lyme Dot Assay (LDA). This test measured whether or not there was Lyme antigen in urine that reacted specifically to rabbit anti-*B. burgdorferi* antibodies. Dr. Stricker stated that the LDA was negative, and this indicated that no spirochetes remained, at least not in Chris's blood and urine. Whether they had morphed into blebs in the far reaches of his brain, lungs, or liver was a question neither he or the test could answer. Chris wanted to stop the treatment immediately. He repeated his contention that he'd never had Lyme disease in the first place. Dr. Stricker advised against halting the treatment. He said he could not cite any studies on the danger of stopping early because there were none. However, he reminded Chris that his recommendation for the three months of treatment had been based on enough life cycles of *Borre-lia burgdorferi* to maximize the chances for success. He reiterated that the original Western Blot Test more than met the CDC's requirements for the diagnosis. By the time we left, Chris had agreed to a compromise. He would terminate the treatment only one week earlier than Dr. Stricker recommended. Echos of conflicts being debated in the wider medical community were re-verberating in our own family.

The myth that Chris still clung to in the face of mounting evidence to the contrary was that he and he alone had made the choice to give up his irrational beliefs. To his way of thinking, drugs or nutrition had nothing to do with it. He was the master of his ship, the captain of his soul. Thoughts determined the quality of his life, not psychotropic drugs, vitamin and mineral supplements, or antibiotics. My comments that the destruction of microbes and the presence of essential nutrients were needed for him to stay on an even keel fell on deaf ears. For Chris, it was "mind over matter." Yet anyone who read Chris's own assessment of his current functioning couldn't help but be impressed at how "quiet" his brain had become. I just hoped there weren't some encapsulated cysts in the far reaches of his body already morphing into spirochetes.

Chris had stayed with a difficult medical treatment, and for that he was to be commended. But instead of cutting his treatment short at the end, as if to say, "See, I never had Lyme disease in the first place," I would have preferred for him to have been more positive about the experience. Maybe he felt he had to win again. I feared that he could be setting himself up once again to lose by winning, just as he had when he'd told me that he'd slept soundly during the night and then mutilated himself after he couldn't function at work.

Chris and I were polarized. The more he tried to convince me of his views, the more I became convinced that Lyme disease and possibly other microbes were playing a central, perhaps pivotal, role in his illness.

When we got home, an email was waiting from Dr. Ritchie Shoemaker, a family-practice physician in Maryland whose groundbreaking work on environmental toxins, among other things, led to his recognition as the Maryland Family Practice Doctor of the Year in 2000. I had written to Dr. Shoemaker regarding a screening test called the Visual Contrast Sensitivity Test (VCS) that he provided at his Web site. This test measured subtle perceptual changes reflecting damage from neurotoxins to the optic nerve. A more precise test is available in a paper and pencil format. Dr. Shoemaker claimed that cytokine (TNF) induced hypoperfusion is caused by neurotoxins which, among other things, are produced by microbes, molds, and pollution. His work with neurotoxins from the pfiesteria algae was leading-edge, as was his work on other neurotoxin-related illnesses such as Lyme disease.

Using a Heidelberg Retinal Tomogram Flow Meter (HRF), which measured capillary flow in the optic nerve head, he reported a positive relationship between TNF-mediated hypoperfusion of cells contained in the optic nerve head and low scores on the VCS. He said the test provided an actual window into the brain since there is a correlation between hypoperfusion in the optic nerve head and the brain. He reported successfully treating a number of neurotoxin-related illnesses, including Lyme disease, with not only antibiotics, but also cholestyramine (CSM), a drug used to reduce cholesterol. This drug binds with neurotoxins.[6] The implications for diagnosis and treatment of Lyme and neurotoxins were enormous.

I had asked Dr. Shoemaker about his Web site and his approach to treating Lyme disease. Here is part of his response:

The answer to your question, what would I be treating that Rocephin did not, is the basis for my work in Lyme. Lyme makes a neurotoxin. In other species, similar symptoms and VCS deficits respond to toxin binding with cholestyramine . Lyme patients ... develop a significant worsening of their symptoms if they jump in and take CSM without first pre-treating with a medication that blocks transcription by adipocytes[7] of a pro-inflammatory cytokine and the receptor of that cytokine (TNF). So what I believe my protocol treats is the very basic mechanism of what I believe is chronic Lyme.[8]

He invited me to call him, so I did. We discussed whether the VCS could actually demonstrate that Chris was "cured." He said that if Chris's VCS were negative, that is, there was no subtle visual impairment, then there was a high probability that any toxins were out of his body. If there were positive results, the toxins were still there whether or not *Borrelia burgdorferi* were still present. Basically, if the VCS were negative, he was probably well. If the VCS were positive, he definitively wasn't well yet.

Chris finally agreed to watch me take the VCS on the Internet. He watched over my shoulder as I took it, telling me how he saw the figures on the screen. The test results showed that neither of us had any indication of any impairment. Chris was better able to see the very faint lines than I was. I hoped that the *Borrelia burgdorferi* and associated toxins were either dead or gone.

Later I queried Dr. Shoemaker in an email as to whether he had ever treated bipolar illness with CSM, given that neurotoxins appeared to be a common denominator for some bipolar patients. He described a patient who first manifested bipolar symptoms after he was exposed to microcystin, a blue green algae. He said that as a result of the CSM treatment, his patient's manic behavior ceased.

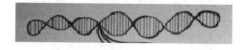

Notes

1. Kersten, A., Poitschek, C., Rauch, S., Aberer, E., "Effects of penicillin, ceftriaxone, and doxycycline on morphology of *Borrelia burgdorferi* antimicrobial agents," *Chemother,* 39(5):1127-33, May 1995.

2. At that time we were still waiting for approval for the MRI. It was not approved. We declined paying for it on our own because, by the time it was turned down, we were already well into treatment. Therefore, we couldn't get any definitive before and after results. In retrospect, we should have paid for it ourselves. In light of subsequent events, proof of a "physical" illness might have helped us get better care for Chris.

3. Lanigan, A.J., "Your Immune System, A Miracle We Take for Granted," from Transfer Factor Resource Page, 2001.
http://www.alphazee.com/t/tf/tf.html

4. Fudenberg, H.H., Demirjian, R., Iversen, P., "Classic infantile onset autism is an antoimmune disease," *Clinical Research (abstracts)* 37(2):556a, 1998.

5. Fudenberg, H.H., "Letters: AIDS Research," *The Scientist* 11(4):13, Feb 17, 1997.

6. Shoemaker, Ritchie, <u>Desperation Medicine</u>, Gateway Press Inc, Baltimore, MD, 2001, 267-270.

7. Transcription involves RNA being synthesized with a DNA template. Adipocyte is a kind of connective tissue cell specialized for the synthesis and storage of fat in animals. In other words, before using the CMS, Dr. Shoemaker blocked the growth of TNF in adipocytes using this medication.

8. Dr. Shoemaker's Web site is at the following URL.
http://www.chronicneurotoxins.com/lymedisease.cfm

22 - Oh, And By The Way ...

Just as I was getting some closure, I stumbled across a new path ... one I hesitated to start down. But though a part of me preferred to ignore it, in the end I had no choice but to follow this path just as I had the others. Whether it led to a cliff, a bog, the moons of Jupiter, or the proverbial treasure at the end of a rainbow, I owed it to my father, to my son, and to myself to complete the odyssey I had started.

My concern was that the path could lead to a place like "The Island of Dr. Moreau." In that movie, based on the classic novel by H.G. Wells, a mad scientist played by Marlon Brando mixes human and animal DNA to create a tribe of hybrid mutants. His tyrannical rule sparks a violent rebellion in which the mutants turn on their creator. What if we ourselves — our bodies, our very DNA — are just such islands, seething with incipient rebellion? What if, in other words, cytopathic (cell-damaging) viral fragments have entered the human gene pool from animals used to develop vaccines? What if these fragments play a role in a wide range of medical and psychiatric illnesses? What if these viruses not only spread from humans to humans, but also cross species barriers as well, like other viruses do? What if humans could infect their pets ... and visa versa?

Dr. Martin's stealth virus

An Australian-born physician and virologist, Dr. John Martin, believes the "stealth" virus is causing the documented increases in psychiatric disorders such as autism and bipolar disorder, as well as playing a significant role in other medical diseases like cancer. Following is the definition appearing on Dr. Martin's Web site:

> Stealth viruses can be defined as a molecularly heterogeneous grouping of atypically structured, cytopathic viruses, that cause persistent systemic infection, frequently associated with neuropsychiatric symptoms, in the absence of significant antiviral cellular inflammation. Stealth viruses typically induce a vacuolating foamy cytopathic effect (CPE) in a range of human and animal cell lines.

According to Dr. Martin, stealth viruses are viral segments which do not provoke the immune system but which nonetheless damage cells by, among other things, causing a metabolic drain. The resulting mitochondria-damaged cells can be significantly impaired or killed.

From 1976 to 1980, Dr. Martin headed the Viral Oncology Branch of the FDA Bureau of Biologics. The mission of this branch was to help ensure the safety of viral vaccines, and especially to consider possible contamination with any viruses that could potentially cause cancers. As part of this work, he found foreign genetic material in polio vaccines that he couldn't explain and that he couldn't get access to because of the proprietary nature of the vaccine technology. He later learned that the FDA was aware that the genetic material may well have come from a monkey (simian) cytomegalovirus (SCMV). Kidney tissues from African green monkeys were being used to produce live polio virus vaccines. Most of these animals were infected with SCMV. A senior administrator who knew of earlier studies pointing to the probable presence of African green monkey SCMV in batches of polio vaccines pointedly told Martin not to worry. "You ingest foreign DNA every time you eat an apple." Dr. Martin worried. He was concerned that the administrator was being overly protective of the vaccine manufacturer. Dr. Martin was not allowed to take his research any further, at least not at that time.

Beginning in 1985, Dr. Martin joined the pathology department of the University of Southern California. He resumed his studies on possible viral infections among patients with complex chronic illnesses, including chronic fatigue syndrome (CFS). Using tissue culture techniques, he isolated viruses from several CFS patients as well as from patients with a wide range of neuropsychiatric illnesses, including autism, bipolar disorder, and schizophrenia. He found that the viruses were not evoking the type of cellular inflammatory response expected for an infectious viral disease. He postulated that the viruses may simply be lacking the antigenic viral components that the cellular immune system would normally target in its defense of a typical viral infection. This concept was embodied in his choice of the term "stealth virus" to refer to a cell-damaging virus that was not being recognized by the cellular immune system. The type of cellular damage caused in tissue cultures by stealth viruses was characterized by the accumulation of lipids (fats) and by the formation of unusual particulate materials. Very similar cellular changes were seen in brain biopsies obtained from infected patients and in the tissues of animals experimentally inoculated with stealth viruses.

Martin's earlier work at the FDA came back into focus when he reported in 1995 that some of these stealth viruses had developed from SCMV. In the *Journal of Clinical and Diagnostic Virology*, he reported that the virus repeatedly isolated from a patient with CFS was unmistakably derived from SCMV. In 1996 he reported in the journal *Pathobiology* his finding of another SCMV-derived virus. This time the virus came from the cerebrospinal fluid of a patient with bipolar psychosis and acute encephalopathy.[1] He reported isolating the same virus from an autistic child.[2] He further stated that he had found a stealth virus originating in an African green monkey in a patient with chronic fatigue syndrome.[3] As with Lyme disease, correlation does not prove causation, but it certainly raised disturbing questions, questions I really didn't want to face.

Other stealth viruses that he isolated did not come from SCMV, illustrating his point that many types of viruses could potentially undergo stealth-adaptation by deleting and or mutating the few critical genes that coded for the antigens recognized by antiviral cell mediated immunity. Dr. Martin was aware that only a few viral components are targeted by antiviral cytotoxic lymphocytes. Unlike antibodies that can be made against many viral components (antigens), the cellular immune system is much more selective and only involves a few viral components.

Over time, Martin had the opportunity to test several patients diagnosed as having chronic Lyme disease. They too showed consistent evidence of being stealth-virus infected. How was this possible? As he continued to obtain DNA sequence data on the SCMV-derived stealth-adapted virus, he found that some of the sequences had come from bacteria. Seemingly, stealth-adaptation not only involved the loss of certain viral genes, but also the acquisition of additional genes. Some had come from infected cells, others had come from various bacteria. It was the presence of these bacterial genes that Martin suggested could account for the positive tests for Lyme disease in patients with CFS, neuropsychiatric and other diseases. Martin uses the term "viteria" to refer to viruses with assimilated bacterial genes. A publication documenting his finding appeared in *Pathobiology* in 1999.

Dr. Martin posted a message on the MMI discussion board in which he presented his opinion that positive Lyme disease testing, including positive Western Blot results could reflect cross-reactivity to stealth viruses. It was my understanding that the Western Blot allowed one to visualize antibodies directed against different viral proteins. I had also understood that stealth viruses did not provoke an immune response. So I wasn't clear how stealth viruses could provoke Lyme antibodies. It seemed to me that a stealth virus that provoked antibodies would be an oxymoron. But that was what Dr. Martin was stating. At least, that was how I understood it. Apparently, the answer is that certain bacteria find a way to infect stealth viruses, producing a new entity he calls viteria, an admixture of assimilated animal and human viral and bacterial genetic sequences. It is their presence that can lead to positive findings of Lyme disease on a Western Blot. I didn't have a clue how one was supposed to differentiate between Lyme, stealth, and the Lyme/stealth viteria.

In 1996, Dr. Martin was invited to speak at the Workshop on Vaccine Safety at the Institute of Medicine of the National Academy of Sciences. He stated that he had detected stealth viruses in CNS-disordered patients, including those suffering from autism, ADHD, aggressive behavioral disorders (in children), schizophrenia and bipolar illness (in young adults), various sensory and memory impairments (in adults), and Alzheimer's disease (in the elderly). He linked these viruses to the undisputed historical cross-contamination of these and other viruses with viruses from other species. He later described outbreaks of a stealth virus in the Mojave Desert and in Tennessee, reporting not only psychiatric symptoms but also examples of patients who had died after demonstrating classical signs of bipolar and other psychiatric illnesses.

The CDC responded with a formal statement. "There is no evidence that polio vaccine, or any other vaccine, has been contaminated with a 'stealth virus.' To our knowledge, existence of this virus as suggested by one researcher has not been confirmed by other investigators."

Soon after the presentation, the University of Southern California, where Dr. Martin worked, banned further investigation into stealth viruses. Either Dr. Martin's work was scientifically suspect, or some kind of cover-up was going on. Maybe no one was interested in letting the proverbial cat out of the bag. Dr. Martin set up his own lab, the Center for Complex Infectious Diseases, where he continues his research on stealth viruses.

If stealth viruses came from other species, and if they were a major cause of bipolar disorder and schizophrenia, among other things, how did these illnesses exist before stealth viruses got into the human gene pool? After all, documented incidents of schizophrenia and bipolar disorder long predate the advent of vaccinations. I believe — and I am no expert here — that Dr. Martin's answer to this objection would be that stealth adaptations from human viruses have been around for a very long time, but that newly formed stealth viruses are accounting for the increasing incidence of these diseases over the last few decades. Over eons of evolution, macrophages in the human body have been routinely engorging themselves on viruses that the immune system determined were a threat. Through a process of natural selection, new viral sequences evolved. These mutated sequences did not provoke an alarm, and were less likely to be consumed by macrophages. Therefore, they could establish themselves and thrive in the bodies of their hosts.

To summarize, if I understood correctly, Dr. Martin was saying that stealth viruses had independently mutated from viruses already within the human gene pool, and from natural cross-contamination such as occurs with viruses like influenza that cross between species. There has been an acceleration of that process though the introduction of these fragments into the human gene pool in vaccinations created from bodily products of other species. In other words, some of the viruses suspected of causing bipolar disorder and schizophrenia were actually mutated viral sequences missing those elements that signaled the immune system that an invader should be attacked by the body's defenses. It was this ability that gave them their name. A stealth virus is defined not by the origin of viral sequences but by the ability of the sequences to evade detection by the immune system. The potential for damage to humans would, among other things, depend on the nature of the particular viral sequence.

When I visited Dr. Martin's Web site, I was, in a word, unhappy. My initial reaction was denial and disbelief. Here I had finally developed a logical basis for a treatment plan for Chris, and now, if Dr. Martin were right, I would have to reexamine everything. I had worked eight months for this? My cognitive dissonance was telling me I couldn't have been wrong. Look how much we "spent" to get here. My mind was already made up. I didn't want to be confused with new facts. I didn't want to have to pursue more leads, raise more hopes, ask Chris to submit to more tests.

Center For Complex Infectious Diseases
Cumulative Double Blind Validation Studies
Viral Prevalence by Category

	Tested	Negative		Positive	
	Total	Number	Percent	Number	Percent
Blood Donors	78	70	90	8	10
Chronic Fatigue	47	2	4	45	96
Psychosis	10	0	0	10	100
Autism	25	5	20	20	80
Lyme Disease	10	1	10	9	90
Multiple Myeloma	30	1	3	29	97

Stealth Prevalence - Courtesy Dr. John Martin

Dr. Martin was suggesting that we got it all wrong. Chris's problem wasn't Lyme disease. It was atypical viral sequences operating in a "stealthy" way. Chris's positive tests were the result of cross-reactivity with these viral sequences. On his Web site, Dr. Martin stated the following: "The pattern of clinical response to antibiotics is more consistent with an anti-chemokine (a type of cytokine) action than to eradication of pathogenic bacteria." Chemokines function like taxis bringing cytokines to sites of lesions or infections.

The chart on the previous page from the Web site at ccid.org displays Dr. Martin's findings from cumulative double-blind testing. Of particular significance is his claim that 10% of symptom-free blood donors test positive for stealth viruses. He reported positive stealth results with the following: chronic fatigue syndrome (96%), autism (80%), psychosis (100%), Lyme (100%), and multiple myeloma (97%). In an email exchange about these findings, Dr. Fudenberg told me that he was skeptical because some years back he had sent ten blood samples from healthy individuals to Dr. Martin, and all of them had come back positive for stealth viruses.

Lyme vs. Lyme vs. stealth

The path we had chosen was already controversial enough without adding stealth viruses to the mix. During the summer of 2001, while I was wrestling with the stealth question, a smoldering debate in the medical community on the issue of the assessment and treatment of Lyme disease was fanned into a conflagration. Lyme-literate doctors (LLMDs) and patients believed that Lyme was being both under-diagnosed and under-treated. Many insurance companies and doctors believed it was over-diagnosed and over-treated and that short courses of treatment were sufficient. They asserted that so-called Lyme patients were either malingering or suffering from psychiatric disorders, although some acknowledged the possibility of a "post-Lyme syndrome." The debate got ugly when one of the pioneers of the "Lyme is under-diagnosed and under-treated" school, Dr. Joseph Burrascano, faced attempts by the New York Office of Professional Medical Conduct (OPMC) to remove his medical license. Those supporting the complaint claimed that extended antibiotic treatment is not only expensive but also unproductive, and sometimes even harmful. And now to add to the confusion, a stealth advocate from the sidelines was arguing that the problem was more likely to be stealth virus than Lyme disease.

Whose data was I to accept? My journey was taking me to medical frontiers where internecine wars for power, control, and, most importantly, money predominated, leaving hapless travelers like myself lost in a barrage of claims and counterclaims. I was in no position to know on a technical basis whether Chris had Lyme disease or a stealth virus, and whether or not either, both, or neither was contributing to his bipolar disorder. And apparently neither was anybody else. If they were, there was so much noise they couldn't be heard.

Treatment of Lyme disease was rarely curative. I asked Dr. Stricker and the nurses at Option Care whether they could guarantee that three months of IV antibiotic treatment would effect a "cure." They said they could make no such guarantee. I was also aware that following completion of the treatment there was no way to accurately test Chris to conclusively demonstrate that Lyme disease was indeed eradicated, even if an MRI had demonstrated reduced white matter hyperintensities. Given that Chris's IV cost $135 a day, I could understand the reluctance of insurance companies to support such treatment, particularly with no assurance of a definitive successful outcome. I learned that there were stealth-like mechanisms within the Lyme spirochete that prevent the immune system from recognizing one of the more common forms of this pleomorphic organism. An s-layer, or slime layer, of glycoprotein, a protein on the outer surface of the cell membranes, acts like a stealthy protection to hide the bacteria from the immune system. This in turn prevents outer-surface protein antigens (OSPs) from attacking.[4] Other forms of the bacteria, however, do provoke immune processes. I wondered if this particular form of Lyme disease was a kind of prototype of a stealth virus. Were stealth viruses also pleomorphic, with certain forms provoking immune responses while others didn't? Why else would bacteria-infected stealth viruses test positive for Lyme disease on a Western Blot? Could Lyme and stealth coexist? In a CFS Radio Show interview on April 11, 1999 with Dr. Roger Mazlen, Dr. Martin stated that when stealth and Lyme coexist in the test tube, the presence of stealth "puts the *Borrelia burgdorferi* into a feeding frenzy." In chat rooms I spoke with patients who told me that Dr. Martin had confirmed they had both Lyme and stealth virus. So why did he state on the MMI board that the Lyme community had it wrong?

I called Dr. Martin, who was kind enough to answer some of my questions on the phone. I had read his Web site, but his model was so novel and his explanations so detailed that I couldn't grasp a lot of what he was saying. He expressed his belief that the Lyme disease community and other groups focusing on such illnesses as chronic fatigue syndrome and fibromyalgia were on shaky scientific footing; he stated that the data supported complex infections and, specifically, stealth viruses as the causes of psychiatric and a host of other disorders.[5] Dr. Martin told me that he didn't accept the diagnoses of either schizophrenia or bipolar disorder. He viewed them as a part of a spectrum of illnesses caused by stealth viruses. He believed that the solution to these illnesses would one day be found through targeting these viruses. He believed that stealth viruses assimilated genetic sequences from *Borrelia burgdorferi*, as well as other microbes. He reaffirmed what I had read, namely, that the resulting viteria caused false positive Western Blot findings.

Dr. Martin agreed to test Chris's blood for stealth viruses. My head was spinning when I hung up the phone. Could it be that the model I had painstakingly pieced together was incomplete or even wrong? When I told Chris of the conversation, he said that he didn't want to have his blood tested again.

When I spoke with Dr. Martin, he said he had been interviewed by medical and science journalist Nicholas Regush for his book, <u>The Virus</u>

Within. He said that several of the cases he had described to Regush as examples of stealth viruses were actually described in the book as cases of HHV-6 virus. Somehow, all this didn't add up. How was a layman like myself to understand, when the professionals seemed to be at such cross-purposes?

Meanwhile, I obtained irrefutable evidence from several sources for the idea of viral cross-contamination. I learned that the Simian Virus 40 had found its way from monkeys into our gene pool, and was considered instrumental in the development of a specific, though thankfully rare, type of very deadly cancer.

Supplements and stealth

If this new bipolar "theory of the week" were valid, it actually would be another argument for the nutritional approach advocated by Truehope as well as the immune-enhancing supplements I tried to get Chris to take. For one thing, Dr. Martin's Web site specifically listed a number of nutrients, such as the B, D, and E vitamins, along with research supporting their role in reducing production of the specialized cytokines called chemokines. Dr. Martin, through a complex alchemy explained on his Web site, stated that reducing production of chemokines through various nutritional supplements, antibiotics, and antiviral medications minimizes the damage done by stealth viruses. I presumed that reducing chemokines also reduced the proliferation of cytokines.

If inadequate nutrition impairs the effectiveness of the immune system, then adequate nutrition would improve it whether or not one could specifically isolate the microbes or combination of microbes and environmental toxins that cause bipolar symptoms. Nutrients could provide the fuel to mount a more effective defense against those viruses that provoke an immune response. Since cells are impaired by the action of a stealth virus and low energy levels render them more susceptible to excitotoxins, then better nutrition could give cells increased energy for managing excitotoxins. And finally, according to Dr. Martin's Web site, nutrients would lessen the production of chemokines. That would mean fewer taxi drivers to move the cytokines to certain areas.

While Dr. Martin's views are controversial and not yet generally known or accepted, I have noticed while researching and writing this book that the number of doctors treating stealth viruses has increased markedly, as has the size of a discussion group called the stealth virus support group. The photo of the unnamed virus from the Stanley Foundation on page 174 looks similar to photos of stealth viruses I would later see at the Center for Complex Infectious Diseases. I also learned from the stealth virus support group that stealth increases cluster fibrin, reduces the viscosity of the blood, and reduces vascularity in the brain.

In <u>The Virus Within,</u> Regush wrote that Dr. Martin's theory of stealth viruses as causative agents of mental illness is similar to the virus model that Doctors Torrey and Yolken are pursuing. Increased incidence of MS with schizophrenia and bipolar disorder lend support to the notion that viruses and/or retroviruses play a role in these disorders. As Regush stated, "The possibility that major disease lurks inside the body, waiting to erupt because of the interplay of viruses that live within us is a frightening proposition."[6]

"Frightening proposition?" Growing up in the 1950s, my greatest fears had been black widow spiders in an old chicken coop behind our house, rattlesnakes in the foothills, and the "Red Chinese." Spiders and snakes I could avoid. But not the Red Chinese. I would imagine my uncle, an avid gun collector, his neighbors and me fighting off waves of communist invaders as they surged through the streets of Fresno. The words "Red Chinese" and the fear that they engendered seem almost quaint today. Now it is terrorists that we fear ... and with reason. But there may be terrorists inside our own bodies. Today's children may have to worry about AIDS, Lyme disease, and what may be the ultimate micro-terrorists: stealth viruses. Where will they hide? How will they arm themselves?

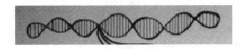

Notes

1. Martin, W.J., "Simian cytomegalovirus-related stealth virus isolated from the cerebrospinal fluid of a patient with bipolar psychosis and acute encephalopathy," *Pathobiology*, 64:64-66, 1996.
2. Martin, W.J., "Stealth virus isolated from an autistic child," *Journal of Autism and Developmental Disorders*, 25:223, 1995.
3. Martin, W.J., "Severe stealth virus encephalopathy following chronic fatigue-syndrome-like illness: clinical and histopathological features," *Pathobiology*, 64:1, 1996.
4. Carrigan, D.R., Harrington, D., Knox, K.K., "Subacute leukoencephalitis caused by CNS infection with human herpespirus-6 manifesting as acute multiple sclerosis," *Neurology* 47:1425, 1996.
5. MMI posters and the CDC point out that no one has duplicated Dr. Martin's work, and he doesn't share his methods. Dr. Martin told me he has given his protocols to public health departments which have not followed through with his recommendations. Some posters at the Stealth Support Group state they were not helped by the Lyme disease model and are now getting help through stealth virus treatment. Also, there is ample proof of cross-contamination from vaccines. In March of 2002, Dr. Martin presented his ideas to the CDC once again, suggesting that they are still open to hearing them, in spite of the increased bioterrorism emphasis.
6. Regush, Nicholas, <u>The Virus Within, A Coming Epidemic: How Medical Detectives Are Tracking a Terrifying Virus That Hides in Almost All of Us</u>, Penguin Books, New York, New York, 2000, 176-178, 209.

23 - Shipwrecked

Around the first of July, 2001, five weeks after Chris completed his IV treatment, he flew to Grand Rapids, Michigan, to visit his ex-girlfriend, Sandy, and the couple, Darren and Mandy, he had known in college. We thought this would be a good way for him to stretch his wings in preparation for his long-term plan to move to Seattle and become self-supporting again. We felt confident he was ready to once again experience being on his own even though we had no proof that the Lyme was gone.

Floundering at sea

Based on his phone calls during the first week, Chris's visit was going well. But on the eighth day, he had an intense discussion with Sandy far into the night about religious issues and their future as a couple. It wasn't the first time. They concluded once again that their differences were too insurmountable for them to have any future together except as friends. Sandy, the daughter of a pastor, held more religiously conservative beliefs than did Chris. Chris told her that he might be a universalistic Christian, a person who believes that God's grace is for all, whether or not they choose to accept it. Sandy replied emphatically that such a belief was not a true Christian belief. The next day, Chris left Sandy's house as planned and went to stay with Darren and Mandy. That night, at his friends' house, he began to obsess about going to hell again. He paced back and forth until morning as his brain drilled down into that all-too-familiar obsessive tunnel vision. He couldn't get away from the thought that he was condemned to eternal torment. He tried watching TV and listening to music, but nothing helped. His old obsessions were back.

The next day, Sandy, Darren, Mandy, and Chris went golfing, but Chris couldn't focus on the game. His friends had to remind him where to go, as well as to stay out of the way of other golfers. They noticed that he seemed distracted.

He called us on July 10. He told us that he hadn't been sleeping for several days and was thinking of coming home early. He said that he had taken 24 supplement pills for two days to try and make up for not taking them. This was the first we had heard that he hadn't been taking the supplements. When I asked how long he'd been off them, he wasn't specific except to say that for two days he'd taken only 8 instead of his usual dose of 16, and he may have missed some days altogether. He was tearful and said he had let us down. His speech was slow, and his concentration seemed impaired. He again reported smells that weren't there, specifically a rotten-egg smell just like he'd experienced before. He said that his skin felt hot. We agreed that he should come home early. Chris had told his friends that he might have to go to the hospital.

Chris's brain was becoming dysfunctional again. I asked what he had been eating. He told me that he was having two meals a day, with cereal and milk for breakfast. The previous night, he'd had pasta for dinner.

The next morning, July 11, Darren called us with some bad news. He had stayed up with Chris until 2 a.m. the night before, but had finally gone to bed. About an hour later, Chris took seventeen 50 mg over-the-counter sleeping pills. When Darren tried to get him up for the flight home at 5 a.m., Chris was slow to waken. Concerned, Darren took him to an emergency room, where they treated him for an overdose and admitted him. The consulting psychiatrist put him on Zyprexa and Haldol and recommended inpatient psychiatric hospitalization. Later, Chris told us that he hadn't taken the pills in another suicide attempt, but had only wanted relief from his growing agitation and inability to sleep.

Gayle and I were stunned. Chris's life had been so stable for the previous eight months while on the IV treatment and the nutritional supplements. Now we felt as if someone had dropped a bomb on us, with the distinct possibility of more to follow.

While in the medical ward, Chris asked to be put in restraints because he feared he would lose control and become violent. After two days, he was transferred to Kalamazoo Psychiatric Hospital.

Had he not taken enough supplements? Had the supplements lost their effectiveness? Had the *Borrelia burgdorferi* morphed into L-Forms, those filaments, cysts, granules, hooked rods and elbows that would allow the microbes to survive the treatment with Rocephin? Had they come back? Was there something else we had missed? I thought of a true story I had read about a man who became psychotic twice in his life, both times after drinking wine he purchased at a particular airport wine shop. Because of the proximity of the two psychotic episodes to his drinking of that wine, researchers traced the wine to a vineyard whose wines were found to contain an excitotoxin unique to that particular vineyard. Had something in Chris's diet similarly triggered this latest episode?

Chris viewed the substance of his discussion with Sandy as the trigger. Clearly, given Chris's history, her comments were ill–advised. But Sandy's comments were no more responsible for his "crashing" than his mother was responsible for Chris obsessing about killing himself by eating oleander leaves simply because of a story she had once told him. A properly functioning brain with adequate nourishment can process such thoughts without imploding.

While Chris focused on his subjective thought processes, I wanted to understand what changes had occurred in his brain. At home, when he was taking the supplements, he had argued with Sandy over the phone about their religious differences without obsessing about them. He'd seen horrible news stories on TV and in the papers without obsessing about them. He'd watched movies I would have preferred he not watch and didn't obsess about any of them. It seemed to me that his brain now lacked the plasticity it had demonstrated while he was at home.

I could have described this setback from a "mental" health perspective. I could say that Chris experienced an unconscious regression in the service of the ego. I could speculate that he had a regressive response to the fantasized loss of the love object. His intrapsychic and interpsychic processes had compelled him to become a helpless child overwhelmed by primordial dependency feelings. But why bother? The person suffering from borderline personality disorder has the same problem as the one suffering from bipolar disorder: low NAA levels suggestive of neuronal death or impairment. Who wouldn't regress when their brain ceased to function correctly? I wondered if he had starved it.

I also entertained thoughts that this bipolar odyssey project of mine, including this book which had grown out of it, was no more than an exercise in need-fulfilling fantasy. I thought of the movie "Awakenings," where a physician finds a way to transform patients from a catatonic-like existence to a life of movement and dance, only to have them return to their previously impaired state. I wondered if Tony had found some way to briefly restore bipolar patients to health only to have them return to their highs and lows. But I had learned too much to turn back. This obstacle was another opportunity to advance. Chris and I had more lessons to learn, from our mistakes as well as our successes.

I emailed Dr. Bransfield and told him what had happened. He suggested that Chris should have a sleep and waking EEG with nasopharyngeal (up the nose) leads to rule out temporal lobe seizure disorder. He indicated that the olfactory hallucinations could have been the result of temporal lobe epilepsy and that he might need Depakote.[1] I shared with Dr. Bransfield a note that I had received from Dr. Cade earlier in my research: "We think within the next year, we will have convincing evidence that gluten and casein are also the culprits in many patients with epilepsy." I told him about Chris's eating pasta before both his fourth episode and this one. I also told him about a friend's adult son whose epilepsy had been controlled by medication yet who had suffered a seizure while taking a bath and drowned; I remembered my friend mentioning to me that her son had eaten pizza for dinner that night. Given that cell inhibition properties are compromised in both seizure and bipolar disorders — that is, neurons fire too easily — I wondered if gluten somehow lessened the effectiveness of neuron inhibition processes in selected individuals. On the other hand, people eat pasta all the time. Hmm ... grasping at straws? Maybe, but it was time to start asking questions again, no matter how farfetched they seemed. There were too many pieces to this puzzle. I would continue to consider as many as possible until I was sure they would not fit.

Dr. Bransfield told me about work being done at John Hopkins University on ketogenic diets, basically diets of protein and fat. He said that these diets were used before the advent of seizure medications and that even now the diet was sometimes more successful than medications. If the effects of diet were similar to the effects of Depakote or Tegretol, then why wouldn't a ketogenic diet be effective for bipolar patients? Conversely, maybe a high carbohydrate diet such as Chris ate, with daily gluten and casein, would not be healthy. I wondered if he was eating foods with a lot of glutamate, an amino acid that, if not properly regulated by the glial cells, can cause both mania and cell death.

An email message from Dr. Bransfield got right to the heart of the matter:

> *My gut feeling is that you probably cannot totally eradicate the Lyme once late stage disease is there. I do feel it is possible to keep it in check. I think putting a stealth pathogen into latency may be the best we can hope for with some of these persistent infections. Think in terms of a herpes infection. You cannot actually eliminate it. These ups and downs are part of the nature of both Lyme and bipolar. Sounds like Chris sometimes is tired of being the patient. When he gets some relief, he wants a break from it, and sometimes this can contribute to a relapse.*

So perhaps Chris's Lyme disease could never be cured, just managed like herpes would be. Failure to stay on top of it with good nutrition, sleep, exercise, and immune-enhancing drugs could cause it to flare up again. Maybe the issue of which came first, the Lyme disease or bipolar disorder symptoms, was just not that important. The body needs to be fortified enough to deal with whatever imbalances exist, whether they are caused by food allergies, Lyme disease, known or unknown viruses, heavy metals, digestive problems, genetic metabolic defects, or microbes yet to be discovered.

I spoke with the founder and president of the Chico Hyperbaric Center, Mitchell L. Hoggard, a pharmacist by training. He said that the presence of neuropsychiatric symptoms in light of Chris's previous Western Blot results was strongly indicative of a recurrence of the Lyme disease. He told me that his son had been wheelchair-bound for 2 years until undergoing 60 antibiotic treatments in the hyperbaric chamber. Since then, he had been symptom-free. Should that be the next step for Chris? But his Web site said that Lyme patients have Herxes during treatment. Chris never had a Herx.

It was time to call Tony. I told him what had happened and asked if he had any experience with a habituation effect, or if the supplements could be putting too much of something into Chris's system. He said they had seen no habituation effects. He said that he and David had conducted an extensive review of the literature regarding the various vitamins, minerals, and amino acids in the supplements and found that even at equivalent amounts of 32 pills a day, there was no evidence of toxic effects, including from the nickel.

He was the most relaxed and confident of anyone I had spoken to. He said that Chris was probably not taking enough supplements. He reiterated that taking 8 wasn't enough, and, if he was exhibiting symptoms, taking 16 wasn't enough, either. He told me that his own son had decided to stop taking the supplements at one point, and a few weeks later had begun getting depressed. He mentioned a woman who had struggled with schizophrenia for 20 years, then became symptom free after eight months on the supplements ... until she decided she didn't need them anymore. It took three months of taking 32 supplements a day for her symptoms to abate again. Tony told me about a church member who, while on a mission trip, was incorrectly told by someone to take the 32 pills in the morning rather than throughout the day. He did this and had both diarrhea and poor absorption. In a few weeks, he became psychotic.

Tony said that he has seen individuals with severe bipolar illness demonstrate the same kind of disorientation Chris felt on the golf course. He said that it was from his brain not having sufficient fuel. I interpreted his statement to mean that Chris may not have been able to utilize the fuel he had due to whatever microbes, antigens, cytokines, or other agents were impairing his digestive and/or metabolic processes.

Tony said, "You know, Dave, I recently had an argument with a physician who accused me of being too simplistic. I told him, 'Hey, when my car runs out of gas, it doesn't work anymore. I put gas in, and it runs.' Chris should be back on 32 pills a day. I personally take 16 tablets a day just to ensure proper nutrition."

When I told him that Chris seemed to feel he was taking a lot even at 16, Tony reminded me that much of the bulk in the tablets is in substances which improve the absorption of the vitamins and minerals.

He said that this crisis provided a good opportunity for what is called an ABA trial. On the supplements, Chris was fine for eight months (A). He "crashed" in 10 days in response to taking a trip, changing his sleeping patterns, stressful discussions, dietary changes, not taking omega-3 fatty acids, and not taking the supplements regularly (B). Since (A) seemed to have worked, and (B) had not, a logical treatment plan would be to put him back on (A) again, or 32 supplements a day, and see the effects. Hence, ABA. Tony recommended doing this before pursuing any further Lyme disease treatment. He predicted that if we put Chris back on 32 supplements a day, he would come around again in less than ten days. I told him that I was sure the hospital would not approve.

On the phone, Chris told his mother and me that he was sorry. He said that he was evil, and that if he were gone, we wouldn't have to suffer anymore because of him. He spoke with slurred speech about how effective the drugs were in calming him down and how the supplements had failed him. He said that Tony was "blowing smoke at me." Chris had never really been convinced of the efficacy of the supplements, perhaps because I was, or perhaps because his brain was too impaired to recognize the effects. In his update in Chapter 20, Chris's cavalier attitude had come through loud and clear.

> *Personally, I am content to just keep taking the nutritional supplements as if they were actually doing something (and they are, because they are loaded with vitamins and minerals that are healthy for me, regardless of whether or not they are helping with the bipolar) and leave it at that. However, my dad has a different opinion, one with which I wholeheartedly disagree.*

After he completed the IV Rocephin, Chris had started to feel more like his old self. He didn't want to be reminded that he still had an illness. If I tried to discuss taking omega-3 fatty acids or taking additional immune-enhancing substances to keep any remaining Lyme disease in check, he would get upset. He had shortened his IV treatment by one week, against the advice of Dr. Stricker, because a Lyme-Dot-Assay panel taken during his treatment showed no indication of Lyme disease, which he interpreted to mean that he'd never had it in the first place. He hadn't considered the possibility that the test results demonstrated the success of the treatment, as far as could be known. In spite of my attempts to convince him otherwise, he had stopped taking the omega-3 fatty acids several months before and only continued to take extra immune-enhancing supplements when I insisted on it, and sometimes not even then. Yet he had been doing so well that it seemed irrelevant to us that he wasn't wholeheartedly sticking to the plan. Seems he felt a need to hold back through partial compliance.

While in Grand Rapids, Chris had diverged even further from the plan. Sandy told me that she had argued with him about taking the supplements, and he had said that he would take him when he needed to. Even at home, Chris took them inconsistently.

Because of this background, we suspected that he had gone off his regular 16-a-day regimen the day he flew out, even though he claimed otherwise. In addition, his eating patterns were very irregular while he was staying at Sandy's house. Eating only two meals a day, one of them consisting of gluten and casein, asssured an excessive amount of opioids. Lack of sleep discipline didn't help.

As the details emerged, I began to realize that Chris's experiences, rather than refuting the effectiveness of nutrients, were actually supporting it, albeit at his own expense. Understanding that my outlook might evolve in response to new information, I concluded that his failure to consistently take the supplements had most likely caused this, his fifth episode. When he'd started to feel "weird," he'd taken 24 supplements a day for two days in an attempt to reestablish equilibrium. As he was feeling a loss of control, he had looked into a mirror and recited aloud, "I am master of my fate, the captain of my soul." This mantra helped him to control his feelings for a short time. But no thoughts from "Invictus" could make up for the deficit of needed nutrients in his brain. In fact, as far as I was concerned, the episode had occurred precisely because Chris had believed that he was the master of his fate and the captain of his soul. His beliefs had consequences. Because of those beliefs, he had not submitted to the discipline required for the regular care and feeding of his brain. His brain chemistry had most likely passed some key threshold due, at least in part, to inadequate nutritional precursors. Chris had never really bought the concept that his mind needed his brain, or that his brain needed supplemental nutrition. That was his father's idea. He couldn't let his dad win. Then again, maybe I was focusing too much on father-son dynamics when, in fact, Chris's brain may have been so impaired from neuro-Lyme disease that the oppositional behavior he had heretofore exhibited may have been both a symptom and a cause of his lack of compliance.

The words that Chris had clung to in his hour of need happened to be the last words a man named Timothy McVeigh shared with the media before his execution — what a chilling coincidence. Simply saying the words of "Invictus" would not make it so, but the promises in "Invictus" could still be fulfilled. To be the captain of his soul, Chris would have to pay a lot more attention to the care and feeding of it.

This excursion away from his home port had demonstrated that his ship wasn't yet ready to sail out on the open seas. Chris needed to maintain the sails, man the bilge pumps, get enough crew rest, and, most importantly, ensure adequate ballast by stockpiling proper provisions for the journey. Otherwise his ship would founder when the first storm came along. But with foresight and diligence, he could prepare himself to weather the inevitable storms ... and sail more smoothly in balmy weather as well.

How did I know my "best" hypothesis was the most reasonable, and not my own cognitive dissonance? If I expended substantial funds to find answers, if I took two years to write a book on nutrients calming the unquiet brain, then how could I admit to myself that I had gotten it all wrong? My own logic would have led me to conclude that all my efforts had been in vain, but for the fact that Chris had not taken the omega-3 fatty acids, Synergy supplements, and other immune enhancing supplements. If he had taken them properly and then "crashed," I would have been forced to conclude that nutrients did not quiet his unquiet brain. However, the reoccurrence of symptoms following his failure to comply with the regimen strongly suggested that nutritional deficits were a key factor. He had unwittingly made it to the "B" phase of the ABA trial, and the data was, unfortunately, impressive.

Another factor that I considered was that Chris was mildly dehydrated even when tested in the hospital on July 12. I had learned from support group members that Lyme patients are less likely to feel thirsty than those with Lyme disease. The humid summer heat and inadequate fluid intake could have been contributory factors in this episode. Also, his urine pH was acidic, 5.5, compared to his normal level of 7.0.

Chris wasn't drinking enough water. His body was in some kind of acid imbalance. QUIN from inflammation creates acid conditions in the body. Add a little Lyme, a fair amount of cytokines, and some QUIN, and the chances of having an imploded brain increase substantially.

Not enough good stuff

I wasn't a specialist in these matters, but it seemed intuitive to me that too much bad stuff was bad for Chris's brain as was too little good stuff. Following is my "backyard mechanic's leave-no-stone-unturned" list of specific factors that could have played a role in Chris's fifth episode.

Not enough good stuff:
1. No omega-3 fatty acid supplements for four months.
2. Inconsistent taking of supplements.
3. Irregular meals.
4. No additional immune-enhancing and anti-oxidizing supplements.
5. Poor sleep discipline, resulting in sleeplessness.
6. Drinking insufficient amounts of water, causing dehydration.

Too much bad stuff:
1. Possible reemergence of Lyme disease from the blebs formed in response to his treatment with IV antibiotics.
2. Exposure to new molds and unknown allergens from humid ecosys-

tem. These mitogens could cause histamine release from mast cells, proliferation of cytokines and neurotoxins, and a cascading increase in protein kinase C.[2]

3. Stressful situations provoking cortisol and ACTH.

4. Delayed food allergies provoking cytokine production and requiring nutritional stores for detoxification, thereby depleting availability for his brain.

5. Exposure to endrin or aldrin. The ELISA/ACT Lymphocyte Response Assay showed him to be strongly reactive to these chemicals. Both are powerful convulsants, meaning that they can lower the firing threshold of neurons. Even though they are no longer used in the United States, they can still be found in trace amounts in foods or drinking water. Aldrin can also be found in homes treated for termites in the past.

6. Exposure to the xylene in auto exhaust. The ELISA/ACT Lymphocyte Response Assay showed that Chris was moderately reactive to xylene, produced from petroleum and found in auto exhaust. Even brief exposure can affect one's ability to perform tasks.

His first episode occurred when he lived near a heavily trafficked street. I noted the smell of car fumes in and out of his apartment. His second episode started shortly after driving five hours in a truck on a freeway. His third episode occurred in Pennsylvania while driving on an interstate freeway heading for Boston. During the fourth episode, he began mutilating himself after walking 8 miles down Highway 20, where the cars were going uphill. (He also had drug withdrawal akathisia.)

When we did fly back from Kalamazoo, we drove from San Francisco to Davis on Interstate 80; Chris reported that his acute sense of smell had returned, even though it had not recurred prior to his discharge from the hospital or during the flight.

During the first five years of Chris's life, when I was a captain stationed at Fairchid Air Force Base, our home was one house away from a four-lane major thoroughfare in Spokane. The drivers would press their accelerators to climb a hill just before our street. I used to wonder if the exhaust I smelled in our front yard where Chris played was a health threat. I am still wondering.

7. Exposure to molds and chemical toxins from the aircraft in which he was flying.

There were two problems. First, Chris's brain was broken. Second, he was receiving drugs for something called "bipolar disorder." These drugs were being administered by professionals who knew little about his unique biological needs and had little inclination to learn more. I decided that if I didn't get him home immediately, they would continue to medicate him, and he would regress as he'd done at Live Oaks Hospital.

Feeling powerless, I decided to utilize my manic inheritance. I would adopt the most grandiose and manic posture I could muster. Minor mania would not do; this situation called for the controlled and manipulative application of major mania. I would become a squeaky wheel. I would light a fire under them ... well, maybe not literally.

I contacted Chris's social worker and doctor and briefed them on Chris's Lyme disease, strongly recommending that he be treated for that and put back on the supplements and fatty acids. They didn't do it. I was not surprised. The social worker asked for a history. I told her I had a 300+ page history that I would be glad to send. She said that would be fine, so I mailed a copy of this book, only with a fictional ending similar to what actually had happened at Live Oak Hospital ... that is, before the peanuts and pills. I wrote a tragic, "more of the same" ending to get their attention in the hope that they would release him and let me bring him home. From observing both my father and son, I learned that as mania takes over, a child emerges who knows others well enough to extort and manipulate, but not well enough to empathize or see the proper social context. I told the social worker that due to circumstances beyond our control, her hospital was now in the book and their actions would help to determine how the book would end. A few days later, I faxed the draft of the new end of the book, along with a summary of events leading to Chris's hospitalization, to Kalamazoo Psychiatric Hospital. So what if the staff talked among themselves about the apple not falling far from the tree? I didn't care. It was mania time. This squeaky wheel was determined to get whatever grease was necessary to get Chris home.

There was a method to my madness. I wanted them to know that Chris wasn't the typical patient, that I wasn't the typical parent, and that we were not going to go along with more of the same, at least not quietly. Furthermore, in my most extravagant of manic fantasies, if they continued with more of the same, I envisioned a future that would not be kind to them. While my internal fantasies were limitless, even so, my rationality prevented me from sharing all of them, such as the following.

The Kalamazoo Bio-Behavioral Hospital of 2016

The staff of the Kalamazoo Psychiatric Hospital in the year 2001 did not suspect that their hospital would be immortalized in a book that would grace the shelves of the Kalamazoo County library 15 years later.

They didn't know that a high school student — let's call her "Jill" — would check out the old book from the library to write a research paper on one of the hot topics of 2016: "The History of Psychotropic Medications."

Jill would read the section about a young man who "crashed" after not consistently taking his supplements and omega-3 fatty acids. She would read about how the hospital had given him psychotropic medications that robbed him of his identity. Then she would ask her mom why they did that to patients back then, and her mom would ask her brother, who happened to be the director of the recently renamed Kalamazoo Bio-Behavioral Hospital. We'll call him "Tom."

And Tom would say in a sheepish way, "But that was how we treated psychiatric patients in those days."

Then Jill would ask, "Uncle Tom, what is a 'psychiatric' patient?"

And he would say, "That's what they used to call patients with bio-behavioral disorders before we knew what caused them. We thought the problem was in their souls, or 'psyches.'"

Then Jill would say, "But Uncle Tom, this book that the man's father wrote is about how nutrients restore broken brains, and you once told us that the first test you perform on new patients is Nu-Tune."

And he would respond, "Yes, our hospital was one of the first pioneers in Nutritional Tune-up Analysis. First we use the Check-Life Test System to check for hyperpolypeptiduria, food sensitivities, nutritional deficits, and any other anomalies. This system was just starting to be produced for law enforcement and medical agencies to assess drug and alcohol involvement from human saliva when this man was hospitalized. After we feed the Check-Life data to the computer, the Nu-Tune program either creates an individualized supplement to correct the nutritional imbalances or recommends filtering either the blood or cerebrospinal fluid to remove the offending toxins. If we need more information, we take a drop of blood and analyze it for 5,000 substances and then design a solution around that. In the old days, there was a saying that some people had "bad blood." Well, sometimes that is true. Anyway, we used to just give everyone the same supplements, but then we found it was more cost-effective and efficient to only supply those that were needed. We find that it helps most of our patients, and it does no harm to the rest. Sometimes we resort to psychotropic medication, but that's very rare now. To be honest, I can't remember the last time we did that. Yes, we could have treated the young man in the book with general vitamin and amino acid supplements from Truehope, and it would have been more effective than the medications, but back then we didn't know what else to do."

And so, Jill and all her classmates who checked out the book for high school research papers would bring shame to the staff at the Kalamazoo Bio-Behavioral Hospital for giving this young man medications instead of the supplements and omega-3 fatty acids whose benefits were widely known even at the time ... in the parallel universe of alternative medicine.

The following is the draft of the end of the book that I did fax to the hospital. I wrote a different spin on H.G. Wells's 1904 short story "Country of the Blind" in order to maximize my manic machinations.

"A nice work of fiction"

The physicians at Kalamazoo Psychiatric Hospital, an old edifice built in the mid-1800s, were not willing to do anything but more of the same. So they got more of the same. After the first few days, Chris came around, likely in response to the too-little, too-late supplements he had taken a few days earlier. But after a week, he became more psychotic, his brain becoming increasingly preoccupied with his "bad" self. The drugs minimized the acute anxiety, but he experienced the same black-and-white thinking. He continued to voice suicidal ideation, to blame himself, to say that he was beyond hope, and to say that even the supplements couldn't help him. His doctor filled him full of drugs that gave his body a metallic odor, caused hypertrophy to parts of his brain, and stressed his liver. His doctors tried to find the right combination of psychotropic medications to restore him to a minimal level of functioning. They wanted to replace his brain impairment with a "tranquilizer psychosis." This is a condition in which the patient is no longer agitated, suicidal, or homicidal. Unfortunately, the patient is also no longer capable of spontaneity or curiosity. He experiences memory and cognitive impairment. He has a waxen facial expression and has lost the naturalness in his physical movement.

There was no way I could convince doctors halfway across the country that Chris had a biological, not a "psychiatric," problem. They wouldn't make the time to hear me talk about elevated acute phase proteins, elevated cytokines such as IL-1, IL-2, IL-6, quinolinic acid, and activation of the hypothalamus-pituitary adrenal axis. His doctor wouldn't even answer my phone calls. What good would it do to share with them almost a year of painstaking research showing that Chris had Lyme disease, mercury and antimony in his system, one of the highest levels for IgG food sensitivities one could have, chemical sensitivities, etc.? How could I tell them that he met the conditions for a disorder that only existed in the minds of the creators and the faithful followers of the DSM-IV? How could I tell them that he met the criteria for a number of biological disorders, the most significant of which was neurologic Lyme disease? My entreaties would fall on deaf ears because the power components of the systems of which they were all a part would call into question their competence if they did anything other than the approved protocols. There would be no chance for a successful challenge to the Orthodox Church of Psychiatry at Kalamazoo Psychiatric Hospital. If they opened their eyes to innovative and powerful ways to help my son, if they deviated from their doctrines, they could dramatically accelerate his return to health. But to do so, not unlike Chris, they would have to face their fears of being cast into the outer darkness, not to mention losing their jobs.

Once upon a time, two mountain climbers exploring remote Hima-

layan regions stumbled upon a pass that wasn't on their maps. The pass led the two men to a lush, green valley. Excited and curious, they climbed down the treacherous, snow-covered mountain as quickly as they could. As they descended through drifting fog, they saw regular patterns of green interlaced with brown lines. Far in the distance was what appeared to be a village. Closer now, they saw farmers' fields and narrow dirt paths. Soon they could make out workers toiling in the fields under the hot sun; the workers were dressed in long, loose robes, earthy brown as the robes of monks, with wide brown hats to protect them from the sun. None of them seemed to have noticed the two men yet.

At last the men arrived on the valley floor close by one of the dirt paths. It was about two feet wide, bordered on either side by clay ridges that stood approximately six inches high. The men noted that the buildings of the village about half a mile away were striking for their absence of color. There was a sort of a grayish-brown hue to the buildings, all of which looked the same. They waved at some workers in the distance, and, receiving no response, shouted a loud greeting. At that, the workers raised their heads and shouted something back in reply. They seemed to be speaking some foreign language unknown to the men. But as their shouts continued, one of the men realized suddenly that he was hearing his own greeting coming back to him, only so distorted in pronunciation as to be virtually unintelligible. Meanwhile, a dozen of the workers were making their way toward the men, walking down the dirt paths in a most peculiar fashion. They shuffled along in two columns of six men each. The leaders carried long sticks, with which they struck the ridges lining the dirt paths, producing sharp clicking sounds at precisely timed intervals. Those following held the back of the robe of the person before them. When the workers had drawn closer, the climbers noted with shivers of horror that all of them had dark, empty sockets where their eyes should have been. Soon the outsiders were surrounded, and the hands of the blind were groping all over their bodies.

One member of this welcoming committee felt the face of one of the climbers. His fingers stopped as he felt the two round protrusions about half an inch up from both sides of the man's nose. A murmur went up from the crowd as he exclaimed something in his own language. The crowd became agitated and, before the climbers could react, bound them tightly. The prisoners were then marched to the village, where they were lowered by a rope into a dark, dry well that was covered with a large stone.

After a hearing by the leaders of the community, it was decided that the visitors, who spoke a strange language and bore even stranger bulges on their faces, were human beings, and not, as some argued, demons who deserved to be put to death at once. But the villagers were not cruel; on the contrary, most of them felt pity for the grotesquely disfigured creatures.

It was not their fault that they had been born that way. They would give the strangers the greatest gift they could imagine. They would welcome them into the village. All that had to be done was to remove those hideous bulging growths on both sides of the bridge of their noses. Then they would fit in just fine. And so it was that the charitable citizens of the Valley of the Blind removed the eyes of the two mountain climbers. And so glad were the mountain climbers for this gift that they remained in the Valley of the Blind, toiling in its fields and tapping their way along its paths, for the rest of their lives.

Winston Churchill once said, "Men occasionally stumble over the truth, but most pick themselves up and hurry off as if nothing has happened." The staff at Kalamazoo Psychiatric Hospital are hurrying off even now without a backward glance.

Now to describe what really happened. Chris was disoriented during his first few days in the hospital, not knowing where he was and unable to relate to visitors. He was lucky to have a doctor who was as responsive as possible given his training. Fortunately, his doctor cut the doses of Zyprexa, Ativan, and lithium when his speech began to slur. Gayle and I stayed in touch on the phone while I tried to orchestrate my — shall we say — unconventional attempt to get Chris released. After eight days, the staff scheduled a hearing that could have committed him for another 60 days. They had already notified Social Security that he would be there for an extended period of time. The day after they received my mini-drama by fax, eight staff members interviewed him and decided that he had improved enough to return home. They decided to postpone the court hearing that could have led to a commitment of up to 60 days.

I hoped that he was receiving special treatment because he was the subject of a book his dad was writing about nutrition and bipolar disorder, and because they knew he had a home where his parents cared for him. Had my little drama done any good? Maybe, maybe not. It made me feel better, and, for my manic persona, that was all that mattered. On July 19, I flew to Grand Rapids, Michigan, picked up a rental car, and drove to Kalamazoo Psychiatric Hospital.

It was time to abandon my hypomanic aspirations. I didn't need them any more. It would have been an exercise in futility, and perhaps even counterproductive, to try to share any of my ideas with the staff. However, I secretly hoped that someone who had at least glanced at the book would have had his or her curiosity piqued enough to ask, if nothing else, where in the world I had gotten such far-out ideas.

The members of the staff I met were cordial. Chris's doctor said that he had read the fax. He complimented me on the quality of my writing and suggested in the casually patronizing way I sometimes suspect is part of the curriculum at medical schools that perhaps I should stick to fiction. I held my tongue with difficulty. A nurse told Chris that she really liked him and hoped he would stay on the medicines in spite of what his father thought. Sandy, whose mother is a psychiatric nurse, reminded me that bipolar disorder has a genetic basis and that sometimes it takes time to find the right medications. Chris, succumbing to what we in the trade call system determinism, suggested that maybe he should stay on the medicines.

In spite of all I had learned, I could feel the system determinism closing in on me as well. Chris's doctor said that he was personally open to the use of supplements and omega-3 fatty acids, but that the hospital had to operate within the parameters of the Joint Committee for the Accreditation of Healthcare Organizations (JCAHO). How could I argue with that?

Fortunately, my worst fears had not come to pass, at least not then. Chris had stopped obsessing about hell, and verbalized a desire to come home. Most important of all, he had slept. His doctor agreed to discharge him to our care, as long as I agreed to make a follow-up appointment at Nevada County Behavioral Health. After one day in a hospital and nine days at Kalamazoo Psychiatric Hospital, Chris was discharged, but not before performing a piano rendition of "Over the Rainbow" during an annual social event at the hospital. One of the staff members shared with me how much his playing had moved her. We flew home.

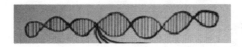

Notes

1. Dr. Ingendaay later made a referral, but the neurologist would not accept it because she wanted more referral information. As I set about providing that information to Dr. Ingendaay, Chris changed his mind about getting the EEG. Chris's epistemology, his world of spirit, of good and evil, significantly impaired our efforts to collaborate on the biology of his illness. With his base line bipolar mindset, he saw any acknowledgment of biological factors as a repudiation of any religious perspective to his life.
2. For details see Appendix 3 - Desiderata and Appendix 4 - Kindling Contributors.

24 - Home Again?

It was not without misgivings that I kept my word and arranged a follow-up appointment for Chris at Nevada County Mental Health. Brainwashed by his experiences in the hospital, Chris was now saying that he wanted to take both the medications and the supplements. The psychiatrist we met with at Nevada County Behavioral Health said that would be fine. I told him that the supplements potentiate the medications and that taking both could be harmful in the long run. I gave the psychiatrist some written material on the supplements ... material, that, not surprisingly, he never got around to reading. Chris and I called Tony to ask what he thought about taking the supplements and the psychotropic medications concurrently. Tony was strongly opposed, saying that it would only make matters worse.

Changing the subject, I asked him how many of his clients had "crashed" on the supplements and why. He replied that none have crashed when they took the proper amounts unless there were extenuating circumstances. Those that did crash took 16 or less a day, oral antibiotics, or Prilosec (Prilosec, an antacid, impairs digestion by disturbing the hydrochloric acid balance). Others had severe diarrhea or constipation, which, because it prevented adequate digestion, resulted in setbacks. He recommended that Chris return to 32 pills a day.

But Chris decided to do it his way. After two weeks of taking 24 supplements daily along with the medications, he reported worsening depression, with suicidal thinking. One day while we were taking a day hike in the Sierra mountains, he told me he was going to start reducing the medications. He did so and soon reported improvement in his mood and thinking.

What now?

Still hoping that the wormlike creatures in Chris's blood were a "one of a kind" for us, and wanting an update on his Lyme disease, I tried to get another dark field microscope exam from New Century, but they expressed some concerns about having their pictures publicized. I wondered why they were not willing to stand by their work.

Chris and I visited Anne Bernard, a naturopath practicing in the Bay Area, to find out if the Lyme spirochetes were still in his blood. She examined Chris's blood, and mine, for comparison, and agreed to give me the pictures for publication. She said the "spirochetes" we allegedly saw at New Century were nothing more than what she called condrits. These condrits signify a problem, but not Lyme disease, which rarely, if ever, can be seen in the blood. This confirmed exactly what Dr. Stricker had already told us. It meant that the initial referral for Lyme disease was bogus, even though the

Western Blot results were definitive — or were they? Ms. Bernard said that Chris's dark field microscope pictures were highly suggestive of excessive protein in the blood, or "leaky gut syndrome." Even though our blood was different, with Chris having more condrits and debris while I had rolleau and stickiness of the blood, both indicated too much protein. The regimen she recommended included daily urine pH checks to measure our progress, alkaline substances to restore proper pH levels, and a regimen to improve Chris's digestive system. This opened up a new area of exploration that would require another book to adequately explore. See Appendix 3 for details.

Meanwhile, I wrote to Dr. Cade to check out the remote possibility that excessive gluten and carbohydrates could contribute to temporal lobe seizure problems by lowering neuron firing thresholds. He wrote back that it could and told me that even though most of his work was with autism and schizophrenia, he had done some informal preliminary studies of blood samples from bipolar patients and had found some interesting gluten/bipolar connections. He asked if we would send samples of Chris's blood and urine to determine if he had hyperpolypeptiduria. See Appendix 6 for details.

Chris reduced his Zyprexa from 15 mg to 5 mg over a six-week period while taking 24 supplements a day. He got a job in sales and told me he was going to stop taking the Zyprexa entirely. I advised him against doing this, reminding him of what had happened just a year ago when he went quickly from 10 mg to none. I had to take my father on an overnight trip to Reno for medical appointments. When I got home, Chris had been off all medications for two days. He was already having trouble sleeping. The night I got home, without telling us, he took 15 mg of Zyprexa to compensate for going off it, just as in Michigan, when he had taken extra doses of the supplements to make up for not taking them. He then began showing symptoms of akathisia. He started to feel suicidal and had to be hospitalized yet again, this time at another hospital in Sacramento, called Sierra Crest. No one thought to give him some Cogentin. Before he was hospitalized he gave a urine sample. The pH was six, acidic.

The first few days at Sierra Crest he kept to himself and would not eat, even though the hospital staff tried to encourage him to. I wondered if in some way he was listening to the wisdom of his body telling him that he needed to let his digestive system recuperate.

In vain, I again tried to have some influence over his care. I told his doctor the history of the current episode and recommended they only continue the Zyprexa, lithium, and Depakote since that had worked in the past. I knew it would be futile to even try to get treatment for his Lyme disease, let alone supplements. I also explained the reasons why I recommended that he be put on a casein and gluten-free diet. I shared a little — very little — of my research. His doctor was sure that the problem was his "bipolar illness" and not valid psychological variables due to diseases or drug effects. It was clear to me that the episode was because Chris prematurely stopped the Zyprexa and suffered discontinuation syndrome, then took too much and suffered extrapyramidal symptoms. The good doctor put his hand on my shoulder and said in a condescending manner, "When your book comes out, I will be the first to read it." I wrote a formal request to have blood taken for Dr. Cade while Chris was in the hospital. My request was denied. The psychiatrist put Chris on 900 mg Neurontin, 1,200 mg lithium, 20 mg Paxil, 20 mg Zyprexa, and 2 mg Cogentin. Chris had won again, but there was no prize, only a huge cost. In response to an invitation from Tony, I decided I could do more for Chris by taking a draft of this book to Tony in Canada than by staying at home and trying to influence those who were not willing to listen to me.

To Calgary and environs

I drove to Spokane, taking Thomas back to college, then driving on to Calgary. While there, I had a very pleasant chat with Dr. Bonnie Kaplan at the University of Calgary. She shared some of her exciting research results and also some of the difficulties of trying to introduce new paradigms of care into her "social system." I was glad to hear I wasn't the only one running into brick walls.

Then I drove to Cardston, a town about 90 miles south of Calgary. As I drove into this small town surrounded by miles of wheat fields and farms, I wondered how in the world a major advance in the treatment of bipolar disorder could have occurred in a place like this, so far removed from academia and health care institutions. Then it hit me. Where else could it have come from but a place so far removed from those institutions? Who else could have developed it but folks like Tony and Dave, who simply hadn't known any better than to come up with such outrageous ideas? Very little health care system determinism out there, just hard-working farmers, ranchers, and hog growers trying to make sure their hogs didn't go crazy.

As I parked in Tony's driveway, he emerged from his house and greeted me warmly. He introduced me to his wife, Barb, and their children. That night, Tony invited me to travel with him and David to Salt Lake City, where they were to meet with officials from the company that manufactures the supplements. The next day, after picking up David in a neighboring town, we headed for Salt Lake. The trip took 11 hours, so I had a total of 22 hours with the two of them to ask questions and share ideas from the book. Not only did I get a chance to tour the plant in Salt Lake where the supplements are made, but I also heard some amazing stories on the trip there and back.

I learned that David — who, by the way, is extremely knowledgeable about nutrition and health — had been through the same experience I was going through. His son had crashed after a two-week period of digestive

335

problems. He also had felt helpless in dealing with his son's psychiatrists, who insisted on using a new drug that made him worse.

I enjoyed hearing of the exciting things happening with the research. These included getting $700,000 from the Stanley Foundation for a research trial in Florida, getting at least $3 and possibly $15 million from the World Bank to finance further trials, as well as Synergy Centers for the homeless, and developing a new powder product to improve absorption. Tony and David also spoke of increasing collaboration with other organizations that were involved in pursuing nutritional approaches for the treatment of CNS disorders. They told me about Dr. Charles Popper of Harvard University. Dr. Popper reported phenomenal success using the supplements with more than 30 patients, including a 10-year-old bipolar son of a physician. The boy's heretofore-unmanageable temper tantrums stopped when he was given the supplements and resumed when he ran out of them. Since he couldn't get the supplements right away, Dr. Popper went to a health food store, where he tried to assemble as many of the ingredients as possible. When he gave these supplements to the boy, the tantrum behavior improved but did not stop. Only after the new supply of Truehope supplements arrived did the boy's tantrums stop completely. In effect, Dr. Popper did an informal ABACB study (A = no supplements, B = Synergy supplements. A = no supplements, C = health food store supplements, B = Synergy supplements). Dr. Popper wrote a companion article published in the December 2001 *Journal of Clinical Psychiatry* along with Dr. Kaplan's paper.

Tony gave me a sample of the new powdered supplements they were developing for those with digestive difficulties. The particle size was half that of the substances in the pills. He suggested that Chris might benefit from this since he appeared to have absorption problems and consequently did not have much of a nutritional reserve.[1] Their ultimate goal was to reduce the dose and increase the absorption for all their clients. Tony talked about a manic bipolar patient who, upon taking the powered form of the supplements, not only slept in just hours, but also rapidly came out of his manic state. Seeing David and Tony restored my sagging spirits.

Blurred vision

My enthusiasm was tempered when I returned to California. After about three weeks in the hospital, Chris was discharged with orders to continue the extensive medications discussed earlier. His thinking and movements were slow. His hands and arms had tremors. He complained of impaired vision. He had a tranquilizer psychosis.

His mom had noticed that his eyes were dilated while he was in the hospital. I suspected that the culprit was Neurontin. I called the county psychiatrist and told him about these symptoms. He stated that the Cogentin might affect the ability of the eye to dilate, but he did not think the Neurontin would. Neurontin is a GABA-like clone. Since it is indicated for seizure disorder, I figured it must have cellular inhibition properties. To this back-yard mechanic, it seemed like a logical inference that it must therefore make the engine (brain) run slower. From my standpoint, the Cogentin and Neurontin were doing a fine job of that. Chris's brain was so slowed down that his eyes remained dilated regardless of the light. Before he left the hospital, Chris had told the staff that his vision was blurry. They uniformly responded by telling him that this was from the medications. There was nothing else to say. It was from the medications. That was all he needed to know.

There was more to this story than just eye problems. According to the Neurontin insert, "During the course of premarketing development of Neurontin, eight sudden and unexplained deaths were recorded among a co-hort of 2,203 patients treated (2,103 patient-years of exposure)." The insert gave no information about the heath conditions or ages of the deceased or provided any symptoms that may have preceded death. Not knowing of any pre-existing conditions with these deaths, I had no option but to suspect that if Chris stayed on Neurontin for a year, there was an eight out of 2,203 chance of his dying. To this backyard mechanic, that meant he had a much better chance of dying on Neurontin than he had of winning the lottery.

When visiting with Tony and David, had I told them that Chris had been started on Paxil after I objected to Prozac. Tony had expressed reservations specifically about Paxil and told me of a class action suit recently initiated over withdrawal problems with the drug. I also learned that in 1998, relatives of a patient on Paxil were awarded $8 million in a wrongful death suit. The patient, with no history of homicidal ideation, had killed his family and him-self soon after his doctor had started him on Paxil. I learned that the drug companies were now calling drug withdrawal "drug discontinuation syn-drome" since drug withdrawal would suggest addiction. By suddenly stop-ping his medicine and then taking too much, Chris had jumped out of the frying pan back into the fire. He was getting "burned," first from his own actions and now from the actions of his keepers.

We started him on the powder supplements and began the process of slowly reducing the drugs, this time under my supervision. I reduced the medications slowly and methodically, cutting by one fourth at a time. I also made plans to let Chris hear from others besides those whose livelihood was based on mainstream paradigms of care. System determinism works both ways.

We are not alone

Dan Stradford is president of Safe Harbor, an organization dedicated to supporting alternative mental health care (www.alternativementalhealth.com). He founded the organization for some of the same reasons I wrote this book. He, too, helplessly watched his World War II veteran father undergo the ravaging effects of mental illness and its treatment. He invited Tony and David to speak at an annual fund-raising awards banquet on September 20, 2001 at the Westin Bonaventure Hotel in Los Angeles. Chris, Ray, and I went to the meeting. Actress Margo Kidder was scheduled to accept an award for her work in alleviating the stigma of bipolar illness and promoting nutritional solutions. However, at the last minute, because of the September 11 terrorist bombings, Ms. Kidder left the LA area to return to her home in Montana. She was mourning the loss of friends and didn't think it appropriate to accept an award at the same time the national tragedy was unfolding. Nonetheless, we had an enjoyable evening and were able to meet other professionals involved in alternative solutions, some of whom were militant in their belief not only that drugs were unnecessary, but that they caused brain damage. Chris and my father had the opportunity to meet and talk with Tony and David. I would have preferred that Chris be more mentally clear for this visit — he was still on large amounts of medications and the supplements — but he and my father said they enjoyed the meeting.

We were 20 minutes from Dr. Martin's office. I suggested to Chris that we pay him a visit to see if we could both get tested for stealth viruses. Chris agreed so we drove the short distance to Rosemead.

Dr. Martin took samples of our blood. Each test cost $250. He showed me convincing evidence that the pair bonds of specific DNA sequences of human patients were virtually identical to the pair bonds of simian cytomegalovirus. Even I could look at pages of "g-a, g-c, t-g, c-a's" and tell if they were identical, or almost identical, or not at all alike. While we were there, a neurologist working with Dr. Martin happened to come in. He interviewed Chris briefly, had him do a few tasks, and concluded that Chris demonstrated subtle neural damage, most likely from a stealth virus. He offered to see him for treatment when the results came back. I was interested, but Chris wasn't buying it.

When I called Dr. Martin a few days later, he told me that both Chris and I had tested positive for stealth virus. The written report stated, for both Chris and me, that the assay showed "the rapid development of a moderate cytopathic effect consisting of vacuolated cells with cytoplasmic inclusions.... The positive culture finding could explain signs and symptoms of a multisystem illness, including neuropsychiatric manifestations. ... An empirical therapeutic trial with close clinical and laboratory monitoring may be advisable." Vacuolated means full of vacuoles, or small air cavities. Cytoplasmic inclusions are nuclear structures found at the site of virus multiplication. According to these tests, both Chris and I were infected with a stealth virus. The report also acknowledged that about 10% of a healthy population also test positive for stealth.

Some weeks later, Dr. Cade's associate, Malcolm Privette, a physician's assistant, called with the results of the Radio Allergo Sorbent Test (RAST) they had administered. Chris had been given a gluten/casein screen to determine the levels of IgG and IgA antibodies against these compounds. Malcolm reported that Chris's level of antibodies against casein was 10,649 in a range from 0 to >9,500, or class 6+, the highest. Normal was 0-100. The level of antibodies against gluten was 2,732 in the same range, or class 2+ of six. Normal was 0-100. His IgA sensitivities to casein were positive; to gluten, negative. These results represented the actual number of antibodies and antigen pairs locked in a death grip in a particular volume of blood. We were looking at a battlefield with, in Chris's case, 10,649 antigen-antibody pairs dueling to the death in the sample measured. The plot just kept getting thicker and thicker. I wondered again if a body awash in antibodies could knock out the GABA in his brain. I surmised that what I had strongly suspected, that Chris should not eat gluten or casein, particularly casein, was true. But the urine sample, taken one week before his hospitalization, did not reveal hyperpolypeptiduria. In fact, peptide levels were low.

From September through November, I continued to very slowly reduce the psychotropic drugs and reminded Chris to regularly complete the Truehope checklist, the scores of which became progressively lower, meaning his symptoms were abating.

By early November, he was down to 0.4 mg Zyprexa a day and a trace amount of lithium. He flew to Colorado to be in a friend's wedding and to sing a song he had composed for it. He was gone for six days and came back in good health, having enjoyed his trip. He had taken at least 24 supplements a day and had stopped all other drugs, including the immune-enhancing supplements, omega-3 fatty acids, and the Zyprexa and Lithium, with no apparent ill effects.

I continued to argue for the maximum prevention regimen. He chose only to take the supplements. Still, he and I sang in Handel's *Messiah* in December. He started a band with a friend. He continued to play the piano in church and sang in the choir. He continued to compose songs, arranging some of them for a high school choir director.

Chris was not manic or depressed as long as he took about 24 supplements a day. Starting in January 2002, he lowered the amount to 16 a day, against our recommendations. But he continued to do fine. He worked at a part-time job. He purchased and installed a surround-sound stereo system for the family ... one that he could afford. He ordered parts to a computer so that he could build his own. He was active socially and seemed to be suffering from none of the side effects he'd experienced while taking psychotropic medications. How long would it last? I didn't know.

From bipolar disorder to syndrome

Is Chris cured? Wrong question. The question isn't "Is he cured?" but, rather, "What would he be cured from if he were cured?" It wouldn't be "bipolar disorder" because there is no cure for bipolar disorder. Besides, that term is a construct having no biological relevance whatsoever. Would he be cured of neuro-Lyme, stealth virus, nutritional deficiencies secondary to malabsorption, food sensitivities, gluten and casein antibodies, leaky gut, and damaged microvilla in the gut; chemical sensitivities such as aldrin and xylene, polysorbate 60 and carbon tetrachloride; heavy metals including mercury and antimony; or high DPT antitoxoid levels? Chris has all of the above, based on various tests he has taken. Would he be cured of GABA-impairing antibodies, parasites, excessive carbohydrates, other viruses, molds, CD 26 impairment, mitogen induced excessive protein kinease C, deficiencies of phosphosulfotransferase, cytochrome P-450 enzymes, or ubiquione (coenzyme Q-10)? How about excessive IL-1, IL-2, sIL-2R, sIL-6R, IFN, and acute phase proteins? What about inadequate glial fibrillary acidic protein, which impairs the body's ability to regulate the excitatory neurotransmitter glutamate? Would he be cured of perfusion defects in his temporal lobes due to Lyme disease? How about high levels of beta-endorphin; cortisol; quinolinic acid, a marker of immunologic activity that has been identified in both schizophrenia and bipolar disorder; or ACTH? All of the above correlate with mania and depression. I plan to explore these questions as well as others in <u>Too Good to be True, Volume II</u>.[2]

We know the answers to some of these questions, but the complete answer to all the factors involved in breaking Chris's brain and giving him bipolar disorder-like symptoms still eludes us. We do know that nutrients have restored him to us and to himself ... as long as he has taken them properly. We hope and expect that whatever protection supplemental nutrients have provided will continue ... again, if he continues to take them in a responsible manner. Given his history we don't think 16 a day is enough, especially without the omega-3 and immune-enhancing supplements. We still advise him to take 24 supplements and two to three omega-3 fatty acids pills as well as the immune enhancing regimen, but he won't do it. Gayle and I are hoping he'll get a chance to test out the new revised flavor-enhanced powdered supplements soon. Less would be required because the particles would be more readily digestible than even the earlier sample he obtained.

This four-generational odyssey will not be completed until I learn exactly how my son's brain was broken. There is talk on chat rooms of a pending foolproof test for Lyme disease. If and when it is approved for general use, we will try to find out if the neuro-Lyme is still playing a role in his illness, as I suspect it is. There is talk of a Dr. Karl Bechter, who has been treating psychosis by filtering the CSF to remove bacteria, endotoxins, inflammatory cytokines, and immune globulins. We will want to know more about that.

I just purchased a book that Glenn Foster told me about called <u>Breaking the Vicious Cycle</u>, by Elaine Gottshall, a nutritionist. This compelling book is about a simple dietary solution to digestive disorders, a solution that allows the body to repair damaged microvilli in the gut. There is a fascinating, meticulously researched chapter on the brain and digestion. She argues and carefully documents that it is not just gluten and casein, but disaccharides and polysacharides that damage the microvilli in the gut. If Chris ever decides to go on the Specific Carbohydrate Diet, he may be able to restore some of his digestive capability so that his gut can absorb more of the mineral precursors needed to keep his brain in top working order.

Both Tony and David continue to search for more effective ways to improve the absorption of the nutrients in the supplements, both through their products and those of others. After this book is published, I plan to look into Primal Defense, a probiotic product designed to restore intestinal flora and trace minerals to improve digestion. David was researching Primal Defense when I visited him in Canada, and I've been hearing positive things about it in the Truehope discussion groups.

Given the potentially lethal nature of bipolar disorder, how could I do anything less than pursue every possibility, keeping an open yet critical mind? As Dr. Bransfield writes in the Introduction to this book, "The most important discoveries in medicine are yet to be made."

There is much more to learn. A number of biological risk factors have already been identified. The sooner patients and their families start insisting that their doctors leave no stone unturned, the sooner these patients will be treated for the biological conditions that are manifested in what I have come to think of as bipolar syndrome. While we search for better questions and answers, we will continue to seek out experts to synthesize what we have learned. We will continue to encourage Chris to take 24 Synergy supplements a day, omega-3 fatty acids, immune-enhancing supplements, and plenty of water. Medications will continue to be ready if needed. But our goal is to treat biologically valid psychological variables by treating the biological anomalies that cause them.

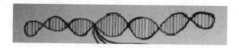

Notes

1. When Chris got out of the hospital, he said he would not take the powder because of the taste.

2. Some of the topics not covered in this book include thyroid problems, excessive kinase protein C, calcium ion abnormalities, anti phospholipid antibodies, increased levels of matrix metalloproteins, and the role of haplotypes, the unique genetic constitutions of individuals. Dr. Shoemaker is conducting some exciting research that points to an association between particular haplotypes and illnesses such as chronic fatigue syndrome, fibromyalgia, and other toxin-related illnesses. This may be applicable to bipolar disorder. Another area for future inquiry is that of glynutritional technology, and a product called Ambrotose.

25 - *Some Paths Less Traveled*

Travelers wanting to get to a destination need to know that the paths they choose will take them there. During Chris's manic episodes, his destination was "truth," but the paths he took on his self-destructive psychotic search led him to a hospital. His beliefs were delusional to be sure, and, further, he saw no logical inconsistency between his being the Antichrist and also being God. Logic was not an impediment to his belief in both propositions because important components of his brain, most probably located in his right hemisphere, were not providing the inputs they normally would have. Chris's epistemology changed as a consequence of the biological processes in his brain. When he came out of his psychosis, his functioning right hemisphere exerted control again, and he could talk of his experiences from a more logical perspective.

Over time, "truth" changes. Each generation has its dogmatic beliefs which are revealed by the light of science and reason to be untrue or less true than had been assumed. Often these revelations are rejected by the established order, which sees in them a threat to social stability, morality, or even belief in God. The history of Darwin's theory of evolution provides perhaps the foremost example of what can occur when a truth revealed by the scientific method crashes head-on into a religious truth. With the advantage of a historical perspective, we can see threads of psychotic thinking in some of the beliefs our ancestors unquestioningly accepted as true.

Evolving "truths"

The 20th century, especially in its second half, saw immense improvements in the understanding and treatment of psychotic behaviors. Instead of ascribing such behaviors to demonic possession, our society learned to recognize them as symptoms of mental illness. It wasn't always that way. In the infamous Salem witch trials of 1692, some unfortunate people were accused of witchcraft and executed, in part because of their strange behavior. It would be more than two centuries before scientists would suggest that the ergot rye mold played a role in the strange behavior of the Salem "witches" as well as the countless victims of European witch hunts. While we know that the basis for the persecution was multifaceted, and included primitive belief systems, we now know that the psychotic-like behavior of the "witches" coincided with wet seasons that were conducive to the development of this mold. Also, many of the "witches" were from the lower social classes, where rye was eaten because it was cheaper than wheat. This indirect evidence suggests that some of the victims displayed psychotic behavior due to the neurotoxin. Yet in Salem, it was a truism that where there were clusters of psychotic persons, the devil was at work.[1] Could there be other assumed truths that we still believe today even though they are not empirically true?

Over time, a paradigm change evolved. Instead of demon possession and witchcraft, those suffering from religious delusions and hallucinations were seen as mentally ill. This was a step in the right direction, but did it go far enough? No one in the United States is executing the mentally ill for witchcraft today, and few attribute bizarre behavior to the influence of literal demons. In fact, when the "mentally" ill act in socially dysfunctional ways, their "mental" illness is often considered to be the cause of, or a mitigating factor in their behavior, rendering them less responsible in the eyes of society, both legally and morally, than a "normal" man or woman who performed the same action might be. How are these people helped? Most often, they are treated with psychotropic medications. The goal is not to identify and treat the primary biological causes of the "mental" illness, but to manage the socially dysfunctional symptoms, sweeping them — and, all too often, the patients as well — under the rug.

The particular constellation of symptoms is not the illness. The illness is the biological anomalies that cause the symptoms. This suggests, for example, that the biology underlying obsessional thinking is similar whether one is dealing with the monomania of the bipolar patient, the automatic negative thoughts of the psychotically depressed patient, or the obsessive thoughts of the obsessive-compulsive disordered patient. To take another example, social unresponsiveness, a kind of functional deafness of both the autistic and the manic, may stem from the same or similar biological processes.

Suggesting that a borderline patient is "regressing in the service of the ego" merely explains behavior based on ego strivings ... whatever those are. Such mentalistic concepts are not reality, but an approximation of reality created by those who develop theories about human behavior. But suggesting that the patient with borderline personality disorder is acting in a regressive way due to an impaired frontal cortex manifested by low levels of NAA is a different matter all together. This implies that either the death or impairment of neurons is one of the underlying biological problems impairing the judgment of the borderline individual. This defines the problem in such a way that specific biological solutions can be utilized once the cause of the diminished NAA is found. Instead of ascribing "mental" illness as the cause of dysfunctional behavior, the theory makers need to be looking at complex infective and environmental interactions that provoke the body's defenses and, in doing so, provoke CNS disorders in those with predisposing genetic traits and/or nutritional deficiencies.

When I began my odyssey to try to understand bipolar disorder, I resolved to do so with an open mind, not an empty head. I had no idea where my journey would lead. I just knew I had to get there ... wherever "there" was. Now, as I approached the end of this stage of my journey, I still wondered where "there" was.

During my lifetime, I had watched my father career from one misadventure to another, independent of whether or not he was taking his medications. In four years, working within the mainstream paradigms, my son had been hospitalized four times in a psychotic state. Although we tried, he was not compliant with his medications, but then, even when he was, the medications didn't solve the hypomania problem, except by provoking severe depression. Physician directed withdrawal from them provoked suicidal and homicidal ideation. He had been unable to complete his college education on time, had broken his kneecap, cut his wrists and his neck, and smashed a rock repeatedly into his head. He had entertained compulsive and repetitive thoughts of killing not only himself, but his family as well. His problems did not disappear when he started taking the Synergy supplements, but when he maintained himself on them he was much improved.

Since Chris had started the supplements and the Rocephin, he was composing music, drawing pictures of people and pets (that actually looked like them), singing in his church choir, attending a church fellowship group. He did not need to be reminded of simple things as he had before these interventions. He had tolerated the Rocephin treatment, even though he was weary of the process and had inexplicably terminated his treatment one week early. With the exception of his setback in Michigan, and his ill fated attempt to withdraw from Zyprexa too rapidly, there was no question that Chris had dramatically improved. He exhibited no signs of mania or depression. He was not hypomanic. While his ability to regulate himself was still compromised, I believe, from the brain impairment caused by neuro Lyme disease, by all the other measures of "there," finding help for my son, we had arrived.

Yet I was just beginning to appreciate the complexity of the undertaking. The odyssey would continue, but this seemed like a good place to pause and reflect on what conclusions I could draw from the journey my family had taken thus far and on how the lessons we had learned could be applied to the broader systems of society of which we are a part.

What would I say to those in the justice system who would allow a hypomanic patient to be falsely arrested for attempted rape, burglary, and sexual assault, beaten in jail, then shipped to a locked ward in a state hospital for sexual offenders where he was drugged for almost two years? What would I say to the education and mental health professionals who routinely viewed drugs as the answer before finding out what the questions were? What could I say to my colleagues who said it was fine to talk about omega-3 fatty acids with staff, but not with patients and their families? What could I tell the mental health professionals who treated a patient through four hospitalizations without learning that he was suffering from neurologic Lyme disease, and then ignored it through two more? What would I say to a psychiatrist who first overmedicated his patient, then abruptly terminated Zyprexa, provoking a psychotic suicidal crisis with self-mutilating behavior? And finally, what would I say to those suffering from CNS disorders and their families?

I would tell them that if their destination is justice and health care systems that protect the public good and restore damaged lives, then many of the paths they have chosen will not lead them there.

To police, jail guards, and judges

One of your fellow police officers once told me that you have the power to make the "crime" seem worse than it is. I told him I already knew that. Try not to be jaundiced by your experiences with the criminal element. Not everyone you come into contact with is a hardened criminal. Some of those you arrest are sick, physically sick in their bodies. Their brains are broken. Ask smart questions. Don't jump to conclusions.

A mom I once knew told her son, while he was growing up, that if he ever needed help, he should go to the police. In the middle of a manic psychosis, he did just that ... and the police killed him. He didn't have a weapon. But the police didn't know how to deal with an unarmed, physically strong, psychotic, six-foot-eight adult man who was out of control. So they shot him. Wouldn't it be easier to execute non-lethal measures instead of the patient?

In my father's situation, neither the responses of the police or the jail guard were appropriate. In Spokane, the police who dealt with Chris worked within guidelines to ensure his safety, as well as their own. They could have easily escalated and made a bad situation worse. Manic patients lack awareness of their personal boundaries and social surroundings. They don't do well in jail or with police. Many guards do not have the sensitivity to distinguish between intentional opposition and mentally ill behavior. Better selection and training of personnel could prevent the grotesque miscarriage of justice that befell my father from happening to some other hypomanic person in the future.

So now you know that I would like to see increased sensitivity and professionalism toward people like my father. Well, keep reading, because that is not the half of it. I am actually more concerned about fundamental belief systems that are manifested in countless ways through your daily operations, to the detriment of the "mentally" ill.

In the justice system, cultural beliefs determine what we do with those who violate society's laws. That is why a higher percentage of criminals are executed in Texas than any other state, and a higher percentage are executed in all the states compared to Europe. While it is possible to understand Scott Thorpe's murderous behavior in Nevada City as a result of mental disease, how do we understand other "crimes" by less flagrantly psychotic persons or by persons who may have heavy metal poisoning, nutritional deficiencies, viruses, subtle forms of brain damage, or complex infectious diseases? Gibran expresses a useful perspective in <u>The Prophet</u>.

> *Then one of the judges of the city stood forth and said, "Speak to us of Crime and Punishment."*
>
> *You cannot separate the just from the unjust and the good from the wicked;*
> *For they stand together before the face of the sun even as the black thread and the white are woven together.*
> *And when the black thread breaks, the weaver shall look into the whole cloth, and he shall examine the loom also.*
> ....
> *And you who would understand justice, how shall you unless you look upon all deeds in the fullness of light?*
> *Only then shall you know that the erect and the fallen are but one man standing in twilight between the night of his pigmy-self and the day of his god-self,*
> *And that the corner-stone of the temple is not higher than the lowest stone in its foundation.* (From THE PROPHET by Kahlil Gibran, copyright 1923 by Kahlil Gibran and renewed 1951 by Administrators C.T.A. of Kahlil Gibran Estate and Mary G. Gibran. Used by permission of Alfred A. Knopf, a division of Random House, Inc.)

In ancient times, the gods were considered to play a major role in the daily life of humans. In our day, we believe the human psyche expresses itself in the will of the person. The concept of "will" assumes a central executive function directed by the "personality" of the individual. Because of this "will," our criminal justice system presumes personal responsibility and accountability for all but the most flagrantly psychotic among us. This belief is anachronistic given what we know today about the human brain. It is interesting that there is no word in our vocabulary like "will-less" or "un-willful" to approximate the concept that a person's misbehavior is not willful. Psychiatry has "ego dystonic," but that still does not convey a lack of personal willfulness. Another phrase is "acting out," but even this connotes an actor who is doing the "acting out." The belief that dysfunctional behavior necessarily is due to willful intent, or what I call the "sin" model, is one of the vestiges from a previous era that our justice system needs to revisit. Individual responsibility is a useful construct, but it has its limitations.

Here is an example. Kip Kinkel, the 15-year-old who killed his parents and two fellow students in Oregon in 1998, suffered severe damage to one of his temporal lobes from a head injury when he was a boy. According to Dr. Daniel Amen, a psychiatrist and a pioneer in the use of the SPECT, whose daylong workshop on ADHD and the brain I attended in the summer of 2000 in Walnut Creek, the pictures from Kinkel's brain are similar to those of other murderers who suffer from explosive violent episodes. Early identification and treatment might have prevented Kinkel from killing his parents and fellow students in Oregon.

Dr. Amen identifies what he calls the "ring of fire" profile corresponding to ADHD and, when more pronounced, bipolar disorder. The "ring of fire" consists of a circle of "hot" areas in the brain, areas that are burning glucose too rapidly. Proper treatment with psychotropic medications results in positive changes in the SPECT. This technology provides a way to assess the effectiveness of an intervention based on biological changes in the brain.[2]

If there were any one American in recent history for whom the word "evil" would apply, that person is Timothy McVeigh. When I saw jail photos of McVeigh, I noticed an area on his scalp where there was no hair, presumably a scar of some kind. I wondered if a brain injury could have played a role in his horrendous crime.

I purchased American Terrorist, a biography of McVeigh by Lou Michel and Dan Herbeck, to learn what I could of this solitary person whose one-man crusade against the U.S. government had taken the lives of 168 people, most of whom he unblinkingly defined as "collateral damage." While some may feel that trying to understand the mental processes of a man like McVeigh is repugnant, given the suffering he caused, I wanted to know more because I recognized in him some of the same hypomanic qualities I had seen in my father and my son.

There was that vaguely apocalyptic "something big" about to happen that McVeigh referred to in letters to his sister. He saw the world in black and white terms. The bad guys were from the dark side, while he was from the good side of "The Force." He was argumentative and could only see his own point of view; there was no room in his brain for any other ideas. He had a Don Quixote-like delusion that his purpose in life was to sacrifice himself and hundreds of others to "right an un-rightable wrong." He handed out pamphlets during the Waco, Texas standoff. He wrote letters to newspapers threatening the "shedding of blood." He believed he would lead a crusade where he would supply guns to followers who would defend themselves against the ever-increasing encroachment of the government upon our Second Amendment rights. He demonstrated tunnel vision by obsessing repeatedly over the government infringing his rights and his need to avenge the Waco incident. He was so rigidly obsessed with the righteousness of his cause that he really was prepared to fight it out in front of the Federal Building and die with his bomb if necessary. He viewed himself as a warrior on a mission; in fact, he grew furious when the prosecutor at his trial accused him of the "cowardly act" of putting earplugs in his ears before setting off the blast. Timothy McVeigh had no followers. While Terry Nickels had supported him early in the process, McVeigh had to coerce him with blackmail to get him to help make the bomb in the Ryder truck. McVeigh's mission was all in his head. If only it had stayed there.

When hypomanic, Chris had a mission to warn humanity about the end of the world. He wanted to forsake college life to get the word out. Something "BIG" was always about to happen. Even when "well," Chris viewed his illness in black and white terms, viewing his spiritual orientation to understanding what had happened to him as the "truth" and my plodding, biologically based research as "false" because it was contrary to his beliefs. Even after repeated incidents in which medications or supplements clearly restored or maintained his sanity, Chris continued to deny that he was physically sick, or, when denial was no longer possible, to minimize the severity of his sickness. My father obsessed about leading a crusade to restore Christian values to the Oregon and California school systems. My son and father, like McVeigh, had no followers, no organization. It was all in their heads. To me, McVeigh's thinking was crazy, even apart from his insane desire to blow up a federal building. I wondered if his defense attorneys, by ignoring the obvious, had given his "cause" more credit than it deserved. This is not to imply that either my son or my father would duplicate McVeigh's behavior. Their personalities, their value systems, their histories are very different from McVeigh's. It is meant to suggest that biologically based hypomanic and obsessive processes, whatever their causes, can produce similar distortions of thinking and behavior. They strongly affect the "will" of the person. To the extent that these distortions are produced by a "broken" brain, one over which the person has no control, biologically mitigating factors exist.

There were questions the book didn't answer. Did the pneumonia McVeigh experienced as a child and possibly after his mother's separation from his father cause his brain to drill down to rigid preoccupations and trap him in his own obsessions? What effect did scarlet fever have on him? What about his four day hospitalization with his sister for an unknown bacterial infection? Why was McVeigh so sickly as a child? What influence did his illnesses have on him? We now know that pediatric autoimmune neuropsychiatric disorders associated with streptococcal infection (PANDAS) are expressed when an environmental trigger, streptococcal infection, provokes obsessive compulsive symptoms in those so genetically predisposed. What kind of HPA activation, if any, was established when bullies stuck his head in a toilet at school? Why was McVeigh described as a "soldier's soldier?" Why did he have so much energy in the Army? Why do the authors refer to his "hyperactive mind"? Why did he feel compelled to push the limits and trespass in Area 51 carrying a rifle? Why did he come so close to killing himself when he got out of the Army? What role, if any, did vaccinations and exposure to environmental toxins such as organophosphates play in his obsessional preoccupation to right the wrongs that were certainly perpetuated by the FBI at Ruby Ridge and possibly at Waco Texas? When he received extensive vaccinations in preparation for his service in the Gulf War, what impact, if any, did these have on his cytokine levels? Did his preoccupation with guns and ammunition expose him to excessive lead? What was his nutritional status? Did he ever receive a SPECT? If so, what did it look like? Would it be similar to those found in patients with obsessive-compulsive disorder, with bipolar disorder, or with ADHD? Would it show brain damage in, for example, the temporal lobe consistent with head injuries? At the workshop I attended, Dr. Amen reported evidence of profound behavioral dysfunction from even the slightest injuries to the head. McVeigh had been knocked unconscious and received a concussion at least once as a child and had received numerous other head injuries over the course of his life.[3]

An even more troubling thought came to mind. Was he exposed to chemical or biological weapons during the Gulf War? According to Dr. Khidhir Hamza, Saddam's bombmaker, Sadam Hussein strategically placed thousands of such weapons in bunkers he knew U.S. forces would blow up, thereby spreading the toxins to the Allied forces.[4]

I wondered why the defense, which spent more than 13 million dollars to defend him, hadn't addressed "mental health" issues — playing the "mental health card," if you will. Perhaps he acted too normally. Maybe he would not have allowed it, since such a defense would have cast doubt on his *raison d'etre*. Based on news reports I had heard on TV, his neighbor in prison, Ted Kaczynski, the Unabomber, had strongly objected to the suggestion of an insanity defense when he was facing trial for his crimes, and he was undeniably schizophrenic.

My point is that individuals like McVeigh need to be studied to better understand how their brains are broken. This is not to suggest that he had bipolar disorder, but I do believe his behavior was clearly obsessive and hypomanic. Maybe he was a "tweener." "Tweener" is a term I picked up from fellow mental health professionals. It refers to the person whose symptoms don't exactly fit the precise criteria found in DSM-IV. "Tweener" behavior may be very dysfunctional yet not meet the exact DSM-IV criteria for a definitive diagnosis. Yet even that term does not do justice to the concept I want to articulate. It implies a diagnosis that fits somewhere between diagnostic categories that exist in the real world. The DSM-IV categories exist only because of a consensual process that declared their existence. If one focuses on biologically valid psychological variables, then the criteria of DSM-IV or the less precise "tweener" categorizations are not even particularly relevant. If McVeigh had nutritional deficiencies, heavy metal toxicity, a chronic infection, or brain damage such as a damaged temporal lobe, he would have had a biological condition causing valid psychological variables that could have been considered a mitigating factor in his defense. We will never know about McVeigh. The evidence is buried. But there will be others.

Finding out if, not to mention how, McVeigh's brain was broken would have been difficult and expensive. It was easier to call him "evil" than to try and understand the biological factors that may have contributed to his ongoing obsessions of perceived wrongs that preceded his irrational, cold-blooded, violent behavior. It was easier to see him as the incarnation of evil than as a tragic example of brain processes gone awry. Destroying the "evil" one doesn't prevent the next McVeigh from taking his place.

Dr. Derek Bryce-Smith, retired professor of organic chemistry at the University of Reading in England, addressed factors which raise inconvenient but important legal questions concerning individual responsibility and guilt that have yet to be acknowledged by legal authorities in an essay entitled, "Crime and Nourishment."

> *The title of this essay is intended to raise the question whether some criminals are suffering subtle forms of malnutrition, or poisoning. Risk factors include lead, mercury, most if not all insecticides, organochlorine compounds, behavior-modifying allergens such as certain food colorants (e.g. tartrazine) and preservatives (e.g. benzoates) and deficiencies of certain micronutrients such as magnesium, calcium, iodine, folate, certain B-vitamins, and particularly zinc.*[5]

Houston resident Andrea Yates was sentenced to life imprisonment in March 2002 for drowning her five children in the summer of 2001.

The murders were a tragedy for Yates's children, her husband, and herself. My only sources for the following observations are various news reports on TV and in the press. Paraphrasing a statement made by her husband on the evening news, "I am angry at her because she drowned our children, but I am not angry because I know it was not her." He was saying the murders were not something his wife would have done. I believe it is highly likely that she had diminished capacity when she chose to kill her children. Her psychotic depression and obsessive delusional thoughts suggest to me that she had a broken brain. I believe, based only on the aforementioned TV news reports and newspaper articles, plus my experiences with Chris, that she was probably incapable of doing anything other than what she did. After giving of her own nutritional stores through five pregnancies, I suspect that her brain was depleted of resources. I can't think of a more intuitive argument for a nutritional deficiency theory of psychosis than a situation like hers where

351

her own nutritional stores were depleted in the creation of not just one baby, but five in a row. I was not alone in asking these questions.

On March 21, Danielle Steel, author of His Bright Light, a true story of her son's losing battle with bipolar disorder that ended in his suicide at the age of 19, wrote an impassioned editorial for a San Francisco Bay area newspaper that circulated at a number of Web sites. Among other things she stated her belief that a determination of sanity was "beyond anyone's wildest imagination." While Yates's crime was clearly horrendous, this author states that Andrea Yates has been failed by the law and the system; in other words, by us.

Yates's psychiatrist reportedly told her to think positive thoughts and not think negative thoughts. If he believed that these comments could have an impact on her psychotic thinking, then he was reflecting a level of cultural insanity at least equal to her personal insanity — and to mine, when I hoped that a constructive written dialogue with my hypomanic son would bring him back to earth. Was it possible that withdrawing from the Haldol exacerbated her illness by provoking a drug discontinuation syndrome similar to what Chris experienced?

My intent here is not to provide a "psychiatric excuse" to minimize or forgive the actions of a Kip Kinkel, Tim McVeigh, or Andrea Yates. Nor is it to suggest that all crimes are a consequence of biological processes that obviate personal responsibility. It is to raise questions that point to new paths.

How many other individuals like Kip Kinkel, Timothy McVeigh, and Andrea Yates are currently going to school, serving in our Armed Forces, and having babies? Before they kill, many could be restored to healthier functioning by screening and treating for head injuries, nutritional deficiencies, heavy metals, and chronic infectious diseases. Applying current knowledge to identify and treat future "American terrorists," school killers, and psychotic mothers could prevent needless carnage in the future. Just providing an improved diet in school and juvenile justice systems has been demonstrated to help academic performance[6] and reduce problem behavior of juvenile offenders.[7]

My Great Aunt Harriet's murder of her son did not impact society as broadly as Timothy McVeigh's behavior. Yet the processes in her brain may have been similar to his.

Chris ran amok against himself; therefore, he could not be prosecuted for his self-destructive behavior. If he had run amok against his employer, his mother, or even me, I would hope, but not expect, that you in the criminal justice system would appreciate the biological processes that can diminish one's ability to be accountable for one's behavior. I would hope, but not expect, that you would understand that people with broken brains can and do commit "will-less" acts. Their broken brains "will" them to do them.

To teachers, social workers, and psychologists

The direct link between nutrition and mental health is becoming increasingly known to the general public but has yet to be understood or accepted by those of us in the education and mental health professions. The public turns to us for help; we stay with our comfortable paradigms; patients and their families develop their own support systems and use the Internet to share what is working for them.

We and those we serve are not experts in the increasingly complex mysteries of the human brain that researchers are continuing to discover. The parents of high-risk youth in Nevada County do not know that other assessment and treatment alternatives are available to them, and, if they did, they have no one to advise them about the relative benefits and risks. Teachers at the schools where I consulted don't teach students about the links between nutrition and mental health or work with parents to support elimination diets for children who needed them. This is not within their educational domain. Those of us providing mental health services are not trained in nutrition and mental health. Many mental health professionals don't even believe in specific meaningful relationships between nutrition and mental health, let alone a relationship between chronic infectious diseases and mental health.

However, there is extensive research that cost-effective interventions like food elimination diets, heavy metal screening and chelation, and nutritional supplementation can help high-risk kids. Don't ignore it. Read it. Some of you still believe, as I did, that kids will perform better through behavioral interventions. Not when their brains are broken.

I worked with a young man diagnosed with both bipolar disorder and ADHD. When he did poorly in school, he would tell himself that he would just have to try harder, as if his difficulties were simply a result of his lack of motivation. One thing he had been able to learn in school was that if he wanted to succeed, he would have to try harder. In fact, for people with his disorder, according to Dr. Amen, SPECT scans have proven that trying harder actually results in diminished blood flow to those parts of the brain needed to concentrate on the task at hand. I recall a meeting where school officials met with my client, his parents, and me. They proceeded to tell the young man that he was going to have to repeat a year in the same grade in the same classroom with the same teacher because he hadn't tried hard enough. It was more of the same again. And we wondered why he threw rocks at windows and got into fights. As long as teachers and parents conveyed to him that he could do better if he only tried, he would only do worse. There is a substantial body of data suggesting that elimination diets, vitamin and mineral supplementation, and having the child listen to Mozart piano sonatas through a headset are more effective in fostering performance than trying to motivate the "will" of an ADHD child.

We prefer to think that our medications, our psychotherapy, our family therapy, our wraparound services, our "next best thing" will fix what is broken. We shudder to think that a real estate manager and animal feed consultant could have developed nutritional solutions for bipolar and other CNS disorders based on the same general principles used by generations of hog farmers to prevent ear and tail biting syndrome in their hogs. We are not open to the idea that nutrients are an effective first line of defense for many suffering from these disorders. Even when we see the data, we are closed to it because of the shame we would feel if it were true.

Our state governments and professional associations have designated various professions to meet the needs of young people and adults suffering from CNS disorders. They have defined and enforced the boundaries of our scope of care. These institutions are not yet prepared to consider the possibility that many of our efforts are tantamount to rearranging the deck chairs on the Titanic ... or, even worse, making room for more deck chairs by throwing "useless" life rafts overboard. They will likely aggressively resist new paradigms of care to protect economic interests and support cognitive dissonance. The argument? So many have done it this way for so long that they couldn't possibly be wrong. It was philosopher Bertrand Russell who said, "The fact that an opinion has been widely held is no evidence whatever that it is not utterly absurd."

Fellow colleagues, wake up and smell the roses. Get smart about the role of nutrition in "mental" illness. You may see this as a threat to your professional identity. I did too. For me, this journey has been a reluctant one, necessitated only by the inability of the old models to help my father and son. So what am I saying, that you should all become nutritional counselors? No, simply that you fully consider the interaction of the person in the environment, which includes the nutrients, microbes, metals, and chemicals our clients take in through water, air, and food. Develop research skills and share them with your patients and their families. Be a biblio-therapist. Leave no stone unturned. Tell your patients about the studies on omega-3 fatty acids at Harvard and the Synergy supplements at the University of Calgary. Tell them how the vitamin and mineral content of their food supply has significantly decreased from 1936 through 1980, some by as much as 20%.[8] Your scope of care is to foster growth and independence, not ignorance and dependency on you.

To doctors and nurses

Dr. H. Hugh Fudenberg, along with some colleagues, wrote the following:

> *We agree and assert that an omission of fundamental impor-*
> *tance exists in the medical literature that has permeated all*
> *of medicine with profound and far-reaching effects on the*
> *quality and cost of heath care. We believe that this tragic*
> *situation may be largely corrected or at least significantly*
> *ameliorated by the proper employment of essential nutrients*
> *adjunctive to conventional care or alone as indicated in the*
> *literature.*[9]

In the introduction to their book, <u>Manic Depressive Illness</u>, published in 1991, Doctors Fredrick K. Goodwin and Kay Redfield Jamison state that their goal is to provide a unifying perspective rather than simply a plethora of information about the causes of the disorder. In my opinion, the research at that time did not support such unifying perspectives. I searched through the index looking for references on signal transduction, cytokines, syphilis, Lyme disease, and nutrition and found nothing. The recommendations in this chapter are based on unifying, if incomplete principles.

The first recommendation is not very sophisticated. Leaving aside all the complexities of bipolar disorder, it seems prudent, though admittedly simplistic, to suggest that this disorder is likely the result of too little of the right things and too much of the wrong things in people with certain genetic susceptibilities. CNS-disordered patients need to get enough of the right things, such as nutrients and water. I am not a physician, but I can guarantee that this will do no harm. Maintaining the health of the tomato plants in my garden with sufficient water and nutrition doesn't guarantee my horticultural success, but it is a good place to start.

Second, when a client like my son meets the criteria for bipolar disorder and has a family history of the same, please attend to the facts of his illness beyond those relevant to your model. Don't squeeze my son's illness into your preconceived mold. Don't jump to the conclusion that infection and environment are not important just because genes are. The client may have a genetic link that manifests bipolar symptoms in response to chronic infection and/or environmental toxins. If you don't ask questions you cannot know for sure if it is the genetic link or the genetic link in response to chronic infections and environmental factors. Routine lab work won't identify this. Viral panels, Western Blots, hair analyses, omega-3 fatty acid tests and others will. When you read that the genetic expression of bipolar disorder gets worse with each generation, remember that pollution levels of toxins such as mercury and chemicals are much higher than one generation ago.

Third, please be open to new models for understanding "mental" illness. Even though in 2002 you are still required to categorize patients with terms like bipolar disorder and schizophrenia in order to get paid for your services, please try not to categorize your patients in your mind this way.

These diagnoses need to be discarded in favor of more explicit biological CNS anomalies that are associated with specific psychological variables. I believe these anomalies will eventually be found to contribute to a wide range of symptoms that overlap current categories and render them obsolete.

Hey, I know I am just a clinical social worker with a checkered genetic past. Still, I am of the opinion that highly respected leaders in your field such as Doctors Goodwin and Jamison got it wrong in their book <u>Manic-Depressive Illness</u>. While addressing the issue of biological specificity they state the following on page 584: "One problem in assessing the diagnostic specificity of these findings [various biological correlates of mania and depression] is that a given measure may differ among subgroups of patients with affective illness, or the findings may vary across different phases of the illness." Of course they do! "Affective illness" is not the illness. They got the cart before the horse. An "affective illness" like "bipolar disorder" is a constellation of symptoms sharing a multiplicity of different biological causes. No wonder the findings vary. You will find the keys to unlock the illnesses in the very biological correlates which you dismiss because the lack of specificity doesn't fit into your affective illness paradigm. The square peg of affective illnesses doesn't fit the round hole of biological causes. Learn from my son's extreme sense of smell. Identify excitotoxins and other environmental triggers. Consider chronic infections. Look for cytokines that are running amok. Facilitate blood flow to his brain.

I know that if you throw away "affective illness" it may be necessary to throw away psychiatry as well. That wouldn't be all bad. Send the psychiatrists back to school to learn about biologically valid psychological variables applied to chronic infectious diseases and drug effects. Train them to become neurologists who can diagnose and treat brain disorders, or, better yet, give them specialized training in gastroenterology so they can assess and treat digestive problems which proliferate in those suffering from CNS disorders. Teach them about nutrition and brain functioning — notice I didn't say "mental" health — so I can confidently send my son to them.

Fourth, psychotropic medicines, while sometimes necessary, keep patients from being curious. They dull the sensibilities and make them overweight and tired. Sometimes they create other symptoms, provoking a kind of self-fulfilling prophecy that often requires more medications. When that happens, and you prescribe new drugs, you really don't know if you're treating the original symptoms or the results of the medications you prescribed in the first place. Instead of adding Wellbutrin, first lessen the Depakote to see if that helps the patient to be less depressed and sluggish. It is more worthwhile to help the patient be in charge of his life than to make him dependent on you. If the patient can get better on nutritional supplements that have a documented track record of efficacy (e.g. Synergy supplements), then use those and use less or no psychotropic medicines.

If you have to resort to medications, more is not necessarily better. The smell test is not very scientific, but if the doses of lithium, Depakote, Wellbutrin, and Zyprexa you are giving the patient cause him to exude a metallic smell and he still doesn't get any better, then please don't do more of the same.

Fifth, even if you have been trained to believe that there is no relationship between food and behavior, have the patient avoid gluten, casein, and other foods while in the hospital. What would it hurt? If that is too much to ask, how about at least keeping the violent patient from foods with high levels of phosphates like soft drinks, processed meats, and those tasty, inexpensive puddings your hospital serves for afternoon snacks? Check out his magnesium, zinc, and trace lithium levels. If they are low, supplement him. Better yet, hire a properly trained nutritionist to be an integral part of your staff. They can do a better job of advising than I can. I am just a social worker.

Finally, while we are at it, let the family be a part of the treatment team. If family members want to contribute to the treatment plan by having the patient take omega fatty-3 acids, applaud them for it. Unless the patient is a diabetic or has bleeding problems, the risk of major health problems from taking 2,000 mg of fish oil is minimal compared to the risks of the medications you are licensed to give patients.

For now, to the extent possible, find out the biological conditions that specifically cause the psychological symptoms and treat those. It will take longer and cost more than the current assembly-line psychotropic medication approach mandated by most managed care organizations, but it will be much more cost-effective in the long run. Think of the long-term cost savings when even a small proportion of the "mentally" ill are able to rejoin society as wage-earning, contributing members. The reduction in long-term disability alone can justify the additional costs of individualized diagnosis and treatment.

I am sorry to be so long winded. I admit I commented that I was making my last or final recommendation. I lied. For years I listened to you when my father and son were ill. Often when I talked, I could tell you were not listening. I knew because you interrupted while I was talking as if what I had to say was of little consequence. I knew because you put your hand on my shoulder and said in a condescending way, "When the book comes out, I will be the first to read it." This is my only chance to make up for lost time, so please bear with me. I really am about to finish. I read a study once claiming that the average physician listened during the first five minutes of an interview, and from then on the patient listened. Please listen to us beyond the first five minutes of the interview.

In closing, for real this time, I will make one more recommendation. Please don't allow yourselves to be bought out by the drug companies. I, too, enjoyed the catered luncheons, the free continuing medical education credits, the cups and pens, the notepads, the umbrellas, the cookies and bagels, and the free ego massages. I know how easy it is to accept their studies and fail to seek out alternative views. I know how easy it is for them to file away unfavorable studies on their products so that the public never sees them. Many of their drugs are highly effective. Some are not. Some are dangerous, particularly when they are withdrawn. Warn your patients about this. There was a provocative editorial in the May 19, 2001 issue of *Lancet.* The writer suggested that the FDA has become a "servant of the drug industry." Is there an "FDA-pharmaceutical complex" similar to what President Eisenhower dubbed the military-industrial complex and warned America against? All of the above can be summed up simply. You've probably heard it before.

Please do no harm.

To CNS patients and their families.

It is terrifying to lose your sense of reality, to feel that the "you" you were is no longer there. Tough on families, too. We have been there and done that. Don't want to do it any more. You don't either. Take charge of the assessment and treatment process. You probably don't have the time to explore the causes of the CNS disorders with which you are dealing, but you can take charge.

You do not have to accept a diagnosis such as "ADHD," "bipolar disorder," "schizophrenia" or even "depression" as the problem. Buy Dr. Gant's book, ADD, ADHD, A Complementary Medicine Solution, and try to show it to your doctor. Buy Dr. Werback's book, Nutritional Influences on Mental Illness, and try and show it to your doctor. Buy Dr. Roger's book, Depression, Cured at Last!, and try to show it to your doctor. Don't do this all at once. If your doctor is not open to listening to new ideas, tell him that you are tired of "more of the same" and leave. That's right, leave. Find doctors who are open to new paradigms of care. There is a growing list at alternativementalhealthcare.com as well as at other sites. Ask your doctor to check out possible biological factors such as heavy metals; food sensitivities; neurotoxins; vitamin and amino acid deficiencies; high levels of vaccine antitoxoids; viruses such as Borna, toxoplasmosis, and stealth; chronic neurological Lyme and other tick-related illnesses, including chronic co-infections with tick-borne as well as other pathogens. These could create a complex reaction from toxins and the immune system that exacerbates symptoms in your genetically vulnerable body. Just because the DSM-IV does not have a diagnosis such as Infectious and Immune Mediated Pathophysiology (IIMP) does not mean that such a disorder does not exist.

Take, for example, the Lyme connection. Lyme disease was discovered in this country just 25 years ago. The *Borrelia burgdorferi* spirochete is very similar in structure and effect to that of a disease that has existed for centuries: syphilis. Interestingly, one of the common presenting complaints of patients with syphilis in the days before early detection and treatment were available was, you guessed it, bipolar disorder. The interest in linking bacteriological and viral infection to "mental" illness is still relatively recent. Stay tuned. Not that many years ago hospitals in the South were filled with patients diagnosed with schizophrenia. Their symptoms were caused by pellegra, a deficiency of B vitamins.

Remember that if your mechanic only diagnoses your car as having a racing engine, he has done nothing to help you understand or fix the problem. Appendix 1 lists some of the paths we took and some resources that may facilitate your journey.

Stay open to new ideas, all the while remembering "caveat emptor"; let the buyer beware. Be open, yet critical. Trust, but verify. Validate the data with your own research as best you can. The Internet already has a lot of the information you need, as well as hype you don't need. Talk with support group members to cut through the latter. Listen to them and read what the posters in the chat rooms have to say. Read the medical literature. Before you act, find a way to determine to the best of your ability if a test measures what the testers say it measures. Find out any risks associated with a treatment method. Learn how well the treatment works from others who had it.

If you are a patient and your family members interpret your difficulties in psychological terms, understand that this may be the only way they can talk about it. When Chris described an inability to talk or his difficulty with directions, we didn't think of "word finding" or "difficulty with directions," the classical symptoms of neurological Lyme. We thought about depression, concentration difficulties, and anxiety.

Trust your instincts. Do not accept "no" for an answer, whether you are getting care from mainstream or alternative medicine. If anyone tells you they have the answer — including this writer, be skeptical. If you feel that the provider has no time to listen to your concerns, or there is pressure to spend more without knowing why, or that your questions are being perceived as irrelevant and slowing the process, then leave and go elsewhere. If you are unsure of the appropriateness of a doctor's recommendation, do not be intimidated, as I was. Or, better yet, keep asking questions even if you are. Respect and utilize helpers, but be cautious of them. If you feel uncomfortable about something, talk to your health care professional about it. If you are a parent and your therapist attributes responsibility for the problems to you, your marriage, or your family system, carefully and non-defensively assess this to see if it rings true. Don't forget that your family could be crazy because one of your members has a broken brain. Remember the "schizophrenogenic" mother story. You and your family decide which providers to select; you process the information; then you make decisions based on that information. You and your family are ultimately responsible for your treatment.

One of my reasons for writing this book was to find out for myself whether or not the claims of Truehope were too good to be true. Based on my research and our experience, I believe that the claims *are* true, even though the phrase "too good to be true" presumes they couldn't possibly be. Such was my orientation when I first encountered the Truehope Web site that claimed to provide nutritional solutions for bipolar and other CNS disorders.

Let me be clear about this. I have seen nothing in a lifetime of living with bipolar disorder that has been as effective as the Truehope supplements. Throughout my life with my father, his moods were generally hypomanic, with severe depression and mania. From Chris's first hospitalization on, we struggled with ongoing hypomanic behavior. The drugs kept him from becoming psychotic, but they also made him depressed and, I am convinced, played a major role in his self-mutilating suicide attempt when he stopped taking Zyprexa. The supplements gave us our son back with normal moods and no drugs.

Does that mean I believe that the supplements are a "cure," and there will be no complications down the road? No, it just means that after some 56 years, I no longer have to settle for non-expectation therapy, or "more of the same." It means that I no longer have to struggle to reconcile complex biological realities with my personal mythology. We are both the creators of our own world and created by it. It means that the precipice dread is moving further into the back of my mind than it has ever been. It is not gone. It will never be gone. If Chris stays on the supplements, it means his brain will have access to chemical precursors he would not have had access to otherwise, irrespective of the specific biological factors which will remain the object of our ongoing inquiries. The supplements have not cured his underlying biological problems, whether they include Lyme disease, stealth virus, leaky gut, or an as yet to be diagnosed brain disorder.

Based on the research and our experience, the Synergy supplements provide a nutritional foundation that effectively corrects some of the biological anomalies associated with bipolar and other CNS disorders. The first two professional journal articles on the Synergy supplements were written by Doctors Kaplan and Popper and published in the December 2001 issue of the *Journal of Clinical Psychiatry*. In that article Dr. Kaplan reported an effect size with the supplements on measures of mania and depression that was greater than .80. This is a level of change rarely found in the literature. It is nothing short of phenomenal, almost, dare I say it, too good to be true!

Effect size measures the breadth of change an intervention causes. To give a hypothetical example, if a person wanted to see how effective a new fertilizer was on the height of sun flower seed plants, he could plant one field without fertilizer and one with it. If the average unfertilized stalks were 10 feet, then a .80-effect size of the fertilized plants would be an average height of 18 feet! An effect size of .30 is considered very good in human research.

But what about all those nutrients? Isn't it too much in the long run? Studies have demonstrated that the amounts of vitamin A, D, B12, selenium and chromium, even at the full initial supplement dose of 32 pills a day, do not exceed established levels of toxicity for those with normal liver functioning.[10] Some warn of the possibility of long-term negative consequences. Even Dr. Kaplan points out that long-term studies assessing possible deleterious effects of the supplements have not yet been accomplished. No solution is completely risk-free. Taking supplements long-term includes unknown risks. Taking psychotropic medications long-term involves known risks.

I would recommend that you discuss with your health care professional the possibility of becoming involved in ongoing self-directed research trials with the staff at Truehope. Before Chris cut back on the supplements, he had been free of all symptoms for eight months by taking the supplements and omega-3 fatty acids. He had no adverse reactions and remained off all psychotropic medications. While subsequent events were to challenge our confidence in the supplements, or, to be more specific, Chris's ability or willingness to comply with the nutritional regimen, in the end, they strengthened our belief in the efficacy of the nutritional approach.

If something sounds too good to be true, it probably is. At least, that was my mind set when I first heard of Truehope. If it were so great, why hadn't scientists discovered it already? The answer might be relatively simple. Mainstream scientists do not consider supplements to be worthy of research because they're not specifically targeted enough. Using a mixture of ingredients is inherently unscientific in that one cannot know which ingredient is the active one. Western medicine is reductionistic. Single relationships are more controllable and measurable than multiple relationships. A product like the Synergy supplements introduces so many variables that a researcher could be criticized for not defining the variables narrowly enough. Is it any wonder that Dr. Kaplan was initially so hesitant to research the Truehope promise? In addition, without a unique proprietary product, the drug companies have no motivation to support and fund vitamin and mineral supplement research. In the previously cited article by Dr. Popper, he stated: "The groundbreaking approach of examining several nutrient ingredients at once, while a violation of our usual tenets of investigation, may present an opportunity to examine how micronutrients might operate in concert."[10]

Does this mean you should just go out and start taking Synergy supplements or some other nutritional approach with a similarly positive track record? I return to Poel's Rule described in the Acknowledgments: "Know what you know, and know what you don't know." While this book is designed to share our family's odyssey rather than to provide individual solutions, some general perspectives might be constructive here.

What if your level of a nutrient were already too high, such as high copper associated with some depressive disorders or a high copper/zinc ratio associated with violent behavior? According to a colleague of mine, researchers at the Nutritional Research Center, founded by Dr. Pfeiffer, have established that some depressed patients have what they call a "high copper" type of depression. The question then would be whether or not the Synergy supplements would increase the copper or if countervailing substances such as zinc, magnesium, and vitamin C which the supplements also contain, would bring the copper or the copper/zinc ratios to within normal limits. Before you went down that path, you would need to determine if you had this problem and, if you did, whether the synergistic effects of multiple nutrients would aggravate or ameliorate it. If you had a disease like Wilson's disease, increased copper could be very dangerous. You would also want to be sure you didn't have any sensitivities to some of the minerals such as iron and/or nickel.

Most importantly, find out through reputable professionals, what is broken before trying to fix it with nutrients. David Hardy tells of a woman who came to him asking to participate in the Truehope research program. She had already been assessed by her doctor, who diagnosed her as having chronic fatigue syndrome. The doctor offered her Elavil. She chose the supplements, and in a few weeks she phoned David with glowing feedback about how wonderful she was feeling. Her energy had been restored. Six months later, she called to tell him that her original symptoms of extreme tiredness had returned. David told her that if her problem was nutritional insufficiency, the supplements should still be working. Since they weren't, he suggested that she see another doctor for further assessment. The woman called back later to report that a new doctor had diagnosed her with cancer. A few months later, she died. This incident points out the power of the supplements as well as the dangers of exclusive reliance on a nutritional solution before a complete diagnosis is rendered. Truehope supplements and the immune enhancing supplements help Chris cope with ongoing long term neuro-lyme and or stealth virus, but they don't destroy the infection(s).

If we assume there are multiple contributors to CNS disorders, then nutritional supplements, while helpful for many, perhaps even the majority, cannot specifically address all of the relevant biological imbalances. The tremendous effect size found with the Synergy supplements does support that nutritional deficits are a major cause of bipolar symptoms. It may be — and I am using arbitrary numbers here — that something on the order of 75% of bipolar disordered patients are in a group that responds solely to nutritional intervention. Yet that group may only include 25% of the biological anomalies, known, or still to be discovered that are responsible for bipolar symptoms. For want of a better word, we could call these the "simple" bipolar syndromes. The other 25% of patients might represent 75% of the known, or still to be discovered biological anomalies that manifest as bipolar syndrome. Perhaps they would respond to specific treatments targeted towards more complex causes such as excessive protein kinase C, Lyme disease, or stealth virus. This is all the more reason why standardized assessment protocols are needed for individuals like Chris, who have been helped by the supplements, but who also have other biological anomalies that require prioritizing, assessment, and treatment. The same logic could be applied to the broader range of CNS disorders. Since nutritional deficits are found to be common for a great many CNS patients, general nutritional support would be needed, as well as targeted treatment for other contributing factors.

Dr. Gant uses an approach that includes nutrients from a company called Nutrenergy. For those wanting to save money, he recommends a relatively inexpensive, albeit less effective, protocol for all ADD/ADHD children. If that is inadequate, he recommends relatively expensive specialized assessments. These assessments are then followed by an individualized nutrient protocol. Similarly, the Pfeiffer Treatment Center at the Health Research Institute creates individualized, customized supplements targeted to individual deficiencies obtained through extensive (and expensive) tests. They do not provide the kind of comprehensive, broad-based nutrient solution such as is found in the Synergy supplements.

The point is to do your own due diligence with your health care provider so that you can do whatever you want in the confidence that you know what you know and know what you don't know. Tony and David prefer that their clients work through their doctors and do not profess to assess or treat medical problems. There are many alternatives from which to choose. There is no one magic answer, and even the good answers are not without some risk. While other vitamin and amino acid supplements may be as effective as the Synergy supplements, I have not discussed them in any detail only because we have not had any experience with them.

Assuming that established economic interests are unable to crush those providing nutritional solutions for CNS disorders, I believe that comprehensive, broad-based supplementation such as is found in the Synergy supplements will eventually provide effective support for the majority of patients. Solutions similar to those of the Bio-Behavioral Hospital of 2016 will eventually evolve and move to the mainstream for those whose bipolar syndrome is based on more complex etiologies.

This will happen faster if patients and their families refuse to accept the status quo. Lobby your congressman for more research into the causes of bipolar syndrome and other CNS disorders. Demand that "psychiatric" disorders receive parity with medical disorders, or, better yet, insist that they be redefined as medical disorders. Alone, one person, one family is powerless. As a part of a grass roots movements families can be very powerful.

As biological assessments and more user-friendly interventions such as nutritional solutions proliferate, I hope that terms like "mental" illness will fade into the history books. I hope that better classification systems will evolve based upon biologically valid psychological variables applied to diseases and to drug effects. It was Arthur C. Clark who wrote, "The only way of discovering the limits of the possible is to venture a little way past them into the impossible."

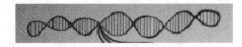

Notes

1. Lienhard, John H., "Rye Ergot and Witches," 1999.
http://www.uh.edu/engines/epi1037.htm
2. Amen, Daniel, "Healing ADD," Walnut Creek, November 17, 2000, from comments during his presentation.
3. Michel, Lou and Dan Herbeck, <u>American Terrorist Timothy McVeigh and the Oklahoma City Bombing</u>, HarperCollins Publishers, New York, N.Y., 2001, xv, 7-116.
4. Hamza, Khidhir, <u>Saddam's Bombmaker</u>, Simon and Schuster, New York, N.Y., 2000, 244.
5. Bryce-Smith, Derek, "Crime and Nourishment," *Perspectives, A Mental Health Magazine*, 1999.
http://mhnet.org/perspectives/ articles/art03964.htm
6. Schoenthaler, S.J., Bier, I.D., Young, K., Nichols, D., Jansenns, S., "The effect of vitamin-mineral supplementation on the intelligence of American school children: a randomized, double-blind placebo-controlled trial," *Journal of Alternative and Complementary Medicine*, Vol. 6(1):19-29, February 1, 2000.
7. Schoenthaler, S.J., Bier, I.D., "The effect of vitamin-mineral supplementation on juvenile delinquency among American schoolchildren: a randomized, double-blind placebo-controlled trial," *Journal of Alternative and Complementary Medicine*, 6(1): 7-17, February 2000.
8. Mayer, A., "Historical changes in the mineral content of fruits and vegetables," *British Food Journal,* 99:207-211, 1997.
9. Fudenberg, H.H., "Neuroimmuno Therapeutics Research Foundation," 2000.
http://www.nitrf.org
10. Kaplan, B., Simpson, S., Ferre, R., Gorman, C., McMullen, D., Crawford, S., "Effective mood stabilization with a chelated mineral supplement: an open-label trial in bipolar disorder," *Journal of Clinical Psychiatry*, 62(12):, 936-943, December 2001.
11. Dr. Popper reported conducting trials of the Synergy supplements with 22 patients (adults, teens and preteens) who met criteria for bipolar disorder. He judged that 19 showed a positive response. Among 15 who were treated with medicines before the study, 11 had been stable for six to nine months on no medications.
Popper, Charles, "Do vitamins or minerals (apart from lithium) have mood-stabilizing effects?" *Journal of Clinical Psychiatry*, 62(12):933-935, December, 2001.

26 - Getting Our Hemispheres To Work Together

In order for the human brain to function properly, both hemispheres need to work together effectively. The right and left hemispheres need to maintain plasticity, the ability to accept inputs and modify responses accordingly. Institutions sanctioned by society to provide services for CNS-disordered patients also need plasticity. As stated previously, the response of the justice system to my father was just as bipolar as he was in his response to it. If our justice and health care institutions function like bipolar patients, how effective can they be?

Plasticity and progress

Dr. Daniel Amen, at the conference I attended in 2000, made the point, in a joking manner, that the modal (most frequently occurring) SPECT finding with physicians is an overactive cingulate gyrus. The cingulate gyrus is a region in the center of the brain that spans from the front to the back. He found that patients with an overactive cingulate gyrus, as revealed in the SPECT, tended to be obsessive and rigid, not the kind of people who enthusiastically embraced new ideas. He painfully discovered this when he began trying to present new findings showing dramatic relationships between SPECT images and psychiatric symptoms. He learned that openness to innovative ideas was not the modal style of doctors.

Now I am the last person to want my doctor to change his mind every time a new theory comes along. I want a predictable, reliable doctor, someone who doesn't deviate from the standard of care, particularly if he or she happens to be a surgeon. But if having a doctor with an overactive cingulate gyrus impairs the introduction of new ideas, what happens when many doctors get together and form associations? Organizational plasticity could be impaired. Research that already exists demonstrating the effectiveness of nutrition as a stand-alone intervention in CNS disorders would be ignored. Maybe this is why drug companies target ads toward consumers when they want doctors to prescribe a new drug, or why new discoveries such as the role of *H Pylori* in stomach ulcers take so long to be accepted. Maybe that is why most doctors are very uncomfortable even talking about nutrients and the brain.

If the APA maintains that the DSM-IV reflects some inherent reality and tries to make the data fit a classification system based on symptoms rather than biology, what will that do for patients suffering from CNS disorders? If the professionals ignore biologically valid psychological variables and fail to apply them both to diseases and to drug effects, where will that leave us? It will leave us with more of the same. It will leave us with psychotropic drugs as the first line of defense against various illness of the soul (psychiatric illnesses) that we still call functional because in the past no one knew what caused them. And lastly, if those who bring disturbing facts to the table are ignored, how will more effective solutions be found? One cannot find a solution until there is an agreement about what the problem is.

Dr. Martin's story illustrates the well-known truth that social systems respond poorly to negative feedback. The FDA, the CDC, and the medical profession as a whole all ignored his findings. If this cat were let out of the bag, additional areas of inquiry might be explored. Unwanted conclusions might follow, the most damning of which is that the AIDS virus may have been caused by polio and/or hepatitis B vaccinations created by using contaminated imported monkeys for development of the vaccines. As Dr. Martin stated, "One would surely not import wild monkeys from Africa, create short-term primary kidney cultures, add a human virus, and administer the crude garnish derived from the virally infected cells to virtually every child in the county. ... Yet this is essentially the situation with live polio vaccine, and comparable arguments can be made for other human and animal viral vaccines."[1]

Whether or not he is correct, it is highly unlikely that the existing power structure will be open to Dr. Martin's ideas. These institutions will not display plasticity when it comes to processing the information Dr. Martin has put before them, unless, that is, as he predicts, stealth viruses find their way to Los Angeles and other major cities in epidemic proportions. The public outcry would then make it impossible for his ideas to be ignored.

The bipolar patient is unable to utilize feedback due to a broken brain. If the institutions established to protect the public and find answers to these complex problems were to demonstrate the same lack of plasticity, people with CNS disorders would neither be properly diagnosed nor treated.

Scientists are beginning to learn what causes CNS disorders. They are learning that the body's immune response to chronic and complex bacteriological and viral infections plays a much larger role in the etiology of these illnesses than has heretofore been recognized. They are learning that a one-size-fits-all model, as appealing as this is to the managed care community, simply does not reflect reality.

An autistic child improves on a diet free of gluten and casein. A bipolar patient does fine on a wheat-free diet until she eats wheat and crashes. A mother who sleeps with her cat develops toxoplasmosis and bipolar disorder. She responds to the Synergy supplements. A sports fisherman is exposed to blue green algae and develops bipolar disorder that is responsive to CSM. A gardener with depression tests positive for organophosphates and later develops Parkinson's disease. A bipolar juvenile delinquent has lead poisoning. Another has mercury poisoning. A bipolar patient has Borna virus while another has neurologic Lyme disease. An ADHD child has a zinc deficiency.

A depressed teenager is deficient in magnesium. A mother with bipolar disorder has coexisting long-term infections. Her son, a difficult child, has stealth virus, and now a brain tumor. A businessman with severe mood swings has an admixture of different components in differing concentrations resulting in a unique set of symptoms. Each person's symptoms are different due to the interaction of multiple infectious and environmental factors and that person's unique genetic structure and nutrition profile.

There is no neat, simple explanation. The "chemical imbalance" theory is not big enough to embrace the variety of biological conditions that cause CNS disorders. When enough biological exceptions are found for the "functional" illnesses of bipolar disorder, chronic fatigue syndrome, fibromyalgia, and schizophrenia, the exceptions become the rule. Then research begins to focus on the biologically valid psychological variables as they relate to both diseases and drug effects. The biological dysfunction needs to be identified and treated, not just the symptoms of the illnesses.

Will future diagnostic and treatment paradigms be based on research or on the cultural biases of unresponsive institutions? Will research follow the money or the science? Unless the public participates in the process, the groups with the most clout will prevail. I would like to believe that Chris's doctor diagnosed his Lyme disease solely on the basis of his symptoms and the Western Blot results. However, the doctor also said that Chris's results more then met the CDC's criteria for Lyme disease and that the treatment was therefore reimbursable. Aren't those criteria just like the DSM-IV criteria, essentially a political statement reflecting the consensus of scientists whose livelihood is based on their findings? How was this any different than another doctor telling us that Chris met the criteria for Bipolar I, and that therefore antipsychotic medications were reimbursable? Based on what I was told and what I have read, I believe Chris has Lyme disease. But, if he and a sizeable number of bipolar patients are in fact infected with a stealth virus, and they lack a powerful lobby to represent them, then they will not have access to adequate assessment and treatment.

Empirically based assessment and treatment guidelines are needed for the biological causes of what I now think of as bipolar syndrome, as well as for a host of other CNS disorders. DSM-IV provided a good start. It replaced words like "hysteric" and "neurotic" with more acceptable, accurate terminology. However, it still fails to provide a comprehensive framework for effective classification and treatment of the biological conditions that cause psychiatric disorders. It sheds no light on the biology of bipolar disorder. There is a diagnostic category called "Mood Disorders Due to a General Medical Condition" as well as "Substance Induced Mood Disorder." The former could include infections, while the latter could include use of or withdrawal from drugs, as well as exposure to toxins. However, these are not specific enough to include the plethora of conditions I encountered in the course of this odyssey, conditions such as Lyme disease, polypeptiduria, food sensitivities, and nutritional deficits. The developers of DSM-IV appeared to me to be more concerned with descriptive nuances than biological causes. DSM-IV labels by description, not biology. While it pays the bills for those of us in the mental health business, it does not provide sufficient plasticity for the future.

When DSM-IV was first published, providers could listen to what some have called the patient's "organ recital" and then count the number of symptoms. If the patient had four pain symptoms, two GI symptoms, one sexual symptom, and one pseudoneurological symptom, all of which had no apparent physical basis, as determined by the clinician, the doctor could render an "objective" diagnosis of somatization disorder. How would a chronic illness like Lyme disease or stealth virus fit into that scenario? What would happen to the patient if no one knew to test for those illnesses and prematurely diagnosed the patient with somatization disorder? After the patient was referred to a psychiatrist and didn't get better, the therapist could in his own mind blame the patient for not being motivated to get well. Academics could write papers arguing that these so-called "Lyme patients" were actually responding to their own psychological problems.

Dr. Loren R. Mosher wrote the following to the APA upon his resignation from that organization: "DSM-IV is the fabrication upon which psychiatry seeks acceptance by medicine in general. Insiders know it is more a political than scientific document. To its credit it says so — although its brief apologia is rarely noted. DSM-IV has become a bible and a money-making best seller — its major failings notwithstanding. It confines and defines practice, some take it seriously, others more realistically. It is the way to get paid."[2]

The street lamp theory of obfuscation

One day, while reviewing posts from the MMI discussion group, I came upon the comments of a Dr. Debra Solomon. I immediately emailed her for permission to use her quote in this book. She responded positively. Her ideas were central to one of the main themes I was trying to get across, that the assessment and treatment of psychiatric disorders need to be viewed in a much broader context than they currently are. Dr. Solomon told of a joke she had heard in her childhood.

A man is walking down the street at night and sees a friend looking for something under a street lamp. He asks the friend what he is looking for.

"I dropped a quarter," replies his friend. "Can you help me find it?"

Together, they look for another fifteen minutes with no sign of the quarter. So the first man asks, "Where did you say you dropped it?"

"Oh, I dropped it over there across the street."
The confused man asks, "Then why are we looking here?"
"Because the light's better here!"
She explained her analogy.

> *What disappoints me about psychiatry these days is that we're*
> *trying to erect street lamps (brain imaging, drug studies) to*
> *shine on the brain to find which neurotransmitters cause*
> *which disorder, whether it's OCD or somatization. But maybe*
> *the missing quarters aren't just in the brain; right across the*
> *street (the blood-brain barrier) is the rest of the body—the*
> *endocrine system, the immune system, toxins, infectious*
> *agents, etc. And it's all connected. Duhhh ...! It's so basic to*
> *our training, every one of us physicians, psychiatric or oth-*
> *erwise, but the triumvirate of managed care, academia, and*
> *the pharmaceutical industry has dumbed down and enslaved*
> *the medical masses ...!*

Her comments did not just apply to physicians. One day, while Lori, Chris's home health nurse, was changing the dressing on his PICC line, I told her about a time when I was "dumbed down." I accepted the word of a medical expert, who, although he was not aware of it, had also been "dumbed down" by the system of which he was a part. I told her how, in 1993, I had unsuccessfully tried to find new treatment approaches to astrocytoma, a type of brain tumor.

Astrocytoma is almost always fatal. My mom had it. It was inoperable. She had decided to forgo treatments and their side effects and spend as much time with her family as possible. By the time she visited us in Alaska, the tumor was affecting her speech and thought processes, primarily with episodes of what we in the trade call "word salad," a flow of words utterly devoid of meaning. My mom and I both believed what we had been told: that any treatment would be worse than her illness, and that her illness would ultimately be fatal. Still, it was difficult to watch her mental status deteriorate so steadily.

In the winter of 1993, I flew down from Alaska and took her to the University of San Francisco Medical Center (USFMC). As the doctor told us of his pending fishing trip to Alaska with his son, he as much as affirmed my mom's death sentence by telling her that there was nothing he could do to help, but that she had a good attitude for having such a serious disease. I asked him persistently and repeatedly if his "gamma knife" treatment, or any other new treatments or clinical trials offered any hope. I asked about alternative treatments. No matter how I worded my questions, the answer was always the same. No, there were no alternatives. The tumor was intermingled

369

with too much of her brain.

On the other side of the family, my mother's stepdaughter, who worked at Loma Linda Medical Center, dealt with her anxiety at my mom's downhill slide by strongly encouraging her to undergo radiation therapy. My mom finally consented, had a brain biopsy, and submitted to a series of radiation treatments that precipitously facilitated her downhill course and led to her death at the age of 74. I couldn't understand the logic of injuring a damaged brain by taking a brain biopsy, then killing more brain cells with radiation. But I kept my thoughts to myself. I wouldn't question my mom's decision to find hope in a hopeless situation, nor would I try to find new solutions. Back then, I still trusted the mechanics.

Some years after her death, I learned about Dr. Stanislaw R. Burzynski, who, for the last 25 years, has been shrinking and curing brain tumors, some of which have historically been 100% fatal. His initial theory was about as unbelievable as the notion that a treatment approach similar to vitamin and mineral supplements for ear and tail biting syndrome in pigs could effectively ameliorate bipolar symptoms in human beings. Dr. Burzynski identified a group of peptides he called antineoplastons in human urine. He noted that healthy people had more antineoplastons while cancer patients had less, suggesting that the peptides may be involved in promoting apoptosis in what were otherwise immortal cancer cells. He determined that antineoplastons are peptides that essentially "tell" the cancer cells to stop growing and start acting like normal cells.

He started producing antineoplastons from urine and then later synthetically manufactured them. His antineoplaston-treated patients began to experience tumor regression for some tumors that had historically always 100% been fatal. Some tumors completely disappeared. The FDA tried to shut him down for years, then took him to trial for various allegations that are beyond the scope of this book. For further information, see The Burzynski Breakthrough, by Thomas Elias. During the trial, it was revealed that if the FDA succeeded in shutting him down, a number of his patients would certainly die. Not only was he acquitted of all charges, but since then, the FDA has sponsored 72 phase two trials for a multitude of cancers, although still imposing highly restrictive conditions.

I learned from the Burzynski patient Web site that two individuals who had been patients at the USFMC had turned to Dr. Burzynski before I took my mother there. One little girl, Crystin Schiff, was totally cured with the antineoplastin treatment. That means her tumor completely disappeared. She died anyway, of complications from her chemotherapy and radiation therapy. Another person, a businessman, opted to ignore the recommendations of USFMC doctors and put his trust totally in Dr. Burzynski. His tumor disappeared, and he became symptom-free.[3]

When I finished telling Lori what happened, she pressed the tape on

Chris's arm and looked up. "You know, we treated a man with an inoperable brain tumor a few years ago using Dr. Burzynski's approach."

"Oh, really? What a coincidence. How did he do?"

"It took a long time of daily infusion of whatever Dr. Burzynski gave him, but his brain tumor disappeared."

If the physician at USFMC had informed us of this alternate resource that had already produced such striking results in two of their former patients, we would have tried to have my mom treated. If Dr. Burzynski had accepted her, based on preliminary results obtained May 15, 2000 from the FDA-supervised clinical trials that began in 1988, she would have had a 63% chance for either an objective response or stable disease. Based on these preliminary results, of the 211 brain tumors treated in FDA-supervised clinical trials, 25 had complete remission, 34 had partial remission (greater than 50% tumor reduction), 73 had stable disease (less than 50% tumor reduction), and 79 had progressive disease. What was even more remarkable was that the FDA required that many of these patients fail chemotherapy and/or radiation therapy before they could be enrolled in the trials, suggesting the possibility of even better responses had they been treated before their immune systems were compromised by traditional cancer treatments. Yet Dr. Burzynski has been professionally ostracized by many in the medical profession. He has been strongly criticized by some doctors on the Internet. They fail to acknowledge that because of his treatments, some children, whose prognosis was certain death, are alive today.[4]

My mom had a favorite saying: "You're down on what you are not up on." The doctor at USFMC was down, "dumbed down," on what he was not up on. Hard to believe that he wouldn't have known about the two cases, especially since the doctors allegedly strongly argued against referral to Dr. Burzynski in both. My mother's doctor was the expert, the one my mom and I relied upon for advice concerning decisions that affected whether she lived or died. Unfortunately, because I trusted him and he was down on Dr. Burzynski's treatment, I did not get up on it. When I didn't get any direction from an "enlightened" institution like USFMC, I decided that nothing more could be done.

Has the oncology industry been shining the light on an adaptation of germ and chemical warfare called chemotherapy and radiation therapy while leaving promising treatments such as antineoplastons in the dark? Has the psychopharmacological industry been shining its light on neurotransmitters while leaving infectious agents, the immune system, and nutrition in the dark? Seems that I had been searching under the street lamp, when I should have been looking in the dark, unexplored areas. If I had explored those dark corners away from the light, my mom might have had a few more years with us.

I will not make the same mistake again.

Beyond <u>The Red Monkey and the American Gulag</u>

In 1986, I started to write a book called <u>The Red Monkey and the American Gulag.</u> The term "red monkey" came from a story I once heard. Apparently, if you paint a monkey red, the rest of the monkeys in the troop will kill it. The book was going to be about all the "red monkeys," such as my father, who languish in literal or metaphorical confinement because the mental health and justice systems fail them. The draft for the introduction was as follows:

> *Small town USA, one of the last bastions of the traditional values that helped make America what she is today. Traditional values. Clear sense of right and wrong. The world is simple, seven streets east and seven streets west. There are good buys and bad guys. It is a clean town. The trash is swept up from the streets. Every morning residents look though clean windows to clean roads and sidewalks.*

> *In this land of liberty and justice for all, there exists a human disposal system similar to, yet different from the Gulag Archipelago described by Solzhenitsyn — more subtle. The American Gulag is a human processing factory that takes human raw material, sorts it, and then disposes of it. Unless you have been there or have known someone who has been there, you would have difficulty imagining that such an institution exists. It starts in school ... .*

I began the book during a time when being tough on crime helped elect politicians even more than it does now at the beginning of the 21st century. <u>The Red Monkey and the American Gulag</u> was the right idea at the wrong time. But the main reason I did not pursue the book is because I found the writing of it to be too depressing. What could I offer except to point out the obvious: The way our society deals with "red monkeys" is deplorable, and something should be done about it? But what? Drug them? Institutionalize them again? I had no solutions. Who would be interested in a book that was not only depressing, but offered no hope? My rough notes stayed on floppy disks for 14 years until Chris's situation forced me to look for new alternatives. I completed this book because I found solutions that gave our family hope.

In this book, I have tried to present objective, real-world findings obtained by researchers all over the globe who are working to solve the puzzle of bipolar and other CNS disorders. I have attempted to shine some light into dark areas far from the street lamps. I am confident that the measured and effective measures we have heretofore taken are the best we can hope for at this time in the real world, where discrepancies exist, where humility and caution are needed, and where my son wants to get on with his life.

In my search for a coherent model for bipolar disorder in my family, I sought to match behavior with biology. I searched for a connection between biologically valid psychological variables and diseases and drug effects. Some of the behaviors included concentration difficulties, problems with directions, word-finding problems, memory problems, abstract-thinking difficulties, poor judgment, interpersonal boundary problems, sleeplessness, psychotic mania, and suicidal depression. Some of the biological findings included inadequate diet, excessive IgG food sensitivities, heavy metals such as mercury and antimony, high DPT antitoxoid levels, *Borrelia burgdorferi* and/or atypical infectious agents, chemical sensitivities, "leaky gut syndrome," endorphins and exorphins, St. John's Wort, excessive Depakote, and Zyprexa withdrawal.

Throughout this process, I found a number of relationships in which there appeared to be little illumination in mainstream psychiatry or medicine. I tried to shed some light on these dark areas. As I finish the book, I have more answers than when I began it, yet I also have more questions. I came upon unexpected discoveries that have helped my family gain essential understandings into the nature and complexity of this illness. While there is much more to be learned and there are no simple answers, I am sure of a few basic facts. Brain and mind are inexorably linked. A broader understanding of "bipolar disorder" is needed. The "disorder" is the behavioral manifestation of specific biological anomalies. Nutrients can play a central role in restoring brains that have been broken from any one of a number of causes, including microbes. Nutrients are not a cure-all. More of the same will result in more of the same.

In the future, if we need to, we will go down some other paths. We may lower Chris's DPT antitoxoid and his mercury and antimony levels.[5] We may stop all gluten and casein. We might identify probiotics and/or pancreatic enzymes to facilitate digestive processes and diminish food sensitivities. We might return to New Century and complete the viral panel — no kinesiology, please.

I have described the experiences of four generations in dealing with behavior that I have come to understand as bipolar syndrome. My family traveled down numerous paths and found novel solutions to a syndrome that probably affected my great aunt Harriet, my grandmother Rose, and definitely affected my father and son. Our journey is not a road map for others, but it does provide a framework for those who wish to have more control over their destiny and who are willing to travel down dark, unlit paths in pursuit of better solutions for what we currently call bipolar disorder, as well as other CNS disorders. Our less-traveled crooked path took us from psychotropic medications to nutritional supplements to food sensitivities to high

IgG levels to Lyme and, finally, to stealth, with interesting side trips along the way.

The right nutrients properly absorbed into the body ameliorate the symptoms of bipolar syndrome and other CNS disorders for a large proportion of patients. I cannot prove that all of the hypotheses in Appendix 1, Diagnostic Resources/Hypotheses for Bipolar Syndrome, are accurate. I cannot prove that they are inclusive, or even that they are conceptualized adequately. There is some overlap in the list. I cannot prove that one particular treatment recommendation generated from one hypothesis will necessarily be effective. There is no "magic bullet." Some of these hypotheses may be proven not to be useful at all, as I initially suspected with Truehope. But to the extent that research demonstrates each separate hypothesis to be valid, then each biological anomaly consistent with that hypothesis would have to be considered a risk factor for bipolar syndrome. Many of these risk factors, such as various microbes, food sensitivities, heavy metals, nutritional deficiencies, and omega-3 levels, can now be measured and then corrected through proper interventions. While addressing one factor may or may not produce symptomatic relief, identifying as many factors as possible increases the likelihood of successful intervention with less or no need for psychotropic medications. The solution is not necessarily in one "cure." It is in identifying and ameliorating the multiple factors that contribute to bipolar syndrome and other CNS disorders.

In the opinion of this backyard mechanic, these risk factors should be in any differential diagnosis of a patient presenting with depression or mania. This is normally not done, and in Chris's case was actively opposed by his doctors, who preferred to treat his "bipolar disorder" with mind-numbing drugs. What could I say? They had the entire medical-university-pharmaceutical establishment on their side.

Dr. Gant, who specializes in the ADD/ADHD and substance abuse populations, uses many of the same diagnostic work-ups that I learned about and obtained for Chris. His focus is on removing toxic substances and restoring proper levels of vitamins, minerals and amino acids. He receives thanks from his ADD/ADHD patients and their families for his revolutionary non drug treatment approach. From his substance abuse patients, he obtains post treatment abstinence from drugs and alcohol approximately three times the national average. In spite of — or perhaps because of — his innovative and effective practices, the OPMC of New York, the same organization that investigated Dr. Burrascano, investigated him. Thanks to his critics, according to testimony he gave at the White House Conference on Complementary and Alternative Medicine Policy on January 23, 2001, "I have endured two interrogations, an office raid, charges of negligence, incompetence and fraud, and eight months of hearings on the charges."[6] He is still practicing medicine; he recently completed a new book on treating addictions; and, last I heard, when I saw him at the Safe Harbor Meeting in Los Angeles, he was initiating litigation against the OPMC for violating their own investigative guidelines. It is sad, but not unexpected, given how systems operate, that those who bring novel and effective treatments to those who otherwise could face the prospect of being a "red monkey" have to put up with such harassment.

One night, several months before finishing the book, I heard on the evening news about a truck driver who had tried to sue the State of California because he had spent so many years of his life in hospitals and jails. He was diagnosed as having bipolar disorder. One of the complaints in his ill-fated lawsuit concerned the months he spent in the "hole" while in prison, presumably for out-of-control behavior. The state rejected his lawsuit because he had improperly completed the paperwork. Shortly thereafter, he drove a commercial truck into the historic state Capitol building in Sacramento, killing himself and causing $13 million of property damage to the building. Some might explain away the behavior as that of a madman. I believe he was trying to tell us something. He was telling us that for him, the system was broken. He was angry, and he was not going to take it any more. My 86-year-old father still writes to the federal courts, the governor, and, occasionally, when we can't intercept his letters, to the president. He continues in his own futile way to try to restore the damage to his self-esteem caused by his bipolar behavior and the reaction of the "bipolar" justice system to it.

CNS patients don't have to lose their will to biological processes that take over their brains. They don't have to exhibit behavior that subjects them to human processing factories where, like products, they are sorted, sent down conveyer belts, then disposed of in various jails, hospitals, boarding homes, and intermediate care facilities throughout their troubled lives. They do not have to become the "red monkeys" of the American Gulag. If they stay the course and don't give up, they can transform their precipice dread into the dizziness of freedom. We did it, and, if we need to, we will do it again.

Hearing the music

The fearfully and wonderfully made human brain is like a symphonic orchestra — not the best analogy, but an apt one. Perhaps a thousand-member symphony would be a better representation of the actual workings of the human brain, though even that falls far short.

In any symphony, a flawed performance by the conductor or one or more orchestra members is likely to result in anything from a mangled but still-recognizable piece of music to utter cacophony. When our brains are broken, they distort our perception of God's creation — indeed, even our perceptions of God, others, and ourselves. When the conductor inspires the orchestra players to perform their best, they create beautiful music. When all the parts of our brains are synergistically working properly, our brains have a fantastic capacity to accurately perceive and interact with the environment around us, as well as to marvel in wonder at that which we can't understand. When our brains are functioning well we can hear the music that music only talks about.

An adequate supply of nutrients to the brain does not necessarily ensure that all the "players" will perform as directed, but it is one essential ingredient without which brain "cacophony" is sure to result for those with a genetic predisposition to bipolar syndrome. Whether that cacophony manifests as mildly irritating "brain fog" or something as devastating as bipolar syndrome is a consequence of the interaction of each genetically unique person with his or her unique environment. Even though we still have a long way to go, the technology already exists for better assessments and more effective interventions.

In the meantime, we will enjoy this rest stop from our four-generational bipolar odyssey before we continue on our way. We will try to keep an open mind and learn whatever we can about innovative approaches to biological conditions that cause or contribute to bipolar syndrome. While we search for more satisfactory answers to increasingly complex questions we will keep trying to assure that Chris takes enough Synergy supplements, immune enhancing supplements, and omega-3 fatty acids to remain stable. If we can get him to stay on his program until we can find the professional expertise to prioritize and attack his numerous contributing biological conditions, then, based on our experience so far, he will stay on an even keel.

Tony and Barbara still have the original bottle of lithium they bought for their son in 1996. It would be great if we could keep the bottles of lithium, Depakote, Wellbutrin, Neurontin, Paxil, Prozac, Haldol, Zyprexa, and Cogentin unopened too.

January, 2002

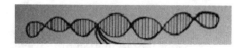

Notes

1. Horowitz, <u>Emerging Viruses: AIDS and Ebola - Nature, Accident or Intentional?</u> Tetrahedron, Inc., Rockport, Mass., 1997, 493.
2. Mosher, Loren R., "Psychiatrist dissolves 35 year association with American Psychiatric Association," December 4, 1998.

http://www.home.att.net/~thesaint/lrm.htm

3. The Burzynski Patient Group Web site, April 16, 2001.
http://www.burzynskipatientgroup.org/

4. Elias, Thomas T., <u>The Burzynski Breakthrough</u>, Lexikos, Nevada City, Calif., 2000, 340-341.

5. Actually, many of the nutrients in the Synergy supplements, such as selenium and others, play a role in helping the body chelate heavy metals. We have not yet measured Chris's mercury and antimony levels to see if this has made a difference, but will in the future.

6. Gant, Charles, <u>ADD and ADHD: Complementary Medicine Solutions</u>, MindMender Publishers, Syracuse, N.Y., 1999, 165.

Epilogue

Life was good. Chris had a part-time job working in a horse stable. He was slowly and carefully putting his computer together. He was increasingly in demand at church, playing the piano and singing solos. He practiced with his band, spent weekends with friends, and was gone a lot of the time, sometimes with his supplements and sometimes without ... more often without. With the help of my editor, I was putting the final touches on the last few chapters of this book. It was easy for Chris, easy for us, to wake up each morning and assume that the complex interplay of biological processes needed to create the daily miracle of normal human consciousness would continue uninterrupted. We had tried to get Chris to take 24 supplements a day as well as to continue with the rest of his regimen. He continued to say that he would only take 16 a day. We had to remind him sometimes to take his supplements, but, in order to encourage him to take responsibility, we did not monitor him on a daily basis.

In February 2002, Chris had a very creative streak. He wrote poems, raps, and short stories. He composed 12 new songs, one of which, an outstanding praise song entitled "Turn Me Around Again," would prove, in retrospect, all too prophetic. One day in mid-February, while driving home from church, he told me how good it felt to have so many activities to look forward to, and that he enjoyed being able to make decisions and act on them rather than feeling paralyzed by his own thinking processes. This normally would have made my heart feel good, but earlier that month, we had bought a family membership in a local fitness center. After Chris and I started working out three to four times a week, I began to notice two things. First, he began demonstrating some hypomanic behavior. He began spending an increasing amount of time at the computer writing short stories and working on a new journal. He was going to bed later, was sleeping irregularly, and was increasingly absentminded about taking his supplements. Second, I began having trouble getting to sleep, a rare occurrence for me, and something I would not have associated with a moderate workout three to four times a week. Since I have friends who sleep soundly after strenuous exercise, I suspected that my paradoxical reaction might stem from my genetic legacy.

As usual, my exhortations for Chris to put more order into his life fell on deaf ears. He had begun pacing around the house as though driven by excessive nervous energy; he told his mom that when he was jogging at the fitness center, he felt like he could run forever. On February 27, I wrote an email to MMI asking if there was a relationship between exercise and hypomania. Here was my query:

As I am finishing up working with an editor on my book, it looks like I will have to write another. There is just too much information for one book.

For example, my son recently became slightly hypomanic after joining and going to a fitness center where he works out pretty hard. Anybody have any experience with exercise and mania? Any good references? I know that long-distance runners sometimes get "punch drunk" from the endorphins they generate, and that they have been known to run into things because of impaired consciousness. I can see how increased metabolic demands, along with leaky gut, could strain a body already minimally dealing with exorphins from undigested gluten and casein, food sensitivities, and various toxins. Could exercise stir up Bb? I was under the impression that exercise and the generation of heat made the terrain for Bb more inhospitable.

He has been on the Synergy supplements for 5 months now and has been doing fine with no meds. So far, this minimal bout is under control, but it does raise more questions, and, for me, brings up the perennial "precipice- dread."

I received a response from Dr. Kinderlehrer, a Lyme-literate physician and MMI member with a background in nutrition and environmental medicine, who had himself suffered from Lyme. Here is his response, quoted with his permission.

Exercise, if vigorous enough, leads to lactic acid production. [Lactic acid is also a mitogen.] *The relative acidity affects the amount of ionizable calcium and magnesium available, destabilizing nerve endings. People prone to panic attacks often describe exercise as a trigger. This can be prevented to some degree by taking calcium and magnesium before exercise. In addition, Borrelia likes acid environments — this is the rationale behind taking hydroxychloroquine, to raise the pH or relative alkalinity. These factors might have something to do with exercise-induced mania.*

Dan Kinderlehrer, M.D.

Dr. Kinderlehrer was suggesting that Chris's exercising may have provided a fertile environment for *Borrelia burgdorferi*. In a subsequent message, Dr. Kinderlehrer told me that he had treated Lyme patients with a combination of Biaxin, an antibiotic, as well as hydroxychloroquine.

Meanwhile, I found a study by Starkie and others demonstrating that significant exercise led to a 21 +/- 4-fold increase in IL-6 mRNA expression(P<.01).[1] IL-6 is the same proinflammatory cytokine implicated in several studies on depression, alcoholism, and anorexia discussed in Chapter 19. I also saw an MMI post referring to a study in which IL-6 was implicated in Alzheimer's disease.

During the last week in February, I showed the message to Chris and suggested that we shouldn't go back to the fitness center until we learn some more about what Dr. Kinderlehrer had written. Given Chris's blind spot when it came to things biological, I was not surprised when he made a discounting, sarcastic remark. I couldn't see taking the car keys, and he would have gone without me regardless, so I went along. At the fitness center, he asked for paper from the office staff so he could write down the raps that came to him while working out.

On March first and second, a Friday and Saturday, Chris played piano at a weekend church retreat where the participants fasted for 24 hours. We made sure he didn't fast. As the weekend ended, he ate some soup made with hydrolyzed vegetable protein, an excitotoxin. The next day, there was a dramatic change. He began talking about a conversion experience he'd undergone during the retreat. On Sunday morning, March 3, Gayle and I became concerned when we observed subtle signs of hypomania in public. In church he smiled a lot and skipped steps while walking up to the piano. Not a problem for most families; for us, a problem.

Concerned, I accompanied Chris to his job at the stable later that afternoon. He acted in a grandiose manner with his employers, telling them that he would bring others to the stable and would sell their horses on the Internet, making them thousands of dollars. Several days later, they terminated his employment.

That evening, after we returned from the stable, Chris started calling friends near and far to tell them about his conversion experience at the retreat. His message was intrusive; he shouted on the phone, as if he couldn't contain his excitement. We could hear the pounding of his feet whenever he walked in the house.

That night we stopped all gluten and casein and put Chris on 600 mg lithium, 1,000 mg Depakote, 10 mg Zyprexa, and 1 mg Cogentin. We insisted he take 32 pills of the supplements daily, along with four 1,000 mg omega-3 fatty acid tablets, lipoic acid, Co Q10, and pycnogenol, an antioxidant. By this time, Chris had developed a nonproductive cough that I suspected was due to allergies from working around the hay; over the next several days, I came down with a bad case of hay fever myself. Thinking that his emerging mania might be related to seasonal allergies, I also gave him some Cold-Eeze, as there is some evidence that it may reduce cytokine levels.[2]

Later that night, Chris tried to buy a plane ticket online so he could fly to Houston to defend Andrea Yates and then sing to her in jail. The next day, he paid $39 on the Internet to find the Yates's address and the phone numbers of her neighbors. He mailed a musical cassette tape our family had recorded for our own enjoyment some months before to the Yates family.

On Monday, March 4, he decided not to take any medications, only supplements. The Holy Spirit would take care of him. We talked with Tony, who took time from filming a Discovery Channel special on the supplements and he agreed to send a sample of their latest powder that was flavor enhanced and had even smaller particles than the previous one he had given us. (We never received it as Truehope had problems with their supplier.) Meanwhile, I had to crush the medicines and put them in the Truehope supplements, not a good way to ensure exactly the right amounts. That night he was singing at the top of his voice at two in the morning. On Wednesday, March 6, he was up early in the morning, dancing around the house. He had his bag packed to fly to Houston, where he still planned to sing to Mrs. Yates as she awaited her trial verdict. Chris refused his medications again, but a phone call with a friend convinced him to take them after all. On Thursday, he telephoned some neighbors of Andrea Yates. That night he slept soundly, only to bound up the stairs early the next morning. He agreed to provide a urine sample to Dr. Cade, so that he could check for polypeptiduria. His urine pH was an acidic 6. By March 8, he was still manic, but not as exuberant. He continued sleeping through the night.

By March 11, he was much calmer, but still perceiving the world in black and white terms. He had been sleeping well for five nights. After taking a nap, he asked what day it was and expressed surprise on learning that it was March already. He asked questions about the winter Olympics, which had long since been over. He was like Rip Van Winkle waking up from a long sleep, surprised to discover a different world.

At this point, we breathed a sigh of relief. In just over a week, by using the medications and supplements, we had stopped Chris's mania. Hospitalization would not be necessary. For the next few weeks, he did very well, with no indications of mania or depression. He walked normally without the pounding gait that had previously reverberated throughout the house. There were no more vocal cord-breaking songs at 2 a.m. He was sleeping at night. He still phoned his friends a lot, and the focus of those calls inevitably shifted to him and his religious experiences, but he was not overemotional. One day I heard him talking on the phone to a friend, saying it might have been his mania rather than God telling him to contact Andrea Yates. I saw that as a good sign.

We were so relieved and emotionally exhausted that we let up on Chris, who, throughout the ordeal, had required continual prompting by us for him to stay on the treatment plan. Now he started to eat gluten and casein again. He refused the omega-3 fatty acids and additional immune-enhancing supplements. He began forgetting to take his Truehope supplements, even though we reminded him to do so. He took his medications regularly, but only because I gave them to him myself.

On April 4, Chris helped our neighbors put a new roof on their house. The neighbor in charge of the project was a hard-of-hearing perfectionist who had a tendency to yell a lot. During the day, Chris was in an environment of mold (the reason for the roof replacement), pollen, and sawdust. These are common mitogens that provoke lymphocyte proliferation. The night after his first day of working on the roof, he was busy at his computer when I brought his medications in to him. I noticed he was writing about being bullied as a child. We talked about his day and he said could handle the yelling because he knew the neighbor was hard of hearing. I did not watch him take the pills. I had been slowly reduced his medications, but after the events of the next day I tried to increase them again.[3]

The next morning found him at the computer. He hadn't slept, nor had he taken his medications or supplements. He skipped breakfast and rushed to the neighbor's to resume working on the roof ... only to come back within five minutes for his shoes, which he'd neglected to put on in his haste. By now, any attempt to keep him from working on the roof, to get him to take his supplements, or even to eat his breakfast was doomed to failure.

The next day, after his second night of not sleeping — again, because he wouldn't take his medications — he started calling friends and telling them that he was the prophet Elijah. When Gayle and I tried to curtail his calls, he yelled at us at the top of his lungs, insisting that he was totally in control. He was angry with us for trying to get him to take his meds and supplements and otherwise trying to restrict him. In retrospect, I should have left him on the higher dosages for a substantially longer period of time.

On Sunday night, April 7, Chris refused again to take either supplements or medications. He told us that God was all he needed, threw his pills on the floor, and said he wanted to go to the hospital where he could launch some sort of "big" movement that would bring the TV and newspaper reporters in droves. We had heard that before. That evening he talked to a crisis worker on the phone, calmly at first, but then, when he didn't get his promised admission, tearfully, and with a great deal of pathos. I took him to a local hospital Emergency Room, where I hoped a crisis worker could get him to take his medicines. To my surprise and relief, the crisis worker did what no one else had been able to do: convince Chris to take his medications. But on the drive home, Chris informed me that he was only going to take them for one night.

The therapist part of me tried to make sense out of the senseless. Maybe for Chris, the choice between being a small, vulnerable, separated "self" and a transcendent being moving toward and joining with the light of God was a no-brainer. From my perspective, like an ill-fated moth, he was again obsessively drawing close to the incandescent light that had already burned him. There had been a moment, I believed, when he consciously chose to stop taking his medications. I believed that he had known perfectly well what the result would be. I tried to imagine what incentive there could have been for him to choose to reenter the psychotic realm. Perhaps it was an oceanic feeling of oneness with others — indeed, with God Himself. Even if Chris's still-incapacitated right brain were to be restored to health, the fear of losing his spiritual foundation could keep him from revisiting the world of reason and logic. Chris wasn't the first to express such fears. Keats once wrote the following in response to Newton's calculations of the orbits of the "heavenly" bodies.

> [The natural sciences] will clip an Angel's wings,
> Conquer all mysteries by rule and line,
> Empty the haunted air, and gnomed mine,
> Unweave a Rainbow. [4]

Perhaps Chris's plunge into insanity was his response to an equation where existence was equal to matter plus time plus chance: the "What is your foundation?" question addressed prior to a previous psychotic episode. He didn't want to unweave the rainbow of his new religious certitudes.

Perhaps he was responding to his mother's and my concerns that since he wasn't sticking to the Truehope/omega-3 fatty acid/additional supplement program, quite possibly his next glass of milk, his next cup of soup, his next glutamate saturated potato chip, — or even a few sticks of sugarless gum — contained just enough high octane glutamate fuel to generate his next manic episode. Based on my research, these fears were not unfounded. Even something as apparently innocuous as glutamate-containing aspartame provoked mania and seizures in a person with no psychiatric history who switched from sugar to aspartame in an attempt to lose weight.[5] However, we had no way to quantify or prioritize the dangers that lurked in his environment, his body, and the refrigerator and cupboards. We already worried about his not taking enough supplements. But what should we worry about the most, mitogens from the horse stable, mold and pollen from working on the roof, antigens from Lyme, or excitotoxins from his diet? Before this episode had started I had located a doctor in San Francisco who I thought could help us prioritize these issues, but Chris had declined to see him. Now, as we found ourselves increasingly taking the responsibility to keep him from becoming manic, Chris became more oppositional.

On the other hand, maybe I was engaging in grand but useless speculations, attributing to him motives and feelings to try to make sense out of nonsensical behavior. Maybe he was suffering from anosognosia, the ignorance of the presence of a disease. Maybe, like the stroke patients discussed in Chapter 15, Chris simply had an impaired brain that was unable to be aware of and maintain itself properly. Maybe my attributional "hunches" were simply a futile attempt to put meaning into what were clearly irrational, inexplicable behaviors reflective of his brain impairment.

By April 8, Chris had gone three days with no sleep and no medications (with the exception of the medications he took as the result of the ER visit described above) and no supplements. That day, Chris was playing ball with two neighbor boys, ages 7 and 9. When the boys threw the ball on the roof of our house, Chris tried to get them to climb up onto the roof from a railing on our front porch. I had been watching. The boys looked scared. I told the boys that they didn't have to do what Chris was asking them to do. Chris, meanwhile, leapt from the railing to the roof and pulled himself up, seemingly without any effort. Then, having thrown the ball back to the boys, he jumped down from the roof, a distance of about ten feet, and called me "Satan." As Chris and the boys walked back to the neighbor's house to resume their game, I went inside and called their mother to tell her that it was not safe for them to be with Chris because of his impaired judgment. I knew that if I had tried to separate them, he would have escalated more. Meanwhile, the boys' father, Frank, who had heard the yelling while working on the neighbor's roof, came out and told Chris to stay away from his boys. Chris picked up a baseball bat that had been on the lawn and said to Frank, "I'll bet you are really scared now." Frank told him to go home and take his meds. Chris came in and told me that Frank was Satan.

Clearly, my son was now a danger to others and to himself. Since he would not take his medications, I took him to Behavioral Health. On the way, he screamed out religious warnings about the terrible fate God had in mind for the sinful citizens of Lake Wildwood. They had ignored God for too long: now it was payback time.

Had Chris's judgment and common sense become permanent casualties of the brain impairment inflicted by neuro-Lyme, previous psychotic experiences, or brain hypertrophy from psychotropic medications? Had his failure to grasp the biological basis of his illness left him increasingly vulnerable to its return? Even when Chris was "well," the issues confronting him were black and white. As far as Chris was concerned, he either had a spiritual malady from wrestling with God, or there were biological causes for his illness. If the former, then he had been chosen, like the prophets of old. If the latter, then God, the source of his personal meaning and significance, was, or might as well be, dead. Chris couldn't see that his illness could have a biological basis without that fact undercutting the existence of God or his ability to have a relationship with God. My attempts to get him to recognize this had only driven a wedge between us. Even as far back as my ill-fated attempts to reach him in a written dialogue, Chris had found my beliefs wanting. Throughout the odyssey, our ability to communicate was hampered by his conviction that my research was somehow a repudiation of his world views, views which had literally been all over the emotional and theological map. His thinking processes were very different from mine. In reality, Chris's problem was simple to state, though hard to understand and even more difficult to fix. His brain was still broken. His black and white thinking was a constant symptom of a brain that was not functioning properly, even when he was free of the so-called positive symptoms of bipolar disorder.

Chris was admitted again to Live Oaks, where they gave him up to 30 mg of Zyprexa a day only to find that his thinking remained psychotic and his speech became even more pressured. Then they treated him with a drug called Clozaril, the indications for which are primarily for schizophrenic patients for whom no other medication has worked. His doctor gave him a new diagnosis, schizoaffective disorder, in my opinion, to justify the use of a drug for which he was a known advocate in the professional community. According to one of the nurses, he gave seminars on Clozaril to professionals around the state. This doctor also ignored Chris's Lyme disease which I believed was continuing to play a role in progressive damage to his brain and judgment, saying that since the drugs treat the symptoms, that was all that was needed. I didn't even try to explain any other conditions Chris had.

The previous summer, when I had shared with Tony our compliance problems with Chris, he had told me about two friends of his, Bill and Harvey, who went hunting one cloudy fall day. During the day, they got separated in a sudden snowstorm that left almost three feet of snow on the ground. By 5 p.m., after searching for hours, Bill finally found Harvey. His friend was calmly sitting in a snow bank. Bill tried to rouse him for the trek back to the car, but Harvey told Bill to go on by himself. He would hike out the next day. Bill could tell that Harvey, whose clothes were wet, was suffering from hypothermia, which has profound effects on judgment. He explained to him that if they didn't get back to the car before sunset, they would both be dead before morning. Harvey refused to budge. Bill knew that he couldn't carry his friend all the way to the car. He also knew that further argument would be futile, a waste of precious time. So he grabbed the nearest stick and gave Harvey a good thwack. Needless to say, that got his attention. Bill then informed him that he was going to get up and walk back to the car even if he had to beat him with the stick every step of the way. He gave him a few more solid thwacks to show he meant it. It wasn't long before Harvey stood up and started trudging through the snow. They reached the car in time and survived.

Chris's mental confusion, his religious preoccupations, and his inability/unwillingness to look squarely at the facts are the same as Harvey sitting there in the snow. His brain was not functioning well enough, even when he was "well," to make the choices he needed to make in order to stay healthy. We can't hit our 26-year-old son with a stick to make him take his supplements and or medications, or to change his dietary habits, but we can do everything possible to make sure that he gets the care he needs.

I made some phone calls attempting to get him admitted into a long-term clinical trial for neuro-Lyme patients currently underway at Columbia University in New York. I set up a future phone consultation with Dr. Rogers, the physician specializing in environmental medicine as it pertains to psychiatric illnesses. I called the Amen Clinic to see about getting a SPECT. I also wanted to get the EEG and MRI. And I had not ruled out a physician specializing in stealth treatment. We would have to take it one day at a time, using whatever sticks we could find to motivate Chris to turn away from that hot incandescent light bulb and toward health.

I began this book on an optimistic note. There are still grounds for optimism. There is a significant and growing body of research demonstrating that nutrients can restore broken brains and that biological conditions which cause behaviors currently classified as mental disorders can be identified and treated. The future is on Chris's side. But the present is not.

After Chris recovered from his acute psychosis, the public guardian, at the request of Behavioral Health Services, put Chris into an intermediate care facility in preparation for their plans to place him under a conservatorship for a year. Maybe they thought Chris needed a good thwacking, too. Seems they wanted to put him into the American Gulag, having concluded that the only problem he had was bipolar disorder. He remained on Haldol and Clozaril, two medications known to reduce NAA in the frontal cortex.[5] By the first of May, Chris, no longer psychotic, tearfully asked officials from the county to let him return home. He acknowledged he had gotten into a power struggle with his parents and said he would not do it again. A court fight loomed. The county officials evidenced no interest in the diagnostic work done outside their narrow world. They didn't believe he had Lyme, and even if he did, it would not make any difference. Maybe they believed that our desire to keep Chris out of the Gulag by finding treatment for his brain disorder made us unfit to care for him. Maybe they think he suffered from a Clozaril deficiency.

We have come full circle, starting with my father's misadventures and his subsequent incarceration in the Gulag, exploring and successfully using alternative understandings and treatments, and ending with yet another hospitalization of my son and attempts by Nevada County Behavioral Health Service to place him under a conservatorship. How ironic that this hospitalization should come on the heels of our first success in treating him at home for a level of mania that was reaching psychotic proportions. If the county were to succeed, we would have no more say in his care. There would be no further exploration into the causes of his illnesses. He would not get the medical care we have been seeking for him. No one would look at his brain, the very organ which is causing him to have these problems.

Chris's insight is impaired because his brain is still broken. Sufficient nutrients restore brain functioning by preventing mania and depression. They alleviate the impact of Lyme disease, stealth virus, and any of a number of already diagnosed conditions he has. They do not heal the brains of these maladies. If the county succeeds in putting him under their care, not only will they relegate him to the American Gulag, but they will also remove his remaining insight just as effectively as the citizens of the Valley of the Blind removed the sight of the hapless mountain climbers. My son would live out his days in the American Gulag, clutching the robes of his keepers who, as they click their way down the narrow paths, will call out "medications" once, twice, or perhaps three times a day.

Chris did not need to be transformed into a red monkey and placed in the American Gulag. It was time to start looking at his brain, something that should have been done after his first episode. For cardiac patients, a physician needs to know as much as possible about the patient's heart if the patient is going to be competently treated. How much more should doctors who purport to treat the broken human brain find out about the specific organ they are attempting to treat? To put it another way, how long would a cardiologist remain in practice if he hospitalized a patient seven times for heart problems and never once actually looked at his patient's heart or obtained any direct information about it?

Of all the contributing biological conditions we have identified with Chris, not one was identified by his treating psychiatrist. Not one has been acknowledged or treated throughout seven hospitalizations. His keepers had their DSM-IV Bible to give them the only truth they needed.

This has been a difficult journey. It remains so. Having to deal with Chris's illnesses is difficult enough ... but now having to deal with my former employers makes it that much harder.

Because of the chronic nature of Chris's illnesses, his impaired judgment and oppositional behavior, my own flawed attempts to maintain his stability, and the rigidity of the health care system, his biological illnesses were winning once again. Until there is comprehensive assessment and treatment for those whose biologically valid psychological variables are manifested in dysfunctional behavior, I fear there is a chance that my son and thousands of others like him will continue throughout their lives to be sorted on assembly lines which will deposit them into the various cells of the American Gulag.

I will do all I can do to prevent my son and others from this fate. As I wait for some illustrations and final proofing for the book, he is in a locked ward at the American River Behavioral Health Center, a facility in Sacramento to which he was transferred. His driver's license has been taken away. He is unable to act independently. He has no say in his medical care. His life is micromanaged by his keepers. He feels desolate and helpless.

I believe that the physicians of the future, hopefully sooner rather than later, will examine their patients instead of their DSMs. I do not expect this to happen to Chris at American River Behavioral Health Center. Right now, the system has all the power. The patient and his family have none, except whatever power comes from knowledge. While the present does not favor Chris, or the thousands like him who, in long lines daily pace down antiseptically clean halls in their twilight world, the future will offer more, if he can hold on long enough. In the meantime, Chris has been forced against his will, as was his grandfather, into the American Gulag, a place where he too, can be drugged and warehoused, not for the temporary relief of his symptoms, but for a lifetime. The longer he is there, the more completely his remaining sparks of energy and light will be gradually extinguished by the incessant actions of the daily chemical lobotomy he is forced to endure and the daily reassurance of his keepers that they know what is best for him.

Only when families and patients refuse to accept the status quo, when they demand assessment and treatment of the causes of these illnesses, will there be a chance that those with broken brains will receive definitive treatment for the biological causes of their symptoms. The promise of life, liberty, and the pursuit of happiness has been denied to certain groups for many years now, not the least of which have been the "mentally ill." It is time for a change.

The odyssey isn't over, by any means. There continue to be important challenges and discoveries, some of which will be discussed in <u>TGTBT, Volume II</u> ... that is, if I don't decide to call it <u>The Gulag Strikes Back</u>. I continue to have confidence in the Synergy supplements and remain firmly convinced that definitive differential diagnoses of biologically valid symptoms of bipolar syndrome and other CNS-disordered conditions are urgently needed, and not just in Nevada County.

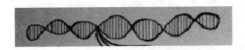

Notes

1. Starkie, R., Arkinstall, M., Koukoulas, I., Hawley, J., Febbraio, M., "Carbohydrate ingestion attenuates the increase in plasma interleukin-6, but not skeletal muscle interleukin-6 mRNA, during exercise in humans," *Journal of Physiology - London then Cambridge*, 533(Pt-2):585-591, 2001.

2. This study showed reductions in a measure of soluble interleukin-1 receptor antagonist, but it was not significant.

Prasad, A.S., Fitzgerald, J.T., Bao, B.F., Beck, W.J., Chandrasekar, P.H., "Duration of symptoms and plasma cytokine levels in patients with the common cold treated with zinc acetate, a randomized, double-blind, placebo-controlled trial," *Annals of Internal Medicine,* 133:245-252, 2000.

3. On March 12, since Chris was sleeping and seemed to be back to his old self, I lowered his Zyprexa to 7.5 mg and Depakote to 750 mg. He continued doing well, so on March 19 I dropped the dosage again, to 5 mg Zyprexa, 500 mg Depakote, and 300 mg lithium. On April 1, I lowered the Zyprexa to 2.5 mg, which I tried to raise to 5 mg on April 5, the day after he said he forgot to take his meds. Everything changed after he started working on the roof of the house. Situational factors could have included the stress of working and following orders for a day, the environmental stresses of pollen and mold, as well as the reduction of one or more medications.

With the perspective of hindsight it is easier to see where a more aggressive intervention could have made a difference, as, for example, not allowing Chris to drive the car to the fitness center, maintaining him on higher amounts of medications longer, insisting he stay with the regimen that had worked. Unfortunately, when Chris "appears" to be fine, it is hard for Gayle and I to be the stern task masters. It is hard to tell a 26 year old what to do when he appears to be in charge of his facilities. When he isn't, it is too late. The emotional exhaustion from dealing with my father's ongoing medical crises also played a role in my reduced vigilance as well.

With all of the "state" biological correlates that accompany mania, such as AP proteins; IL-2R; lymphocyte proliferation; an increase in protein kinase C and other protein kinases, glutamate, excitatory G proteins etc., one would think that a test could be developed that could predict the risk of having an episode. If we had "ammunition" to suggest he was close to going over the edge, we could use that to motivate compliance with the regimen.

4. Keats, John, "Lamia," lines 234-237, <u>The Poetical Works of John Keats</u> (Cambridge Edition), rev. P.D. Sheats, Boston: Houghton Mifflin, 1975, 156.
5. Walton, R.G., "Seizure and mania after high intake of aspartame," *Psychosomanics,* 1986: 27:218-20
6. Bustillo, J.R., Lauriello, J., Rowland, L.M., Jung, R.E., Petropoulos, H., Hart, B.L., Blanchard, S.J., Keith, SJ., Brooks, W.M., "Effects of chronic haloperidol and clozapine treatments on frontal and caudate neurocemistry in schizophrenia," *Psychiatry Research*, 107(3):135-149, 2001.

Appendix 1 - Diagnostic Hypotheses/Resources

Bipolar as well as other CNS disorders are associated with and caused by a number of biological anomalies. Most likely, these are genetic in origin and occur from the interaction of genes and environment. A few of the brain anomalies associated with bipolar symptoms include low GFAP, high protein kinase C, high G proteins, excessive VMAT2, low ubiquinone cytochrome c reductase core protein 1, low GABA among a 40% subset of bipolar patients and low NAA. Some of these anomalies, as, for example, low NAA may be a result of treatment or exacerbated by it. These CNS disorders are also associated with and caused by environmental factors. With the left brain hope that these hypotheses, or, risk factors, can guide effective treatment decisions and the right brain caveat that correlation does not prove causation and that those who know far more than I rightly claim to know a lot less about the exact biochemical abnormalities that have yet to be identified, the following hypotheses represent the "nurture" side of the nature/nurture debate:

1. Carbohydrate Excess

Resource: I found some testimonials of bipolar patients praising a low carbohydrate diet, but no sites claiming effectiveness of such a diet for bipolar symptoms. I found several sites supporting low carbohydrate, high protein diets such as the Atkins, paleolithic, and ketogenic diets for the general public, one of which is listed below.
Phone: None
URL: http://mercola.com/article/Diet/carbohydrates/paloelithic_diet.htm
Dx Test: None
Dx Cost: None
Tx: Low carbohydrate diet
Tx Cost: Minimal
Hypothesis: Carbohydrates destabilize glucose levels. Low energy supplies contribute to hyperpotentiation of neurons such as is found in bipolar disorder.
Evidence: The brain uses 25% of the glucose available to the body. Bipolar patients have higher rates of diabetes than the general population. Their brains do not regulate glucose metabolism well. During a manic episode, glucose burns too rapidly in parts of the brain while the opposite occurs during depression. Russian scientists have found that fasting alone has been curative for mania and schizophrenia.[1]

During Chris's psychotic episodes, he almost always experienced olfactory hallucinations and behaved in ways consistent with what some characterize as temporal lobe epilepsy. Symptoms of this disorder include olfactory hallucinations, self-destructive and irrational behavior, hypergraphia (excessive writing) and hyper-religiosity.

Since seizure medications are often effective with bipolar symptoms, it is only logical to infer that if there were such a thing as an anti-seizure diet, such a diet might prove similarly effective. There is such a diet, the ketogenic diet developed at Johns Hopkin's Medical Center before the advent of seizure medications. For some seizure patients it is more effective than medications. It consists of high protein, fats, and low carbohydrates.

When Chris was hospitalized for depression and agitation, he did not want to eat. Perhaps his body was telling him that it needed a rest from the carbohydrates he had been ingesting. Rather than viewing such "fasting" as a sign of pathology, perhaps it should be viewed as an attempt by the body to heal itself. Note that there are no tests or resources for this hypothesis. There is no money to be made from this one. Maybe the old adage is correct and the best things in life are free.

Comments: Dr. Amen recommends a high protein, low carbohydrate diet for individuals with prefrontal cortex and temporal lobe problems, or those with cognitive difficulties and mood swings. Proponents of the paleolithic diet point out that historically, thousands of generations evolved on a hunter-gatherer diet that was free of grains, processed foods and sugars while only 500-1000 generations evolved and adapted to an agricultural diet of corn, wheat, and, in this century, processed foods.

2. Chemical Sensitivities

Resource: Doctor's Data
Phone: (800) 323-2783
URL: http://www.doctorsdata.com
Dx Test: Chemical Sensitivity Blood Test
Dx Cost: $500
Tx: Chemical Desensitization
Tx Cost: $840

Hypothesis: Environmental insults provoke chronic activation of the body's defenses, increasing cytokines and inflammation.

Evidence: A subset of Gulf War Syndrome patients had diminished executive functioning and low NAA, as do patients diagnosed with bipolar disorder. Among other things, they had been exposed to organophosphates. Chris's test results showed strong reactions to aldrin and endrin and moderate reactions to xylene, carbon tetrachloride, and polysorbate 60, suggesting chemical sensitivities. For the body to detoxify various pesticides and chemicals, nutrients are required. The detoxification process results in depletion of vital precursors of brain chemicals.

Comments: Aldrin/Endrin desensitization sets cost $70 per treatment at New Century Wellness Center. We did not pursue this, but gave Chris supplements which included vitamin C, selenium, and other vitamin and minerals known to detoxify the body.

3. Childhood Vaccinations
Resource: New Century Wellness Center
Phone: (775) 826-9500
URL: http://www.lonezone.com/2000/catalog/i/cwc01.html
Dx Test: Vaccination Panel
Dx Cost: $450
Tx: Anti DPT toxoid, Anti MMR toxoid, etc.
Tx Cost: unknown
Hypothesis: Vaccine antigens provoke cytokine production and tissue inflammation. Thiomersal in vaccines is suspect.
Evidence: Dr. Tang claims to have helped many patients with bipolar disorder by reducing their antitoxoid levels. Some studies show correlation between vaccination and the onset of autism while others don't. There is more research on a vaccine-autism connection than a bipolar connection, but similarities between the two conditions suggest that vaccinations may play a role in the development of bipolar syndrome as well.
Comments: Chris's DPT antitoxoid, the only test we had done, was 10 times normal. The panel contains tests for DPT, bartonella, pertussis, tetanus, mumps, rubeola, rubella, enterovirus, and polio. We opted to focus on leads that appeared more compelling and had more research to support them.

4. Food Sensitivities and excitotoxins
Resource: Great Smokies Diagnostic Laboratories
Phone: (800) 522-4762
URL: http://www.gsdl.com
Dx Test: Food Antibody Assessment (IgG and IgE)
Dx Cost: $160
Tx: Avoidance of offending foods, rotation diet, and zinc. Various enzymes and digestive aids may improve digestion and reduce food sensitivities. Foods such as MSG, aspartame, hydrolyzed protein are to be avoided.
Tx Cost: unknown
Hypothesis: Some foods provoke excessive defensive responses, contributing to cytokine proliferation. Glutamate-containing foods can overwhelm impaired glial cells lacking in GFAP, causing excitation and cell apoptosis.
Evidence: Signal transduction is viewed as one of the primary methods of causing mania, seizures, neurological illnesses. Bipolar patients have more allergies and food sensitivities. Delayed response to sensitive foods creates an overall heightened state of immunity in the body, resulting in activation of cytokines and utilization of brain chemical precursors for detoxification rather than supplying the brain with needed nutrients. Glutamate regulation is en-

ergy-intensive. Excessive unregulated glutamate stimulates neurons to death.
Comments: Tony Stephan said that zinc in the supplements helped some users to overcome certain food allergies or sensitivities. For example, one patient taking Synergy supplements was able to eat oranges without pain. There are various products to reduce food allergies, but we did not explore this, viewing the food sensitivities in the context of poor digestion and already existing chronic immune activation. Digestive enzymes and an alkaline diet are presumed to counter some of these effects, though this is an area that requires due diligence by the consumer.

5. Gluten, Casein, Polysaccarides, Disaccarides

Resources: Dr. Robert Cade, Elain Gottshall, M.S.
Phone: 352-392-8952 (Dr. Cade)
URL: http://www.paleodiet.com/autism/cadelet.txt
Dx Test: Radio Allergo Sorbent Test (RAST) for blood, High Performance Liquid Chromatography (HPLC) for urine
Dx Cost: RAST $99; HPLC unknown
Tx: Casein and gluten free diet, Specific Carbohydrate Diet
Tx Cost: minimal
Hypothesis: Gluten and casein contribute to an excess of opioid-like peptides that directly correlate with the pathology of autism and schizophrenia. There may be an inverse relationship with mania.
Evidence: Dr. Cade reported in personal correspondence to me that in preliminary studies, low HPLC scores correlate with mania, high scores with depression. These results were counterintuitive for me, as I had speculated that the same mechanisms by which high gluten and casein contributed to seizure disorder might contribute toward bipolar disorder symptoms, specifically mania. Dr. Cade did find that exorphins are consistently elevated in patients with epilepsy and that both the frequency and severity of seizures decrease as the HPLC scores become normal.

Chris's score on the Radio Allergo Sorbent Test (RAST) for casein was 10,649. Average is 100. For gluten, it was 2,732. Average is 100. Chris had exceptionally low polypeptide levels, according to Malcolm Privette, associate of Dr. Cade. These low levels were consistent with Dr. Cade's preliminary findings that bipolar patients have low scores during mania, high scores during depression. Therefore, I suspect that the counterintuitive findings from Chris and Dr. Cade's manic patients suggest that the antibodies generated for the successful regulation of exorphins (hyperpolypeptiduria) may come at a substantial cost both in terms of energy and the depletion of vital nutrients. If the body did not have to mount such defensive operations, then the corresponding increases in cytokines and antibodies would not occur.

Nutritionist Elain Gottshall reports that avoidance of casein and gluten does not go far enough in allowing the body to heal damaged microvilli in the intestines. This damage comes from gliadin fractions that likely penetrate the intestinal cell membranes, then reach the underlying layer of white blood cells, causing an immune response. In addition, she cites evidence that polysaccarides and disaccarides also damage the microvilli, and that avoidance of gluten and casein is not enough for those suffering from Crohn's disease, ulcerative colitis, celiac disease, and the malabsorption that is found in a large number of psychiatric patients, and which often plays a primary role in their illness. In order to repair the intestine, she recommends the Specific Carbohydrate Diet during which the only allowable sugars are monosaccarides (honey) for at least one year after cessation of symptoms.[2]

Comments: Dr. Richard Kunin, an othomolecular psychiatrist, suspected that Chris had intestinal enteropathy not only from the RAST and IgG results, but also from his physical exam. Both malabsorption and food sensitivities could be clues to leaky gut. According to Anne Bernard, Chris's dark field microscope findings also support this diagnosis. Werback describes a case of exacerbation of bipolar depressive symptoms after a patient ate foods containing wheat.

Schizophrenia rates rise in cultures recently introduced to wheat. Some have claimed that these rates are higher in cultures with less historical exposure to wheat such as Northern Europe vis a vis the Middle East. The presumption is that evolution has selected out those who had psychotic reactions to wheat over time, thereby lowering the incidence rate. I couldn't find any studies corroborating this.

6. Inadequate Immune System

Resource: GNLD
Phone: NA (local distributors)
URL: http://www.gnld.com
Dx Test: Dr. Stricker's specialized T-cell test is one test to measure the functioning of the immune system. There are others as well.
Dx Cost: unknown
Tx: Enhance immune system
Tx Cost: $200 per month

Hypothesis: Responding to antigens requires adequate nutritional resources to mobilize the body's defenses and remove byproducts generated in defensive operations.

Evidence: Activation of the immune system, particularly cytokines, has multiple effects on the CNS. Immune system abnormalities have been found in bipolar disorder. Chris has extremely high antibodies to foods, especially casein and gluten. The immune system has powerful influences on all major CNS disorders. IL-1 and IL-2 are generated by the body's immune system to deal with threats. IL-2 given to humans causes behavioral and cognitive abnormalities found in major depression and schizophrenia. If one accepts the premise that antigens, whether identified or unidentified, require a robust response from the body's immune system, then strengthening the immune system would be a logical treatment option, unless such enhancement facilitates the development of antibodies which can actually harm the organism. While the safest approach would be to prevent exposure to the antigen or mitogen in the first place, facilitating a smart, efficient immune system with the correct nutrients would facilitate a healthy, rather than an out of control immune response. For example, zinc is known to reduce inflammation caused by the immune system in response to antigens. In addition, depletion of nutrients for defensive operations lessens bioavailability of choline and inositol, two of many essential precursors for proper brain functioning.

Comments: Glen Foster recommended the following immune enhancing regimen to help Chris deal with Lyme disease: buffered C, Carotenoid Complex, co-enzyme Q10, lipoic acid, and vitamin E. He told me that the same recommendations would be true for any chronic infection in which the body's immune response needs to be enhanced.

7. Infectious and Immune Mediated Pathophysiology (IIMP)

Resource: None
Phone: None
URLS: www.actionlyme.50megs.com/index.htm
       www.mentalhealthandillness.com
Dx Test: NA
Dx Cost: NA
Tx: Treat the chronic infection(s), boost the immune system
Tx Cost: Unknown

Hypothesis: Chronic known and unknown infections, alone or in combination, provoke the body's defensive operations, increasing cytokines and creating brain inflammation, vasculitis, direct cell injury, inflammation, toxins, autoimmune reactions, and excitotoxicity.

Evidence: Known conditions associated with bipolar syndrome include *Borna* virus, toxoplasmosis, *Bartonella, Borrelia burgdorferi,* babiosis, and stealth viruses. Mitogens are known to provoke a cascade of signaling molecules such as protein kinase C which is targeted by lithium to reduce mania.

Comments: Presumably, cytokine levels would be one measure of such cytokine mediated illnesses. The concept of IIMP provides a broad class for illnesses yet allows for specificity of symptom expression. Instead of imposing a label like "bipolar disorder," for example, a physician might label the illness as "Infectious and Immune-Mediated Pathophysiology, subtype Neuroborreliosis (IIMP-nb), manifested by bipolar syndrome." The advantage of IIMP is that the illness would be conceptualized as a CNS disorder with psychiatric manifestations, not as a psychiatric disorder per se. That disorder would then be treated. This concept has not been articulated, let alone accepted by mainstream psychiatry or medicine. However, evidence suggesting immune dysfunction in schizophrenia continues to accumulate. Dr. Bransfield posted a message on MMI of a study in which celecoxib (Celebrex), an anti inflammatory drug was more effective as an add-on therapy for treating schizophrenia than Risperidol alone.

8. Mercury, other heavy metals

Resource: Great Smokies Diagnostic Laboratories
Phone: Patients are not encouraged to call. Need referral from physician who can access the facility.
URL:http://www.gsld.com
Dx Test: In addition to hair analysis, there are the Urine Toxic Element Test ($100) and the Chemical Sensitivity Blood Test ($500).
Dx Cost: $150
TX: Chelation with DMSA, DSMA
TX Cost: unknown
Hypothesis: Mercury binds to sulphur-bearing proteins and has been associated with bipolar disorder, other psychiatric illnesses.
Evidence: Sources of mercury can include immunizations, dental fillings, fish, water, and air. Vaccines provoke cytokine release. According to Dr. Fudenberg, immunizations have been shown to reduce production of liver enzymes, phosphosulfotransferase and the cytochrome p450 family, impairing digestion, detoxification, and depriving the brain of needed precursors to first and second messengers. Mercury impairs the ability to digest gluten and casein, leading to proliferation of exorphans. It also results in antibodies to brain proteins such as tubulin, present in almost all cells, including neurons.

There is general agreement in the scientific community that thiomersal should not be in vaccines. It is still present, though it is scheduled to be removed — eventually. In 2002, a class-action lawsuit was initiated based on previously secret, unpublished CDC data reporting a definite relationship between vaccinations and autism.
Comments: Analysis of Chris's hair showed both mercury and antimony contamination, but the Urine Toxic Element Test by Doctor's Data did not confirm either. For heavy metals, hair analysis is better than blood. A recent article in *JAMA* noted inconsistency in hair-analysis results. However, differences between blood, hair, and urine can be explained by the type of mercury compound being tested. Firms such as Great Smokies Diagnostic Laboratories are reputable. Some labs engage in unethical practices in which they promote products based on their alleged findings.

9. Neuro-Lyme disease

Resource: LLMD, IgeneX

Phone: (800) 832-3200

URL: http://www.igenex

Dx Test: Western Blot, C-6 Peptide Elisa (new test by Speciality Labs)

Dx Cost: $155

TX: Daily IV Rocephin IV X 3 months

TX Cost: Worst case scenario, IV treatment, $135 a day

Hypothesis: Chronic Lyme disease manifests through a number of organ systems causing rashes, joint pain, arthritis, and AV heart block; sometimes the sole manifestation can be neuropsychiatric illness.

Evidence: Treatment of schizophrenic and bipolar psychoses with antibiotics has been effective. A group of patients suffering from major mental disorders, including, but not exclusively limited to, bipolar illness, have almost twice the incidence of antibodies to Lyme disease as a control group with no psychiatric diagnoses. Doctors specializing in Lyme disease treatment have noted that an exceptionally large percentage of their patients manifest bipolar symptoms and improve on antibiotics. Chris tested positive for Lyme disease, with 6 bands in his Western Blot. His grandfather, with three positive bands, was suspicious for Lyme disease; five bands are necessary to meet CDC requirements for the diagnosis. False negatives are more prevalent than false positives, but false positives do exist.

Comments: Rocephin is the most effective antibiotic but it often does not kill all spirochetes because of their pleomorphic characteristics. This often is a chronic disease. IgeneX is well spoken of by Lyme patients. However, in 2002, government reviewing authorities reported that IgeneX had poor quality control, prompting some in the Lyme community to suggest conspiracy theories by anti-Lyme professional and insurance interests. Critics say that IgeneX gives doctors and patients the answers they seek. The Lyme community stands by IgeneX, while the CDC and broader medical community continue to harbor concerns. Lyme patients can't get needed treatment because of negative findings. Critics say that patients "shop" for the diagnosis and that treatment itself is dangerous. Stony Brook Labs is being used for the Colombia neuro Lyme study because it is thought to be the most rigorous, and least likely to give false positives. This may be good for research, but not for neuro Lyme patients needing care. According to Dr. Kathy Corbera, Coordinator of the Lyme Disease Research Study, the new Peptide Elisa C-6 test is more accurate than the Western Blot. No test is foolproof.

10. Neurotoxins

Resource: Dr. Ritchie Shoemaker

Phone: (410) 957-1550

URL: http://www.chronicneurotoxins.com/lymedisease.cfm

Dx Test: Visual Contrast Sensitivity Test (VCS)

Dx Cost: online screening $8, in office $30

Hypothesis: Lyme disease, pfiesteria, and chronic fungal syndromes produce neurotoxins that create symptoms by, among other things, stimulating cytokine production. Optic nerve functioning is compromised sufficiently that the VCS can identify patients affected by the neurotoxins. According to Dr. Shoemaker, the Heidelberg Retinal Tomogram Flow Meter provides an assessment of global brain hypoperfusion by providing assessment of the extent of hypoperfusion in the optic nerve.

Evidence: So-called "post-Lyme syndrome" may in fact be a result of neurotoxins that remain even after the *Borrelia burgdorferi* are gone. These neurotoxins can be effectively treated with a toxin-binding drug called cholestyramine, or CSM. This drug filters the offending neurotoxins out of bile in the lower intestine. Dr. Shoemaker claims that the VCS is a better test for confirming the presence of Lyme neurotoxins than any measure of blood or urine. His claim that Lyme makes neurotoxins has been disputed by some, but he reports positive results with his patients.

Comments: The patient takes the VCS online, or a more precise version in an office setting, then arranges treatment through their doctor with Dr. Shoemaker. A more sensitive test to assesses brain hypoperfusion is the Heidelberg Retinal Tomogram Flow Meter. A follow-up unpublished ongoing study at family practice sites in 16 states and four foreign countries, reports a 92-percent improvement rate in more than 400 chronic Lyme patients.

Near the end of his IV treatment, Chris took the VCS online and passed it. According to Dr. Shoemaker, this meant there were no neurotoxins impairing his optic nerve. Critics say that his data has not been published and that there is no evidence of a neurotoxin from Lyme disease or pfiesteria in the peer reviewed literature. Dr. Shoemaker reports successfully treating a patient who first exhibited bipolar symptoms after being exposed to a particular algae.

11. Nutrition Deficiencies

Resource: Truehope
Phone: (888) 878-3467
URL: http://www.truehope.com
Dx Test: bipolar disorder symptoms
Dx Cost: NA
Tx: Vitamin/minerals/amino acid supplements
Tx Cost: $110 per month

Hypothesis: Inadequate supply and/or absorption of needed metabolic precursors predisposes the brain to either acute or sub-acute delirium, which can provoke both mania and depression.

Evidence: To date, the majority of bipolar patients on the Truehope regimen show improvement with either no psychotropic medications at all or substantially less than they had needed prior to taking the supplements. Two studies establish efficacy with adults and youth. Double-blind studies are underway. The literature supports positive effects from specific nutrients, suggesting a synergistic effect when many of these nutrients are taken together. A study published in the December issue of *Journal of Clinical Psychiatry* reports not only significant improvement in patients, but also an effect size of .80, a result rarely obtained in human research.

Comments: There is an initial intake of 32 Synergy pills a day followed by 16 or more a day, depending on needs. There is no research on possible excessive accumulation of particular minerals such as nickel and germanium, both of which can have toxic effects. David Hardy explains that the particular form of nickel and germanium is not harmful in the amounts taken in the supplements. Dr. Tang of New Century claims that "allergies" to supplements will diminish their utility. Tony Stephan has found no negative accumulative effects from any of the substances in the supplements. When Chris took the recommended amount, there were no signs of mania, hypomanic behavior, or depression, whereas he had been hypomanic when taking psychotropic medications. When he cut to 16 a day or less, his symptoms returned. A new powder will hopefully reduce the need to take so many pills a day. Digestive problems should also be addressed if they exist.

12. Omega-3 fatty acid deficiency

Resource: Great Smokies Diagnostic Laboratories
Phone: (775) 826-9500
URL: http://www.gsdl.com/
Dx: Essential and Fatty Acids Analysis (RBC)
Dx Cost: unknown
Tx: omega-3 fatty acids
Tx Cost: $15 per month

Hypothesis: For starters, omega-3 fatty acids reduce cytokines, facilitate circulation, create healthier neurons, and reduce brain inflammation. Omega-3 fatty acids inhibit delta-5 desaturase which is active in converting linoleic acid to arachidonic acid which is then converted to inflammatory compounds associated with depression.

Evidence: Historically, changes in dietary intake from omega-3 fatty acids to omega-6 fatty acids have been associated with greater incidence of major depression. Numerous studies point out the need for fatty acids in the American diet, not only for the brain, but also the heart. A double-blind study at Harvard demonstrated convincing evidence of the efficacy of omega-3 fatty acids in treating bipolar illness. Previously rapid-cycling patients who took them in addition to their regular medication had significantly fewer episodes than the control group. The fatty acids were well-tolerated. Omega-3 fatty acids, like lithium and valproate appear to inhibit receptor-linked G protein signal transduction pathways.

A double-blind placebo-controlled study with 40 severe schizophrenic patients over 12 weeks showed that the addition of omega-3 fatty acids to regular medicines demonstrated a significantly greater reduction of both positive and negative symptoms compared to the placebo group. Dyskinesia scores were also more favorable.[3]

Comments: The purity of the products and concentrations of eicosapentaenoic acid (EPA) and docosahexaenoic acid (DHA) vary widely. Fish oil, as opposed to salmon oil, contains oils from bottom fish that may or may not be as pure as the more expensive salmon oil. Dr. Stoll has a proprietary fish oil called Omega-Brite, which is much more expensive than standard omega-3 tablets. Glenn Foster's company, GNLD, makes a very pure salmon oil. Glenn cites research from Tufts University that the GNLD product exceeds stated EPA and DHA standards, while other products contain much less than is state on the bottle, due to degradation. Flax seed and flax seed oil are good sources of omega-3 fatty acids. Diabetics and those with bleeding problems should check with their physician before starting this supplement. Eating salmon increases omega-3 fatty acids, but, with the advent of mass production of salmon through grain fed farming, the omega-6 levels are increasing in those fish to the detriment of omega-3 fatty acids. One other caution is in order. Eating a lot of fish increases the risk of excessive mercury intake.

13. Stealth Virus
Resource: Dr. John Martin
Phone: (626) 572-7288
URL: http://www. ccid.org
Dx Test: Stealth Virus test through Dr. Martin
Dx Cost: $250
Tx: Nutrition and antiviral TX
Tx Cost: unknown
Hypothesis: The human gene pool has been contaminated by virus segments from other species through a process of mutations and adaptations accelerated by vaccinations. These cause CNS disorders, cancers, among other things.
Evidence: Dr. Martin isolating simian cytomegalovirus from autistic and bipolar patients, both of whom he has successfully treated with nutritional and antiviral treatments. By definition, a stealth virus does not initiate an immune response because it is not recognized by the body as foreign. Dr. Martin states that 100% of psychotic patients test positive for stealth. Only 10% of healthy patients test positive. This would mean that the odds that stealth virus is involved in bipolar syndrome are much higher than even Lyme disease. Also, according to Dr. Martin, stealth virus impairs CD26 molecules, which, among other things, cause digestive impairment in autistic children. While he agrees that wheat and gluten play a role in CNS disorders, he says this is due to impairment of CD26. Both Chris and I tested positive.

Comments: Dr. Martin claims that cross-reactivity of stealth viruses may be causing false positive Western Blot results, leading people to get treated for Lyme disease instead of stealth virus. He believes that the effectiveness of antibiotics in treating Lyme disease stems from suppression of chemokines, not the destruction of spirochetes. If his ideas were to gain acceptance, there would be widespread criticism of the FDA and CDC for allowing animal viruses to become a part of the human gene pool through vaccinations.

14. Viruses
Resource: New Century Wellness Center
Phone: 775.826.9500
URL: http://www.lonezone.com/2000/catalog/i/cwc01.html
Dx Test: Viral Panel
Dx Cost: $450
Tx: homeopathy
Tx Cost: unknown

Hypothesis: Here are some of the viruses that can impair brain functioning, resulting in symptoms of bipolar syndrome: Epstein-Barr virus, cytomegalovirus, herpes simplex virus, *Varicella Aoster* virus, *Borna* virus, HBLV (or HHV-6), toxoplasmosis, *Bartonella* (cat scratch disease).

Evidence: Correlation has been found between these viruses and bipolar illness. Human cytomegalovirus is high in bipolar patients, as well as those with schizophrenia. Other viruses have been shown to coexist with bipolar illness. Epidemiological data from population studies and seasonal variation of illness suggests a positive correlation between exposure to viruses and bipolar illness. Also, Stanley Labs has obtained images of brain tissue from the post-mortem brains of bipolar and schizophrenic patients that are highly suggestive of viral damage, even though they couldn't identify a specific virus. Increased toxoplasmosis antibodies are found in bipolar and schizophrenic patients. Toxoplasmosis is a disease carried by cats; exposure to cats is associated with both schizophrenia and bipolar disorder.

Comments: We did not do the entire viral panel.

Notes

1. Gottschall, Elaine, <u>Breaking the Vicious Cycle — Intestinal Health Through Diet</u>, The Kirkton Press, Baltimore, Ontario, Canada, 1994, 43-60.
2. Cott, Allan, "Controlled Fasting Treatment for Schizophrenia," *Journal of Orthomolecular Psychiatry*, 3(4):301-311, 1974.
3. Emsley, R., Myburgh, C., Oosthuizen, P., van Rensburg, S., Randomized, placebo-controlled study of ethyleicosapentainoic acid as supplemental treatment in schizophrenia, *American J Psychiatry*, 159:1596-1598, September 2002.

Appendix 2 - Psychotropic Drug Withdrawal Log

September 29, 2000 - Chris comes home from the "Cuckoo's Nest," having received the usual typical psychiatric treatment, along with some nutritional snacks. He takes 15 mg of Zyprexa, 100 mg of Wellbutrin, 1,500 mg of Depakote, and 300 mg of Lithium. We add to that two 1,000 mg Omega-3 fatty acid pills and 32 Synergy supplements. He wanders from one task to another. He walks with me and doesn't have a whole lot to say. Has trouble navigating, relying on me for turns in the road.

September 30 - Chris sees a cantaloupe growing in the garden and comments, "I didn't know that cantaloupes grew on vines." Later, while playing some basketball, he can't seem to put enough power into the basketball to hit the rim or backboard. In contrast to his manic periods, when he walks fast and in front of others, he now walks behind me. He watches the movie "Lorenzo's Oil" this evening and tentatively asks, "Isn't that the actor named Nick Nolte?" Says he is feeling a little tired today.

October 2 - After trying to get Chris to help in my research, I realize he is unable to participate. His speech is slurred slightly.

October 4 - We go to see Dr. Ingendaay, an internist and also a provider of alternative medicine. See Chapter 17.

October 7 - We take a walk. He still complains of feeling tired, but stated that he would feel that way anyway because he has nothing to do. He describes feeling depressed whenever he is around people who seem to be relating to others and enjoying themselves. Says he feels trapped. Feels he can't communicate with others and that he never has been able to. Says he still has suicidal thoughts but has no intention of acting on them. Contracts not to harm himself. Says the fantasy of hurting others has gone away.

Tony calls and talks to Chris and me. Chris tells him how he is doing. Tony says that if Chris were his son, he would take him off one-third of the medications now because his only symptom, aside from the depression, is tiredness. He suggests that taking him down by one-third might help prevent an ADR. Chris agreed to this, and we cut everything by one-third starting tonight.

October 8 - Says he slept well and had an okay day.
October 9-10 - He goes with his grandfather and me to the VA Hospital, where, at the Hilton, he wins $20.00 with one quarter. About time he had a

change in luck! Saves $13 of his winnings instead of giving it all back to the hotel. Appetite is good. Still concerned about gaining weight. Eats very fast, as he always has. He is starting to talk about things with a lot more interest and confidence. We talked about "The Jerk" and now it would be fun to see this classic Steve Martin comedy again. After he takes his medications, he is still very tired. When he sees something on TV that is funny, he laughs.

October 12 - Ray, Chris, and I drive to Napa today. See Chapter 1.

October 13 - Chris reports having two dreams. In one he finds a fortune in dollars in a garbage can. In another he dreams he is watching old people ride a Ferris wheel that is going very fast.

October 15 - Today he fixes a bicycle tire, a project he had started before his hospitalization and abandoned.

October 17 - Today, after talking with Tony, Chris and I decide to reduce his medications by another third. Tony told us they had reduced the protocol withdrawal rate to one month and that excessive delay in reducing the medications ran the risk of causing an ADR. It is hard to believe that seven weeks ago Chris was walking down the road in a psychotic state. Now he is getting into the stock market; Wants to buy some options. Still tired and sleepy when he gets up. I heard him singing the other day.

October 20 - Still reports feeling about the same, going back to bed when he wakes up with nothing to do. However, he helps get an appointment for his grandfather at the VA, arranges for records to be sent to various providers; he is taking more responsibility for his affairs. Tonight he went with us to Elizabeth's basketball game. Afterward the game he sat in the car with some teenage girls and sang with them. We went to McDonalds, where he made a comment about biting the skin off his thumb that has been numb since the injury. I was surprised that he talked about this so openly with others nearby. Also, he quietly sang to himself for a few minutes. I am worried because he is expressing his thoughts without the social inhibition. This is not hypomanic — yet. I ask him to put out his medications for two weeks. When he first came home under heavy medications, he couldn't do it. Now he can.

October 21 - Today on our walk, he as much as told me not to be his therapist. He said he resents my intrusive questions about suicide. I point out that talking about suicide does not cause it, but not talking about it can. I tell him that sometimes when depressed people are coming out of depression, they can become suicidal, and it was important for him to be open about this. He says he is bored talking about it, so I do not press him further. Chris starts running up a very steep hill, leaving me behind. Later in the day, he makes a cake for his mom's birthday.

October 22 - I am concerned because he went to bed after 12 when he had agreed to be in bed by 11:30. I wake him at 9:00 a.m. He says he doesn't appreciate me doing this. Looks like he wants more autonomy. On the other hand, he may be getting irritable, one sign of pending mania. I tell him, "You know, Chris, it wasn't me a few weeks ago walking down the road wanting to kill myself." I tell him that the approach we are taking is a departure from accepted guidelines for bipolar treatment and we need to do everything to give the supplements a chance to work. Lack of sleep discipline has always preceded a manic episode.

When he does get up, he is more cordial. That afternoon, Gayle and I go with him to Nevada City for errands. As he walks, I have to move out of his way to keep him from walking into me. When he was hypomanic, Chris would walk to his own rhythm and others would have to adjust to him, be left behind, or get out of the way. He also sings to himself during the day. Gayle and I talk about how we see him. He appears to both of us to be more confident and self-assured. Yet we aren't sure how to take these improvements, fearful of his becoming hypomanic again.

October 28 - Reduced medications by another third. He did not take the medication during dinner and, when reminded by both of us, said that he forgot it but was going to take it later.

October 29 - We take a walk and get into an argument over stocks. I comment on his irritability, and he admits he has been feeling more irritable lately, primarily over my treating him like a teenager, as, for example, my complaining about his sleeping schedule. I tell him again that the supplement program is contrary to all psychiatric practice guidelines, and, if we are going to give it a chance, he needs to stay on a strict sleep schedule. Chris responds by saying that if the supplements were going to work they are going to work. He is becoming more independent. I feel I am in a double bind. He needs regular sleep, but he resents my efforts to assure this.

November 8 - Today Chris decides to stop all the medications. I expressed reservations, even though Tony had supported his withdrawing faster. It has only been five weeks.

I talked to personnel from New Century Wellness Center. The technician said that bipolar illness could be caused by many things, including autoimmune processes, Epstein-Barr syndrome, toxoplasmosis, and responses to food and air particles. They don't use supplements, claim good success with their homeopathic approach. I make an appointment for December 4.

November 10 - Chris and I drive to Sacramento to see Matt for the weekend. Whew! What an experience. I wouldn't want to do it again. See Chapter 17.

November 20 - Chris calls Matt, but his phone is disconnected. Concerned that Matt may have harmed himself, he calls his estranged wife and leaves a message to find out what had happened to him.

November 21 - Chris has been off the meds for 13 days now. Has written some beautiful tunes and composed words to go with them. Dr. Ingendaay says Chris's hair sample came back with high levels of mercury and antimony. She can get him started on a protocol to remove this.

When we walk now Chris talks a lot less. Before, he would talk about himself. Now he talks about whatever subject comes up. He is more private and resents questions about his mental status or how he is doing. He is reading novels now and sharing them with us.

Tonight Chris returns a book to Steve and Debbie. While there, he calls Gayle and tells her that Steve had invited him to go and watch him mix a CD. I was concerned because he didn't say when he would be coming back. Last time he went to Steve's house, he ended up by the side of the road, bleeding profusely. Gayle says we can't control his life any more. He comes home late, but he does come home.

November 29
Chris and I drive to the New Century Wellness Center for two days. See Chapter 18.

December 2
Chris tells Gayle and I that he felt his bed shake during the night. I am concerned that this could be a recap of his "the bed is shaking because of the devil" routine from his first psychotic break. I am pleased to learn that an earthquake registering 4.8 on the Richter scale, with an epicenter about 24 miles north of our home, struck during the night. Recovery involves Gayle and me, mostly me, learning to get over our precipice-dread, being able to trust that our son is back. He has lost the 25 pounds he gained from Zyprexa during his hospitalization. He is in much better physical and mental shape compared to when he came home.

Appendix 3 - Desiderata

In writing this book I obtained information from various scientists and providers of care as well as from the literature. I tried to clearly and objectively represent these points of view even though some of the viewpoints were mutually exclusive. This section will clarify the issues, and, where possible resolve conflicting information I obtained.

Olfactory hallucinations?

Dr. Fudenberg's affirmation that Chris's olfactory hallucinations could be due to sulphur compounds flowing through his bloodstream conflicts with Dr. Bransfield's notion that temporal lobe excitation could be the cause. My subsequent research on the connection between temporal lobe excitation and olfactory hallucinations supports Dr. Bransfield's view. Learning of Dr. Tintera's assertion that adrenal insufficiency causes a 100,000-fold increase in smell and taste sensitivity offers another explanation. Could there be a relationship between adrenal insufficiency and temporal lobe excitation? During his early manic episodes, Chris not only had olfactory hallucinations, but also had tremendous sensitivity to smells and tastes, so much so that he couldn't stand to be around food. By the way, glutamate, one neurotrasmitter involved in G protein mediated signal transduction abnormalities, also increases sensitivity to taste and smell. While I do not profess to know the answer, I believe this information should be a part of any thorough workup. Any physician claiming to have the expertise to help my son should know how these unique symptoms relate to his medical condition. My best layman's estimate is that low energy supply in the brain causes a kind of cell hyper-potentiation that can lead to kindling, powerful colors, smells, and, in more extreme cases, seizures. So much for clearing up this one. Maybe the correct answer is "all of the above."

Wormlike creatures: Lyme spirochetes?

According to Michael Coyle of Nulife Sciences, a company that sells dark field microscope systems and provides training in how to use them, he has never, in his 15 years in the field, seen Lyme spirochetes in the blood. He has only seen corkscrew-shaped Lyme spirochetes in tissue and cerebrospinal fluid. He says the generic name for the wormlike creatures we saw at New Century is protits. Protits are protein particles. Mr. Coyle did affirm that protits in the blood are an indication of a problem, just not Lyme disease. He consults with an alternative health magazine that recently published pictures purporting to show Lyme spirochetes in the blood when, in fact, they were a type of protit called condrits. He told me that after he read the article, he registered a strong objection with the magazine. He says that because the science of dark field microscopy is in its early stages, there is much misunderstanding; when people make unsupportable claims, they diminish the credibility of the science and provide ammunition to critics, of which there are many.

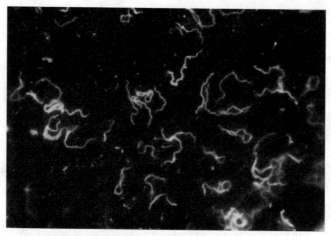

Borrelia burgdorferi in a tick, Ixodes scapularis
Courtesy of Dr. Willy Burgdorfer, Rocky Mountain Laboratories,
Hamilton, Montana 59840

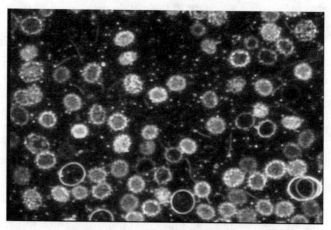

Chris's blood taken 8/15/01 with wormlike microorganisms
Courtesy of Ms. Anne Bernard, Naturopath

I told Mr. Coyle that the staff at New Century refused to release the original dark field microscope photos because they were concerned that the images might be misunderstood. I told him I was looking for another resource for a dark field microscope exam, and he referred me to naturopath

Anne Bernard in Petaluma, California, who has worked with him in his training programs for three years. On August 15, 2001, Chris and I went to Petaluma to have our blood examined. I gave Ms. Bernard a brief history of events and some of the lab data we had collected, including Chris's low urine pH when he was hospitalized in Michigan. What we learned was nothing short of extraordinary.

In the top photo, opposite page, the characteristic shape of the Lyme spirochete is apparent. On the bottom of the same page is a dark field microscope photo of Chris's blood after the blood cells were crushed. The slender threads do not look at all like the Lyme spirochete as seen in the previous photo, but they do look like the substances we saw at New Century. According to Ms. Bernard, these threads are condrits and ascits, pleomorphic microbes existing in various forms in everyone's blood. These microorganisms change shapes and functions based on the terrain of the body. The form they are in reflects one's overall health. They are said to originate from one of two funguses that exist in all life forms, either Mucor Racemosus Fresan or Aspergillus Niger. They have morphed into wormlike shapes because the particular terrain of the body is conducive to this form of the organisms. The longer strands are the condrits; the shorter ones are ascits. Believe it or not, according to an article written by Michael Coyle in Explore, Vol. 10, number 3, 2001, the condrits copulate and within seconds morph into the shorter and fatter ascits. At one time one could see this microscopic X-rated spectacle at http://www.explorepub.com/index.html. Now one would have to obtain the article from that site.

Ms. Bernard stated that the particular frequency and form of the condrits and ascits were probably due to Chris's excessive acidity and high protein levels. Further evidence for the high protein levels is the cluttered background visible in the photo, which she said was indicative of undigested or partly digested protein-based microorganisms. According to Ms. Bernard, this is characteristic of "leaky gut syndrome." If this is true, it would lend support to the idea that undigested proteins play a role in provoking Chris's psychotic behavior.

So, these wormlike microorganisms were not the Lyme spirochete! Chris was right after all. Was he also right about not having Lyme disease? Since the condrits in Chris's blood look totally different, Dr. Tang's original interpretation of the dark field microscope images was clearly incorrect. If Chris's six bands on the Western Blot are proof positive for Lyme disease, then her incorrect interpretation still led us to a correct diagnosis.

Dr. Tang did say that the wormlike creatures only looked like spirochetes, and that more tests would be needed to determine if Chris had Lyme disease. She said it was rare to see spirochetes in the blood, but if she knew what they looked like, she presumably would have said they were condrits, not spirochetes. Also, Ms. Bernard concurred with Dr. Tang that white blood cells were being invaded and killed by something, either a spirochete or a virus, as the following pictures allegedly illustrate. These photos were taken almost four months after Chris completed his IV treatment. Dr. David Dorward from the NIH Rocky Mountain Laboratories found that *Borrelia burgdorferi* are known to thrive in and destroy lymphocytes (white blood cells). When they depart the cell, they are cloaked with cell remnants like a "wolf in sheep's clothing." If Chris's lymphocytes were being destroyed, that could be the reason why. [1] According to Ms. Bernard, the photographs below show white blood cells that are dying. She estimated that about one half of them were dying through some kind of "parasitism" of unknown origin.

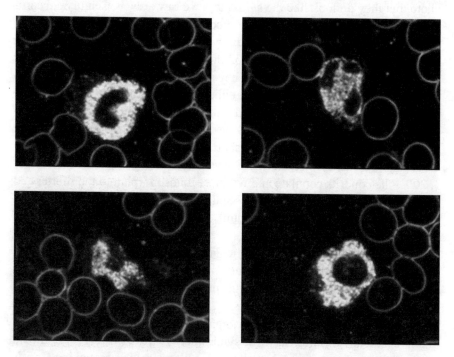

Four pictures said to show damage to Chris's white blood cells

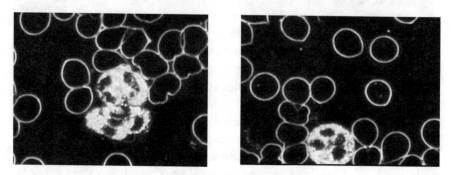

Author's allegedly healthy white blood cells

Another finding reported by New Century from tests on the blood drawn during our November 29, 2000 visit was a low lymphocyte count. It was 8.6, when the normal range is 24-44. By the time Chris saw Dr. Stricker, the count was up to 29.7. Unfortunately, we did not get either pictures or lab data upon completion of his IV treatment. Therefore, we had no way to compare either the pictures or lab data.

I had asked to have my blood examined to show support for Chris and also to better understand any differences in our blood. I did not have any particular health concerns, but, since Ms. Bernard had graciously agreed to allow me to use the photos in this book, I thought that a visual comparison would be instructive, especially if I had the "wormlike" creatures as well. My photos did not show any condrits or ascits, but I did have a massive case of what Ms. Bernard called "rouleau," rows of blood cells clumped together. This suggested to her that I ate excessive protein or digested protein inadequately. She said this could be due to a strong acid balance throughout my body. I told her I had been losing weight on a GNLD protein drink called GR-2 Control to which I added sesame seeds for texture. She said that could have given my body too much of an acid balance.

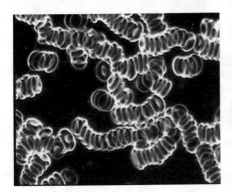 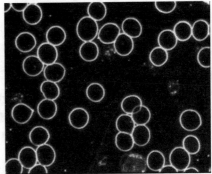

Author's blood taken 8/15/01 and 12/1/01

Ms. Bernard recommended the following for both of us: Digest and Protease, digestive enzymes; Emerald Greens, an "Herbal Superfood"; Cell Food, a water surfactant; omega-3 fatty acids; flax seed oil; and Alkalizer, a source of electrolytes and acid-balancing substances. By restoring enzymes, electrolytes, and a proper pH balance, she said these products would aid digestion. For Chris, she specifically recommended 5HTP and d-Lenolate, an olive leaf extract. She told us she had successfully treated a bipolar patient by giving her 5HTP along with the same enzyme and electrolyte restoring treatment she was recommending for us. Since we believed the Synergy supplements had the necessary precursors, we declined the 5HTP. (Later, Tony said that was a good idea, as too many precursors could have provoked

411

mania.) Chris agreed to take the olive leaf extract to counter whatever was "parasitizing" his white blood cells. Ms. Bernard said that she had cured her mother of hepatitis C using d-Lenolate. According to Ms. Bernard we did not have to know what we were treating. Lyme or stealth — it didn't matter.

I followed most of her recommendations. Chris did not take the digestive aids but did take the d-Lenolate. Meanwhile, he continued to reduce his Zyprexa, working his way down to 5 mg daily. Then he abruptly stopped that drug. As reported in Chapter 23, he then crashed and was hospitalized for several weeks. In retrospect, I made an error by encouraging him to take the d-Lenolate when he did. Though there was good evidence to suggest that this crash occurred from abruptly halting the Zyprexa, taking the d-Lenolate before he was off all medications raised the remote possibility that his crash could have resulted from the die-off of bacteria, a Herx. We should have changed one variable at a time, not two.

Three months later I saw Ms. Bernard again. Chris would not be involved. She took new photos of my blood. I felt a strong sense of accomplishment when I saw the contrast in the two images. I had changed my lifestyle, and the rouleau had vanished! The high protein shakes and pills I had taken from GNLD, and perhaps the sesame, had caused it. I am not qualified to assess the veracity of dark field microscopy, nor can I assess the degree to which the art and science is practiced by professionals or charlatans. However, I can make several unequivocal observations.

First, the tremendous differences in the 20 pictures taken of Chris's and my blood intuitively suggest that those differences mean something. Second, my test showed abnormal blood cells that became normal after I changed my diet. Third, Chris's RAST results, IgG food sensitivity results, and the protein in his blood all support "leaky gut" syndrome. His pictures showed many more particles of presumed protein origin than mine did. Therefore, it would be reasonable to expect that if he were to change his diet or improve his digestion, he could actually see improvements in his blood and that this might could prevent further psychotic behavior. If Ms. Bernard were right, then massive amounts of undigested proteins were contributing to his bipolar symptoms.

I wondered why assessment and treatment for bipolar syndrome couldn't be like this. The patient is symptomatic and takes tests that demonstrate biological anomalies; the patient is treated; the symptoms go away; further tests show that the anomalies are corrected. As Bill O'Reilly of *The O'Reilly Factor* would say, "Tell me where I am wrong."

Oh, by the way — again, if Dr. Martin is correct, then Chris's Western Blot constituted a false positive and the treatment of Lyme disease was unnecessary. Dr. Martin says he has found that among his stealth patients they often test positive for such things as HHV-6, Lyme disease, cytomegalovirus, hepatitis C, chlamydia, and streptococcus.

Lyme disease or atypical stealth virus?

I phoned Dr. Martin to get his feedback on some of the hypotheses I was exploring. He said that casein and gluten do play a role in autism, but the reason is that viruses inhibit the CD26 molecule and that affects digestion of these substances. Dr. Martin said that while there can be additive factors such as diet, chemical sensitivities, and various types of algae and molds, the central problem with many psychiatric illnesses is atypical stealth viruses.

I told him about Chris's psychotic episode after cutting back on the supplements and the dark field microscope findings suggestive of compromised white blood cells. Dr. Martin said that Lyme disease and stealth viruses can coexist, but that many "Lyme" patients are being distracted from the real problem, atypical stealth viruses that don't provoke an inflammatory response. He said that *Borrelia burgdorferi* would have grown in Chris's blood culture if it had been there. He said that we need more doctors who don't "miss the boat" and label patients with bipolar disorder or Lyme disease. He gets calls from parents who are convinced that their child has Lyme disease when most likely they have an atypical stealth virus. He told me of a young man who had been in institutions most of his life due to behavioral problems. The young man now had a glioblastoma, a brain tumor, and his mother was trying to get him into Dr. Byrzynski's treatment program. Dr. Martin said that an atypical stealth virus caused both the behavioral problems and the glioblastoma. Not having heard of Dr. Burzynski's work, Dr. Martin was critical of him. I told him the positive things I had heard.

This backyard mechanic was in no position to rule on the accuracy of any diagnoses given by the experts. The bipolar disorder perspective did seem the most impractical since other perspectives pointed toward causes for which there existed definitive, possibly curative treatments. My task was complicated by the fact that those who advocate a particular viewpoint gained financially by convincing others of its merits, whether the viewpoint involved is bipolar disorder, Lyme disease, stealth viruses, excessive proteins and condrits, "leaky gut," or nutritional deficiencies. The stealth virus approach at least offered something the Lyme approach didn't: a way to assess virulence after a treatment regimen. But regardless of the elusive objective truth, as far as mainstream medicine was concerned, Chris and I were on thin ice with neuro-Lyme, thinner ice with stealth virus, up to our necks in cold water with dark field microscopy, and going under with nutrition. Maybe all the perspectives had some truth. Maybe instead of "either or" it should be "both and." If only doctors got paid for getting people well instead of just treating them.

A role for pH monitoring?

Regarding Dr. Whiley's book, <u>Biobalance</u>, I did not go into pH in very much detail. According to an online book entitled <u>How We Rot and Rust</u>, the ability of the body to assimilate minerals is related to pH level.[2] Minerals on the lower end of the periodic table can be assimilated in a wider pH range, while those higher up the scale require a narrower range. For example, sodium and magnesium can be absorbed within a wide pH range, while zinc, copper, and iodine require much narrower ranges. As one moves up the periodic table toward the heavier elements, assimilation is impaired by increasing acidity. This would suggest that either increasing the minerals available through supplements or improving the body's ability to absorb minerals by, among other things, reducing acidity could increase absorption of important brain chemical precursors. Also, as the body becomes more acidic, there is an increase in free calcium in the blood taken from the bones. This backyard mechanic found this information to be very interesting given that elevated intracellular calcium ions are associated with mania, and calcium channel blockers have been successfully used in research settings to treat mania.

Kill the bugs or alter the terrain?

In the late 19th century there was a historic debate about the nature of bacteria that has profoundly affected our medical practices today. Pasteur said that bacteria were in a constant form and did not change. Bechamp said they were not in a constant form and they did change, hence, monomorphism vs. pleomorphism. Although a layman's response to this necessarily incomplete description of this debate might be "So what?" actually the implications of these two foundational points of view are significant. Do we kill the cancer cells with chemotherapy or do we use antineoplaston peptides to communicate to the cancer cells to stop proliferating and start acting like normal cells? Do we poison the small cell lung cancer or do we communicate with the neuropeptide receptors on the cancer cells and instruct the macrophages that mutated into cancer cells to mutate back to macrophages?[3] Do we use antibiotics to kill Lyme disease or do we create an environment in the body where the Lyme disease is unable to thrive? Pasteur is alleged to have said on his deathbed, "the microbe is nothing, the terrain is everything," but, even if he did, his monomorphism was already dominating the medical establishment and has done so to this day.[4] It is beyond the scope of this book to delve into the complementary and alternative medicine practices that have evolved from the pleomorphic perspective. Suffice it to state that there are many who incorporate complementary and alternative medicine into their practice such as Dr. Gant and some who exclusively work from within the perspective such as Anne Bernard. I have not given the pleomorphic perspective the attention it deserves, because of space limitations in this book, and also the difficulty of learning one more new paradigm. However, the following does utilize both a pleomorphic and a systems perspective.

Consider the human body and the lakes of Florida. Do they have anything in common? They both have a terrain. In <u>Desperation Medicine</u>, Dr. Shoemaker reports research demonstrating that the yearly use of agricultural fungicides that contain large amounts of copper and other pollutants has irreparably damaged the terrain of the Florida Everglades. Cylindrospermoposis, a toxic, copper-resistant blue-green algae now thrives, killing pelicans, alligators, and fish, and sickening people exposed to it. Killing this algae, which has already taken over a number of lakes in Florida, is impossible, as is binding the toxins with CSM, which, though theoretically possible, is not practical. Reestablishing a healthy terrain to the extent possible is the only solution, even though that might be prohibitively expensive and involve dredging the lakes to get rid of the muck and its associated chemicals.[5]

After my visit with Ms. Bernard, I wondered if what Dr. Shoemaker was saying about larger ecosystems applied to our own personal ecosystems as well. Our personal terrain must be restored to health in order for harmful microorganisms to fade into the background. Maybe the issue is not so much killing the microbes as it is providing a terrain that is not conducive to their growth and development.

Antibiomania

Sometimes it takes the professional journals some time to catch up with what's happening in the real world. Since I first met Tony, he had told me several times of the risks oral antibiotics posed for bipolar patients taking the Synergy supplements. But I never had any official proof that I could point to when talking to doctors. In the February 2002 issue of *Journal of Clinical Psychopharmacology*, there was an article entitled "Antimicrobial-Induced Mania (Antibiomania): A Review of Spontaneous Reports." The authors reported on the same phenomena that Tony had told me about. They found the risk minimal, but the population studied — 82 cases reported to the World Health Organization — was not drawn from bipolar patients, and consisted only of cases officially reported.[6] Here is another example of biologically valid psychological variables resulting from drug effects. There may be patients misdiagnosed with bipolar disorder who had antibiomania.

Lithium, Tamoxifen, Haldol, and Clozaril

Lithium exerts a modulating influence over both high and low levels of glutamate, the excitatory neurotransmitter, in the synapse of the neuron.[7] In addition, Tamoxifen, like lithium and Depakote, decreases protein kinase C, which is believed to directly regulate and correlate with neurotransmitter activity. Tamoxifen, a breast cancer drug decreases protein kinase C more efficiently than either lithium or Depakote. Dr. Husseini Manji reported the results of a pilot study using Tamoxifen for mania, reporting positive results in six of seven patients. All five male patients responded.[8] If Dr. Manji's research is replicated, then Tamoxifen would appear to be a much more effective targeted treatment than either lithium or Depakote.

Now for the bad news. Haldol and Clozaril both may be responsible for the reduced NAA seen in the brains of schizophrenic patients.[9] In other words, the treatment, and/or the disease may be causing some of the brain deficits that have been known for years. There are studies showing the efficacy of Clozaril with treatment-resistant bipolar disorder. At one time, frontal lobotomies were pretty effective in controlling uncontrollable patients too.

Notes

1. Grier, Tom, "Motile Menace," Lyme Alliance Web site
http://www.lymealliance.org/research/grier/grier_3.php
2. Here is a comprehensive overview of a perspective initially developed by German professor Guenther Enderlein, whose ideas were based on the work of Bechamp. http://www.biomedx.com/microscopes/rrintro/rr4.html
3. Pert, Candace, <u>Molecules of Emotion: The Science Behind Mind Body Medicine</u>, Touchstone, New York, 1999, 170-173.
4. Enby, Erik, <u>Hidden Killers: The Revolutionary Medical Discoveries of Professor Guenther Enderlein</u>, Semmelweis-Institut Hasseler, Hoya, West Germany, 1990, 15-18.
5. Shoemaker, Ritchie, <u>Desperation Medicine</u>, Gateway Press, Baltimore, MD, 168-193.
6. Abouesh, A., Stone, C., Hobbs, W.R., "Antimicrobial-induced mania (Antibiomania): a review of spontaneous reports," *Journal of Clinical Psychopharmacology*, 22(1): 71-81, February 2002.
7. Nonaka, S., Hough, C.J., Chuang, D., "Chronic lithium treatment robustly protects neurons in the central nervous system against excitotoxicity by inhibiting N-methyl-d-aspartate receptor-mediated calcium influx," *Proceedings of the National Academy of Sciences,* 2641, March 3, 1995.
8. Bebchuk, J.M., Arfken, C.L., Dolan-Manji, S., Murphy, J., Hasanat, K., Manji, H. K., "A preliminary investigation of a protein kinase C inhibitor in the treatment of acute mania," *Arch Gen Psychiatry* 57(1):95-97, 2000.
9. Bustillo, J.R., Lauriellol, J., Rowlad, L.M., Jung, R.E., Petropoulos, H., Hart, B.L., Blanchard, J., Keith, S. J., Rooks, W.M., "Effects of chronic haloperidol and clozapine treatments on frontal and caudate neurochemistry in schizophrenia," *Psychiatry Research*, 107(3):135-149, 2001.

Appendix 4 - Kindling Contributors

There is substantial evidence that bipolar symptoms are caused, in part, by defects in signal transduction mechanisms. These include irregularities in, among other things, calmodulin, G proteins, protein kinase C and protein kinase A. Signal transduction is a cascade of processes by which hormones or neurotransmitters interact with a receptor on the surface of a cell. That interaction initiates complex processes that can lead to alterations in cell functioning such as a change in the amount of second messengers as, for example, calcium ions, which in large amounts can kill brain cells. Signal transduction defects also change cell functioning by increasing glucose up-take. Mitogen activated protein kinase (MAPK) cascade is one type of cascade; there are others. Signal transduction defects probably result from the interaction of many abnormalities.[1]

Another way to conceptualize signal transduction defects is to describe it as kindling. Kindling is a process in which brain functioning is altered due to repeated electrical or chemical stimulation. Over time the brain becomes more sensitized to the stimulation, leading to lower thresholds being needed to provoke either a seizure or a manic episode. This is why it is so important for patients to maintain their treatment regimen in order to prevent repeated episodes. Though originally used to describe a process leading to seizures, the term is also used to describe the process leading to an episode of mania. The brain loses control over its own thought processes.

Evidence of kindling may be something as ordinary as having trouble sleeping. Lack of sleeping can initiate the kindling process. The person can't stop thinking. For most of us, lack of sleeping is an inconvenience. For the bipolar patient, this inability of the brain to turn itself off can lead to psychosis. Here is a short list of some of the factors that can play a role in kindling:

From personal observations

Consuming coffee; soft drinks with caffeine or sugar; high glycemic foods such as melon, orange; beer
Strenuous exercise during the day, especially a few hours before bed
Intense concentration 1-3 hours before bed (e.g., writing software code)
Lack of sleep
St. John's Wort

From research

Inadequate nutrients (e.g., magnesium, zinc, B vitamins)
Inadequate omega-3 fatty acids
Stress-related hormones such as ACTH, cortisol, beta endorphins

Antigens (antibody generators) from Lyme disease, viruses, etc.

IgE allergies

IgG food sensitivities

Quinolinic acid

Glutamate in foods such as MSG, hydrolyzed protein, aspartame

SAMe

Most antidepressants and withdrawal from some antidepressants

Cocaine

Alcohol

Mitogens (mitosis generators, substances which cause lymphocyctes to undergo cell division) such as:

•Chemicals - organophosphates, endrin, aldrin

•Plants and food[2] - pokeweed, marijuana, potatoes, barley, wheat, corn, chicken, beans[3]

•Endogenous - lactic acid

Notes

1. Bezchlibnyk, Y., Young, T.L., "The neurobiology of bipolar disorder: focus on signal transduction pathways and the regulation of gene expression," *W Can J Psychiatry*, 47(2), March 2002.

2. A number of foods cause the body to activate its "Department of Defense" by, for example increasing mitosis of lymphocytes. For more information on specific mitogens from foods see the following URL:

http://www.er4yt.org/Education/Lectins_In_Food.html

3. One of the sources of phytohemagglutinin is beans. See Chapter 19 for further discussion on the relationship between phytohemagglutinin and the lymphocyte proliferation seen in mania.

Appendix 5 - Dr. Kaplan's May 2001 Presentation

Effective mood stabilization with a broad-based nutritional supplement: 20 adults and children

Presented at the Society of Biological Psychiatry,
Annual meeting, New Orleans, Louisiana, May 4, 2001

Bonnie J. Kaplan[1], Ph.D., J. Steve A. Simpson[1], Ph.D., M.D., Richard C. Ferre[2], M.D., Chris P. Gorman[1], M.D., David McMullen[1], M.D., Susan G. Crawford, M.Sc.[1]

[1]Calgary, Alberta, Canada;
[2]Salt Lake City, Utah

Abstract

a) Background: Some research on nutrition-mood interactions has employed single ingredients (B vitamins, DHA). We are evaluating a broad nutritional supplement (primarily trace minerals).

b) Method: The supplement contains dietary nutrients, primarily minerals. Eleven adults (aged 19-46) with Bipolar Disorder (I, II, and NOS) were followed for an average of 44 weeks. Nine children with mood/anxiety disorders (aged 8-15 years) were followed for an average of 14 weeks. Assessment at entry and post-treatment used the Hamilton-Depression Scale (Ham-D), Brief Psychiatric Rating Scale (BPRS), Young Mania Rating Scale (YMRS), Child Behaviour Checklist (CBCL), and Youth Outcome Questionnaire (YOQ).

c) Results:

For the adults, paired t-tests showed treatment benefit on all measures: Ham-D (M=19.0 to M=5.4, $t(9)=5.59$, $p<01$); BPRS (M=35.3 to M=7.4, $t(9)=2.57$, $p<.05$); YMRS (M=15.1 to M=6.0, $t(9)=4.11$, $p<.01$). Psychotropic medications decreased significantly from an average of 2.7/patient at entry to 1.0/patient at follow up ($t(10)=3.54$, $p<.01$).

For the <u>children</u>, treatment benefit was also significant. There were lower scores for the CBCL: withdrawn (t(8)=3.79, p<.01); anxiety problems (t(8)=2.97, p<.05); social problems (t(8)=2.89, p<.05); thought problems (t(8)=3.67, p<.01); attention problems (t(8)=3.85, p<.01); delinquent behaviour (t(8)=3.71, p<.01); and aggressive behaviour (t(8)=3.46, p<.01). The YOQ and the YMRS also showed significant improvement: t(8)=5.97, p<.001, t(3)=4.54, p<.05, respectively.

<u>d) Conclusion</u>: In some cases, the supplement has entirely replaced psychoactive medications. Side effects have been rare, minor, and transitory. This nutritional supplement is an effective treatment for mood instability. A randomized, placebo-controlled trial in adult Bipolar I Disorder is underway.

Appendix 6 - Communications with Dr. Cade

July 17, 2001
Dr. Cade,

I am the person still finishing the book called *Too Good to be True; Nutrients Quiet the Unquiet Brain-A Four-Generation Bipolar Odyssey*. I wrote you in April. This note is to thank you for the feedback and the research papers on your work. I made the changes you recommended.

I was intrigued by your statement that gluten-casein may be the "culprit" in epilepsy. If this proves to be true for seizure disorders, could it not also be true for bipolar, since both seizure and bipolar are characterized, in part, by compromised cellular inhibition processes?

My son had a setback after taking a trip and not taking his supplements regularly. He is hospitalized now. Dr. Bransfield, a private practice psychiatrist who wrote the introduction to the book, suggested he get an EEG since he consistently has olfactory hallucinations when becoming psychotic, but only then. Other indications of temporal lobe issues include sudden mood swings, aggressive non-provoked behavior, and disorientation.

A few years ago, a friend of mine lost her adult son after he drowned from a seizure while taking a bath. He was diagnosed with epilepsy, but it had been managed effectively with medication. That night he had pizza for dinner. Could the hot bath and the gluten in the pizza have been a fatal combination for him? I know it sounds far out, but my son ate pasta on the day before two major psychotic episodes. Of course, people eat pasta all the time, and I might be grasping at straws, but, as I say in the book, there are so many pieces to this puzzle, none should be left out, no matter how farfetched. If you found a link between gluten and casein and seizure disorder, this could be another of those "too good to be true" findings that could apply to bipolar.

I am sure your plate is full, but I was wondering if you or others have considered looking for a relationship between gluten and casein and bipolar illness? I know it is a long-shot, but to me it seems like an intuitive step. In Werback's <u>Nutritional Influences on Mental Health</u>, he tells of a bipolar patient who did great off wheat and became psychotic on it. She had an IgE reaction. Was it idiosyncratic, or did the gluten lessen the effectiveness of cellular inhibition processes?

David Moyer, Lt Col, USAF, Ret
LCSW, BCD, ACSW

Several weeks later, Dr. Cade responded as follows:

Dear Mr. Moyer,

The answer to all your questions in paragraphs two and four is yes. I am quite interested in doing an HPLC on your son's urine and plasma if you could send me samples.

Gluten produces a whole series of morphine-like products, as does casein. These exorphins have a direct effect on the brain.

Sincerely yours,

Robert Cade, M.D., LLD
Professor of Medicine and Physiology

October 2001 update:

After I received this response, I called back and talked to one of Dr. Cade's staff members, Malcolm Privette, a physician assistant. He said that Dr. Cade had been researching this topic and had, in fact, already found patterns of hyperpolypeptiduria that are associated with bipolar disorder! I asked about the cost for the lab work. He said the urine test would be free, even though it cost them between $1,500-$2,000. He said the blood work would cost us $99.00 since it is sent out to a private lab. Malcolm was not sure how much longer the university would fund these exploratory studies. Their priority has been investigating the influence of casein and gluten on schizophrenia and autism.

I had somewhat sheepishly made a speculative, intuitive leap into the unknown ... only to find that Dr. Cade had already made the same leap and was studying it. What is the moral to this story? Never stop asking questions, no matter how far-fetched they may seem.

Later, Malcolm informed me of the results of both the urine and blood tests. The HPCL (opiate-like peptides) test, based on a sample of urine obtained prior to Chris's hospitalization for drug induced agitation and depression, showed a very low level of the suspect polypeptides. The RAST, a blood test that measures antibodies to casein and gluten was obtained after his discharge from the hospital. It demonstrated a high antibody response to both casein and gluten. The normal range for IgG antibodies to casein is 0-100. Chris obtained a score of 10,649! The normal range for IgG antibodies to casein is 0-100. Chris obtained a score of 2,732. Malcolm told me that 5 of the 6 measures taken were significant, and that Chris should not be eating casein, gluten, or even soy milk. He also said that they have used an animal pancreatic enzyme obtained by prescription called Creon for those who are unwilling or unable to completely abstain from wheat and milk products.

April 2002 update:

After Chris's manic setback in March, I sent a urine sample to Dr. Cade's office. I spoke with Malcolm and he again told me that the HPCL scores were negligible. For the second time, Chris again had low levels of these opiate-like peptides, suggesting that his defensive system was successfully binding with them. I told him that Chris's mania had ceased at home on, among other things, a gluten and casein free diet, but that he became psychotic again after returning to his old diet and not taking the medications and supplements. Conversations with Malcolm and correspondence from Dr. Cade indicated that they have found that excessive peptides are present in autism, schizophrenia, the levels correlating with the positive symptoms of schizophrenia and severity of autistic behaviors. Based on his preliminary studies, when a bipolar patient was manic, there was low HPLC, when depressed, high HPLC, or polypeptiduria. Here are some quotes from Dr. Cade's July 10, 2002 letter.

"Fifteen to twenty years ago when we could only measure total peptide content of urine by Sephadex filtration (HPLC was not available at that time) we studied a small number of manic-depressives and schizophrenic patients over several years. ... Total polypeptides in urine were elevated when the patients (bipolar) were depressed and were low when the patients were manic." He then explained how they couldn't tell if the peptide decreases were exogenous peptides from milk and wheat because they did not have the HPLC. "With HPLC we may be able to find an answer."

"I don't have the answers to your questions about epilepsy. I can tell you that exorphins are consistently elevated in patients with epilepsy and that the frequency and severity of seizures both decrease as the HPLC becomes normal."

He encouraged me to continue to send urine samples to see if the peptide levels change based on changes in Chris's moods.

I was initially disappointed to learn that my intuitive simplistic casein/gluten-hyperpolypeptiduria-mania-seizure symptoms connection was wrong. It appeared as though a casein/gluten-hyperpolypeptiduria-depression connection and a casein/gluten-hypopolypeptiduria-manic connection may be correct. These hypotheses raised other possibilities that might explain impaired neuron functioning. But this was an area where a little knowledge could indeed be dangerous.

I knew that G proteins exist in receptors and that when a ligand such as a neurotransmitter binds to a receptor this starts complex processes inside the cell. I knew there were many different kinds of G proteins, including an excitatory one that increased during mania. I knew there was a direct relationship between certain G proteins and positive symptoms of schizophrenia, autism and mania. So why would high G proteins and high HPLC correlate with the positive symptoms of schizophrenia and autism? Why would high G proteins and low HPLC appear to correlate with mania? Why would high G proteins and high HPLC appear to correlate with a depressive episode. Did these patterns even exist?

There were so many processes that could be linked together. It seemed to me that bipolar syndrome and other CNS disorders must result from multiple failures of complex homeostatic mechanisms influenced by a plethora of genetic and environmental factors. But even understanding the processes that are already understood by scientists was beyond my understanding. Speculating would not give me any answers, but we would keep sending samples to Dr. Cade in the hope that he and his colleagues could find it useful in their ongoing research.

Appendix 7 - Chris's Bipolar Puzzle

This section summarizes pieces of Chris's bipolar puzzle I was able to identify throughout this odyssey.

Overview of episodes of illness age 21-26
Legend for charts

Mood:

1 - Major Depression - self destructive, psychotic (hospitalized)
2 - Minor Depression - loss of confidence, difficulty functioning
3 - Base line (creative, disorganized, memory problems)
4 - Hypomanic (boundary problems, overly talkative, little sleep)
5 - Manic - emotionally volatile, grandiose
6 - Psychotic - delusional, danger to self or others (hospitalized)

Psychotropic Medications:
1 - No medications
2 - 1/4 medication
3 - 1/2 medications
4 - 3/4 medication
5 - Full medication

The above categorizations are general, as the types and amounts of medications changed considerably. The depression noted in June and July, 2001 occurred after he started taking 2,000 mg of Depakote daily. The decrease in medications shown in August 2001 represents stopping Zyprexa, as repeatedly recommended by his psychiatrist. This decrease precipitated suicidal behavior. The decrease before the 6th episode is from Chris reducing only his Zyprexa too rapidly. In April 2002 Chris stopped all medicines and supplements. This data is based on informal monthly assessments.

Supplements:
1 - None
2 - Inconsistent (<16)
3 - 16-24
4 - 24-32
5 - 32

Comments:

1. Data on taking additional immune enhancing supplements, including omega-3 fatty acids, lipoic acid, Co Q10, buffered C, and vitamin E, are not listed because Chris would not take them on a regular basis. He took them consistently January through April 2001 and early March 2002, sporadically at other times.

2. Because the data is reported monthly, the chart does not show the time lag between moods, medications, and supplements. The increases and decreases in the supplements and medications preceded the mood changes. The last chart shows two data entries per month. Also, an elevation on mania does not preclude depression, including suicidal depression, but mainly describes the primary focus (i.e. grandiose delusions, pressured speech, etc.).

1998

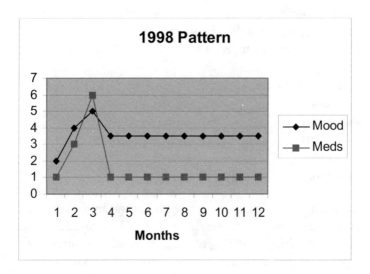

1 - To England for Jan Term.

2/1 - Inability to talk, feelings of depression.

2/2 - Three tablets daily of St. John's Wort.

2/6 - Delusions of the end of the world. Smells sulphur. Amazed at intensity of colors, sounds. Responds to 5 mg Zyprexa, outpatient care. Two weeks later, back in college, stops medications against advice of psychiatrist.

3/15 - Hospitalized for two weeks after delusions returned.

6-8 - Stopped meds; worked during the summer selling books door to door.

9 - Completed senior recital and was awarded BA in music composition.

1999

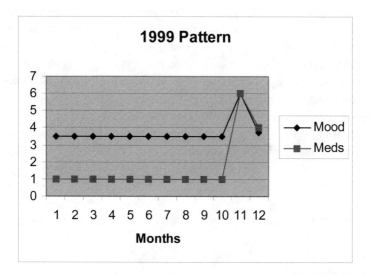

3/98 - 11/99 Worked several different jobs, including the summer book sales job back East.

11/12 - Admitted involuntarily to Sacred Heart Hospital in Spokane for mania and delusions. Smelled sulphur. Remained hypomanic even though I stayed with him through Christmas and made sure he took his medicines.

2000

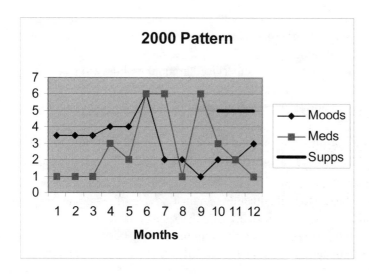

1 - New job selling cell phones. Top producer in office by March. Still off medications.

4 - Hypomanic again as evidenced by excessive journal writing and religious discussions at work. We take him home, ensure he stays on medications, but he remains hypomanic.

6/15 - Chris says he will take his medications and insists on selling books again. We reluctantly agree. After training, he drives with fellow sales persons towards his assigned territory in Pennsylvania.

6/21 - Takes medications inconsistently. Becomes delusional again while driving. Is admitted to the University of Pennsylvania Medical Center in Hershey, Pennsylvania. While under the influence of Haldol, he breaks his kneecap doing flips. He flies home. Hypomanic behavior continues. Psychiatrist increases Depakote to 2,000 mg a day. Chris becomes depressed, confused.

8/14 - Doctor recommends stopping Zyprexa cold turkey. I object to sudden stop. We cut back for two weeks; Chris has more energy.

8/26 - Doctor insists Chris stop Zyprexa "cold turkey." We comply with doctor's recommendation.

8/29 - Chris tells me he slept when he didn't, then, after incident at work, he walks down Highway 20 and impulsively cuts his throat and wrists, and hits his head with rocks. He is admitted to the hospital for 1 month with homicidal, suicidal ideation.

9/1 - I explore Truehope.com, talk with Tony, and order supplements.

9/15 - Chris, doing poorly, is committed for another 30 days. Gayle and I start bringing in four supplement "snacks" a day.

9/20 - We get permission for him to take 3,000 grams of omega 3-fatty acids pills a day.

9/26 - Chris begins making friends with patients and relating to them; he is no longer obsessed about the good/bad Chris. Chris's doctor decides not to keep him for the additional days.

9/29 - Chris is discharged. Begins supervised gradual withdrawal from medications while taking supplements.

10-12 - We seek out additional medical opinions. Lyme and other anomalies are found.

12/1 - Chris is off all medications and doing fine. For the first time in a long time, he does not demonstrate any hypomanic behavior.

2001

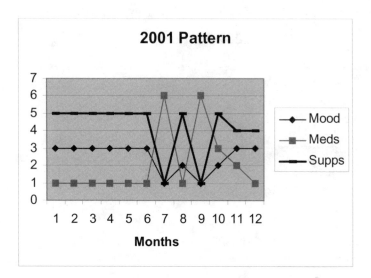

3-6 - Completes IV Rocephin treatment, stopping one week short because he decides he didn't have Lyme disease.

7 - Flies to Michigan to visit friends; inconsistently takes supplements; becomes obsessed and depressed. Takes OD to sleep. Hospitalized.

8 - At home, takes both medications and Synergy supplements on advice of his psychiatrist and against advice of Tony and myself, and gets more depressed. After two weeks on regimen he begins cutting medications on his own. Reports feeling better. Against my advice, he stops Zyprexa at 5 mg then takes 15 mg promoting akathisia. Hospitalized again.

10 - I supervise slow withdrawal from medications without incident.

11 - He flies to Colorado and sings a song he composed for a friend's wedding. He is off all medications without any difficulty and doing fine. Taking 24 supplements a day.

2002 - biweekly chart

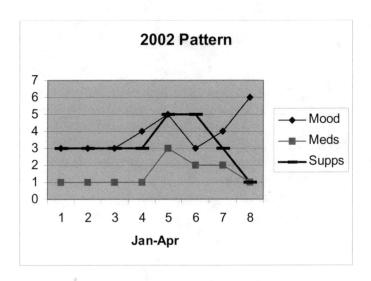

2002 Pattern

Legend: Mood, Meds, Supps

X-axis: Jan-Apr

1 - He starts taking 16 supplements a day without apparent problem and begins smoking again. We suggest he stay at 24-32 a day and advise against smoking. Starts part-time job. Begins working out in a fitness center. Becomes hypomanic.

3/2 - After strenuous fitness center work-outs and eating hydrolyzed protein, an excitotoxin, he becomes manic. We eliminate all gluten and casein and put him on 10 mg Zyprexa, 1,000 mg Depakote, and 600 mg lithium. He takes 32 supplements a day in addition to the immune-enhancing supplements and 4,000 mg of omega-3 fatty acids daily. He refuses to take medications and I crush them and put them into Synergy supplements which he still agrees to take. A few days later, a friend talks him into taking the medications again. He begins to sleep again, forestalling another hospitalization. After about a week of "home hospitalization," he returns to his old self. He returns to eating gluten and casein and manages his own supplements as I slowly cut medications. He chooses not to take omega fatty acids or the immune enhancing supplements, and becomes inconsistent with the supplements again. I tried to increase medications after Chris becomes hypomanic three weeks later.

4/5 - After "forgetting" to take his medications which were given to him, Chris then refuses medications and supplements. Hospitalized April 8 after three nights of not sleeping.

Madly in love and lethargic in London

Chris's first episode coincided with an intense romantic attachment. At first he felt "high" from his love interest. Dr. Amen tells of a SPECT he gave to a man with no psychiatric history who agreed to be a test subject after the man had just fallen passionately in love. Dr. Amen writes that the man's SPECT looked like "he was taking cocaine." He reported that activity to the right and left basal ganglia was so intense that it almost resembled seizure activity.[1] Chris, too, was "madly" in love. However, his romantic feelings gave way to feelings of depression and inadequacy.

Surprisingly, falling in love has something in common with obsessive compulsive disorder (OCD). Both conditions are associated with a narrowing of the focus of consciousness. Both young people who are intensely in love and those who suffer from OCD have low levels of serotonin. Lovesick young people who thought about their loved one for 4 hours or more daily had a 40% average drop of serotonin in their blood compared to controls. OCD patients had similarly lowered levels of serotonin in their blood.[2] After a year, when the initial infatuation was past, the serotonin levels of the lovers returned to normal. One member of the research team, Dr. Hagob Akiskal, of the University of California, ventured a hypothesis on the evolutionary significance of this phenomenon: "Without intense emotion, no one in his or her right mind would fall in love and have children."[3] There is profound simplicity in the phrases "madly in love" and "crazy for you." Had "falling in love" driven Chris mad? Had low serotonin levels narrowed his focus and worsened what had appeared to be a normal "where am I going after college" mild depression? Had his obsessive religious preoccupations been caused or exacerbated by low serotonin levels? Could his serotonin levels, already compromised by Lyme disease, nutritional deficits, or genetic factors, been further impaired by strong feelings of infatuation?

What about his sleeping patterns? A sudden change from the jet lag after his return from England could have contributed. One night without sleep had to potential to provoke a manic episode.

Wehr reports on the successful treatment of a bipolar patient by regulating sleep. For several years, the researchers helped a rapidly cycling bipolar patient maintain a rigidly self-enforced schedule of bed rest in the dark for 14 hours per day, later reduced to 10. The authors concluded that "fostering sleep and stabilizing its timing by scheduling regular nightly periods of enforced bed rest in the dark may help to prevent mania and rapid cycling in bipolar patients."[4] DSM-IV reports the same thing. Irregular sleeping can provoke bipolar disorder, while regular sleep can help to manage it. There could have been a jet lag effect both going to and coming from England.

Losses and other provocations

In one chapter of the book <u>Mania, an Evolving Concept</u>, I found writings by a psychoanalyst who pointed out that depressive or manic attacks are precipitated by the loss of the all-important love object. The patient feels rebuked or not appreciated.[5] Chris and his girlfriend had broken up. Maybe the stress of that could generate cortisol and/or beta-endorphins. I had been a bit skeptical of psychoanalytic doctrine ever since I'd had to regurgitate it for tests in a human growth and behavior class in graduate school. Even then I considered psychoanalytic theory to require a certain degree of religious-like faith, but I could not deny that Chris had lost a recently acquired "love object."

Cultural factors had also played a role in the etiology of Chris's illness. The 20th century was drawing to a close. A number of doomsday cults had emerged. The Heaven's Gate cult had committed mass suicide so they could hitch a ride on a passing comet. Japanese religious extremists had killed subway passengers by releasing lethal gas into subways. Chris had been studying eschatology, the study of the end of the world, a subject that has fascinated religious leaders and mystics since the time of Christ. The Y2K panic was a part of his cultural milieu. The craziness in the culture as reflected in the general climate of millennial disaster provided some of the raw material for his psychosis.

Stresses had preceded the first two episodes. In the first, his girlfriend Joan had broken up with him. In the second, he had tried to convince his new girlfriend, Sandy, to adopt his religious views. Chris had a tendency in his relationships to either lose himself or try to dominate his partner. He would dance to the girl's tune or attempt to make her dance to his. It was "either or," not "both and." He couldn't master the normal give and take that couples have to develop in order to be with each other and still maintain their separate identities. But didn't all relationships have conflict? Why couldn't he handle it?

Before he took the St. John's Wort, he was experiencing depression and manifesting some psychotic thought processes in his journal. Already depressed and obsessive from low serotonin, he may have inadvertently triggered his initial manic episode by taking the St. John's Wort, which had flooded him with serotonin through its MAO-inhibiting properties. Then, after the Zyprexa adjusted his brain chemistry, he improved dramatically, only to become psychotic when he stopped taking the Zyprexa. What role had withdrawing from Zyprexa played in his subsequent episodes?

The first, third, fourth, sixth, and seventh episodes in which he was hospitalized all occurred within days or weeks of going off the Zyprexa: the first and third on his own initiative, the fourth on his doctor's orders, the sixth and seventh on his own initiative, though I had slowly cut back before he refused to take them prior to his seventh hospitalization. The first hospital episode had been less than two weeks after stopping Zyprexa.

The second episode could not have been related to medication issues because he had been mildly hypomanic for a year and a half without medications. A number of different sources agree that the time between a patient's first and second episodes of bipolar symptoms is the longest, often in a range of around 24 to 30 months. Chris went 18 months before his second episode. The natural progression of episodes is for decreasing time between subsequent episodes, often with a tendency toward seasonal patterns in the spring and fall, which Chris has demonstrated.

The third had been less than two weeks after stopping or erratically taking Depakote and Zyprexa.

Regarding the fourth episode, Chris had been improving for two weeks as we slowly reduced the frequency of the Zyprexa rather than stopping it entirely as Dr. Lund recommended. Four days after complying with Dr. Lund's recommendation to completely stop, Chris had been overcome by obsessional thoughts: frightening fantasies of killing his family that had led him to attempt suicide rather than harm anyone. It was obvious that withdrawing from the Zyprexa had played a role in these episodes, but what role, exactly, was less clear. What was responsible for transforming my son from a gentle, thoughtful college graduate to a person afflicted with akathisia and obsessed with thoughts of killing himself so he wouldn't harm others? Was it his illness, his medications, or his withdrawal from the medications? For a social worker used to finding dynamic meanings in behavior, Chris's homicidal and suicidal ideation was baffling. Neither he nor I could find a clue as to why he would feel homicidal or suicidal, that is, unless it was simply mindless rage at his own powerlessness over the total transformation of his personality: rage that needed a target. But that notion seemed inadequate to me. For one thing, Chris wasn't even angry at Dr. Lund, whose ill-advised recommendations had led to his self-mutilating behavior. The most reasonable explanation was that his impaired brain was further damaged by rapid withdrawal of Zyprexa. Then there was the question about his smoking just before his fateful walk down Highway 20.

Research by scientists at Brookhaven National Laboratory in New York suggests that cigarette smoking may slow the breakdown of dopamine. This could lead the average person to experience pleasurable feelings not just from nicotine, but from increased dopamine as well. The researchers found that smoking reduces monoamine oxidase inhibitor B (MAO-B), an enzyme that breaks down dopamine in the brain. MAO-B ensures that excess dopamine and other neurotransmitters are broken down or taken back up and stored in the neuron. If dopamine remains free in the brain, it can send spurious signals. Smokers had an average of 40% less MAO-B, and this was presumed to increase their dopamine levels.[6] Could smoking just two cigarettes have increased the amount of free dopamine in Chris's brain enough to push him over the edge? By the way, Zyban, a chemical relative of Wellbutrin is effective for smoking cessation because of its dopamine increasing properties. And what about the chronic effects of the approximately 300 addictive agents the tobacco companies put in cigarettes to ensure that the customer comes back for more? What about the nutritional price paid by the body to detoxify these chemicals? What happens when choline is diverted from producing precursor chemicals for proper brain functioning in order to remove the toxins?

Before his fourth episode, there was a surge of emotion when his employer had sworn angrily at him after being awakened from a nap. Could cortisol, beta-endorphins, adrenaline, or noradrenaline increase that fast in response to perceived threats? Could a particular neural pathway have been overly responsive to the stimulation that quickly? Was Chris like Phineas Gage, the famous quarry worker in the 1880s who survived a rod through his brain, only to be permanently afflicted with uncontrollable impulses? What had propelled Chris to become so emotional and so driven as to take a cigarette from his employer? Given his history, taking the cigarettes would have to be considered highly ego-dystonic behavior.

Finally, I had learned from email correspondence with Dr. Bransfield that Lyme patients reacted adversely to drops in barometric pressure. In contrast to the preceding weeks of Indian summer, the day that Chris had run amok was overcast and cool, without a hint of a breeze, a low barometric pressure day.

Post Synergy episodes

The fifth episode, which occurred while Chris was visiting friends in Michigan could have been due to a number of factors, although his inconsistency in taking the supplements was probably the primarily factor. Chapter 23 explores a number of environmental factors that could have played a contributing role, absent an adequate nutritional defense.

The sixth episode occurred following his return from Michigan. It occurred because Chris chose to stop the 5 mg Zyprexa despite my advice to the contrary. There is a remote possibility he had a Herx to the olive leaf extract, but, given that he did not have such a reaction to IV antibiotic treatment, I don't think that was likely. He then took 15 mg Zyprexa after becoming symptomatic with sleeping problems and akathisia. When I monitored the withdrawal over a two-month period, he made the transition to the supplements without any difficulty, just as he had after the fourth episode. His trip to Colorado in November to sing at a friend's wedding was a success. From September through the middle of February, he was fine.

The seventh episode, discussed below, may have started as a result of excessive exercise, excitotoxins, and situational stress. The first signs I saw of hypomania preceding the seventh hospitalization occurred in the middle of February 2002, after Chris and I had begun exercising at the fitness center. Since January, he had cut his daily dose of supplements to 16 — when he took them.. These factors and his exposure to mitogens at the stable may have contributed to his mania in early March. Tests performed at the time showed that his urine pH was acidic at 6. I didn't know the precise relationship of urine pH to venous pH, except that the appropriate range of urine pH was about 6.5 to 8.0. For the first time, we were able to manage at home with dietary changes, including 32 supplements a day, the immune-enhancing supplements, and psychotropic medication. Chris started sleeping again, and both his emotional high and his nonproductive throat-clearing stopped. Even though his March mania had cleared at home without hospitalization, we were overcome by events on the 5th of April.

What caused the April meltdown that resulted in Chris's seventh hospitalization? Insufficient supplements? From the middle of March on we continually reminded Chris to take 32. He took 16 ... when he remembered. We were so emotionally exhausted from Chris's home hospitalization and my father's ongoing health problems, that we were not as vigilant as we had been when he was manic. Inadequate medications? Possibly? In retrospect, I should have tried to keep him on the higher doses longer. Even though his manic behavior had ended, the "state" elevations of AP proteins and cytokines that accompanied his "home hospitalization" had clearly not yet been fully resolved when he either forgot or refused to take the medications. Perhaps I should have insisted he take them when I gave them to him. Chris needs custodial care when he is impaired, but he balks at it when he is stable, or at least is acting stable, whereupon we try to give him space.

There were other possible confounding factors.

1. He continued to work out at the fitness center after being warned of Dr. Kinderlehrer's comments about Lyme disease and exercise.

2. He returned to eating gluten and casein. With his high RAST scores his body was using resources to detoxify the antigens in the casein and gluten byproducts, thereby lessening resources availability for proper brain functioning. I knew from my research that an excessive number of antigen-antibody pairs impaired brain functioning, probably from excessive IL-1 and IL-2 which occurs as the body defends against antigens.

3. Chris worked with a loud and controlling neighbor. This might have stimulated excessive cortisol production. After working on the roof, Chris didn't take his medications and stayed up all night writing about being bullied as a child. That night, the turning point, he either forget or chose not to take his medications. He had said he would take them.

4. He was exposed to pollen from trees and molds from the roof. His throat-clearing, which had subsided after his March mania had resolved, returned with his April mania. He had two red streaks on both sides of his nose

as well as extensive acne on his back and neck. I have been told by a Lyme patient that they often have inexplicable rashes and acne.

5. He probably did not drink enough water when he worked on the roof. He rarely drank enough water, even when we reminded him.

6. I expect he has Lyme-related multiple perfusion defects in his right temporal lobe. Even though the supplements helped him avoid mania and depression, he still had ongoing memory and navigation problems. He demonstrated some of the symptoms of temporal lobe problems, including excessive religiosity. An EEG, SPECT, PET and/or MRI was no longer an elective option; adequate diagnostic information about Chris's brain was a must. A qualified medical professional needed to assess his brain, and specifically his temporal lobes.

I had read of temporal lobe dysfunction, variously called temporal lobe psychosis, temporal lobe transients, temporal lobe seizure disorder, and partial complex seizures. The exact terminology was unclear, partly due to ongoing controversies. The idea had originally come from Dr. Bransfield, due to Chris's smelling sulphur. In addition, Chris had numerous symptoms suggestive (according to several authors I had read) of a temporal lobe dysfunction: non-amnesic violent episodes, ecstatic facial expressions not unlike what I described in the "God's Palace" section of this book, hypergraphia (excessive writing), ideational viscosity, and excessive religiosity. The extreme self-centeredness Chris exhibited then was classic for temporal lobe dementia. His lack of awareness of his illness was not unlike patients with lesions in their right hemisphere. I found a photo on the Internet that made another compelling argument for looking beyond his "psychiatric" disorder. See photo insert, Lyme hypoperfusion defects.

A professor at the University of California at San Diego, Dr. Vilayanur Ramashandran, whose work was discussed in Chapter 15, conducted a small preliminary study on the relationship between temporal lobe epilepsy and religion. He found that about 25% of patients with temporal lobe epilepsy were obsessed with religion. Exposing both temporal lobe epilepsy and a healthy control group to a series of spoken neutral, profane, sexual, and religious words, he found that the subjects without temporal lobe epilepsy responded to sexual and profane words while a significant number of the temporal lobe group responded to religious words only. Interestingly, healthy religious people did not respond to the religious words.[7]

Chris's experience was not unlike his grandfather's. Both had religious delusions. Ray saw bright lights. Chris smelled sulphur. Was I looking at variants of the same process in Ray and Chris, neurons running amok in their temporal lobes?

There were two huge pieces to the puzzle: *Borrelia burgdorferi* and the mysterious stealth virus. I knew they were big pieces. I didn't know how big, or, for that matter, how they fit with each other or with the other pieces. Maybe the *Bb* attached itself to a stealth virus. Whatever the case, my research had lead me to the inescapable conclusion that some infectious disease, either Lyme, stealth, or other infection was a contributing, if not the central factor in Chris's illness. Chris and I had both been bitten by ticks in Little Rock, Arkansas. But where did the stealth virus come from? Had vaccines caused it? Why was Chris symptomatic while I wasn't. Was there a stealth virus "big picture" I was missing that could account for the breast cancer of both my parents, my mother's fatal brain tumor, and my father's and son's bipolar symptoms?

When I was a boy, I used to try and relate my father's episodes of mania and depression to life events such as my sister's graduating from high school and our family leaving our country home and moving into town. It was a primitive attempt. I'd never been able to find a paradigm that made sense. There was nothing to grab hold to.

Now, a father myself, I was still looking for explanations, only I had more data to guide me. The model I was using was to identify psychological effects from illnesses and drugs. Patterns were there, even though my understanding of them was still limited. This backyard mechanic, combining his research with his experiences with Chris, came to the following treatment-related observations and hypotheses:

1. Zyprexa prevents and stops psychosis, but not hypomanic behavior.

2. Sudden withdrawal from Zyprexa is dangerous, possibly more so than bipolar syndrome. Cutting back slowly over a 2-3 month period works for Chris as long as he takes 24-32 Synergy supplements daily.

3. Depakote in large amounts (2,000 mg) makes Chris depressed.

4. If an EEG demonstrates temporal lobe problems, he will either have to follow a ketogenic diet, or if such a diet does not resolve it, may need Depakote or other seizure medication, in spite of long-terms risks such as liver damage.

5. Seasonal allergies and ingestion of excitotoxins probably play a role in his mania, the former by stimulating excessive cytokine production and mitogen activated protein kinase, and the latter by overwhelming Chris's already compromised glutamate regulatory ability. Mechanisms for this could include low GFAP in glial cells, reduced energy in mitochondria from Lyme disease or stealth virus, or inadequate nutrition from digestive problems and/or utilization of his limited nutritional stores for detoxification processes.

6. Synergy supplements (32 a day) maintain stability and potentiate medications. So far, every time Chris had regressed had been when he had failed to take enough supplements (16 or less a day) and the omega-3 fatty acids. While some patients recover from psychosis from supplements alone, we

haven't see this with Chris. This may be because we have never had the opportunity to exclusively use the supplements when he crashes.

7. Chris's inability to maintain himself on the regimen is likely due to cognitive deficits from an ongoing infectious process and his body's defense against it or repeated episodes of mania. This impairment not only compromises his ability to take pills, but also his ability to regulate his sleep, his eating and drinking behavior. Whether supplements or medications, or both, he needs to consistently take them in order to remain stable. For any effective treatment program to work, there must be consistent compliance.

Some may see this "backyard mechanic" approach to bipolar illness as speculative, especially since the ideas reflect the "leave no stone unturned" approach I used throughout this odyssey. The ideas above are based on a central idea in this book that is not speculative. It is very simple. There are psychological effects from biological illnesses and anomalies as well as from drugs.

I wonder what could be learned if families kept detailed records on the factors which appear temporally related to episodes and if that information was put into a huge database? Pieces of this puzzle may be routinely ignored by patients and their families because of their belief that genetic factors alone are responsible for an illness labeled "bipolar disorder."

Notes

1. Amen, Daniel G., <u>Change Your Brain Change Your Life</u>, Time Books, New York, N.Y. 1998, 86-87.
2. "Scientists put love under the microscope," *The Age*, March 1, 1999. http://www.theage.com.au/daily/990301/news/news20.html
3. Marazziti, D., Akiskal, H.S., Rossi, A., Cassano, G.B., "Alteration of the platelet serotonin transporter in romantic love," *Psychol Med*, 29(3):741-5, May 1999.
4. Wehr, G.A., Turner, E.H., Shimada, J.M., Lowe, C.H., Barker, C., Leibenluft, E., "Treatment of rapidly cycling bipolar patient by using extended bed rest and darkness to stabilize the timing and duration of sleep," *Biological Psychiatry*, 43(11):822-8, June 1, 1998.
5. Aleksandrowicz, Dov R., "Psychoanalytic studies of mania," in <u>Mania, an evolving Concept</u>, Robert H Belmaker, and H.M. van Praag, (eds.), Spectrum Publications, Jamaica, New York, 1980, 316.
6. "This is your brain on nicotine," 2001. http://whyfiles.org/024nicotine/brainscan.html
7. A review of "God and the Temporal Lobes of the Brain," a talk given by Dr. V.S. Ramachandran as part of the program "Human Selves and Transcendental Experiences: A Dialogue of Science and Religion," presented at U.C. San Diego, January 31, 1998, Reviewed by Norman Hall, February 16, 1998.

Appendix 8 - Summary of Lab Work

The following lab results are summarized here to illustrate the complexity involved in ferreting out physical anomalies that contribute to bipolar syndrome. Since this is a work in progress that could be characterized as two steps forward and one step back, it is not meant to provide, or even suggest, a definitive profile for bipolar syndrome. However, these tests are a crude example of the kind of lab work that is needed to discover the biological factors involved in valid psychological variables such as severe mood swings. I would not be surprised to learn that the actual working biological diagnoses will be unique for a good many patients heretofore diagnosed as having bipolar disorder. Perhaps when the technology improves sufficiently so that definitive diagnoses are available, computerized algorithms can match symptoms with these biological anomalies so that clinicians can customize solutions. In the meantime, we continue to provide nutritional support while we search for the health care professionals who can construct the big picture for Chris using, in part, the following pieces of the puzzle we have found.

Kunin-9 (8/2/2002) plus other tests done before publication
IgM Anti myelin associated glycoprotein antibody (MAG) 84 (range 0-50)
IgA MAG 24 (range 0-20)
IgG Tubulin antibody 79 (range 0-60)
The above are thought to be a response to exposures to various heavy metals such as mercury and antimony.
IgG Glutamate Receptor Antibodies 13 (range 0-10)
IgM Glutamate Receptor Antibodies 15 (range 0-10)
These are thought to result from compromised blood brain barrier.
Carnitine Serum 31 (range 35-67) This is probably due to the antipsychotic medications he had to take.
Monocytes 10.7 (range 2-9%) This has consistently been high and suggests infection. When monocytes increase so does TNF.
LDL 136 (62-130) Lipid accumulation is found with stealth virus.
CHOL/HDL 5.6 H
WBC 3.87 (range 4.3-10.80) The lower WBC is likely from the Clozaril.
Total NK subset CD57+ 27 (range 60-360 mm3) In November 2001 while taking the supplements it was 100.
B. Henselae Ab IgG (Bartonella) is 64, or out of range.
Additional analysis will be in my next book.

Nuclear Medicine Report (SPECT) See Color Insert, page 205.

Radio Allergo Sorbent Test (9/19/2001)

      G Casein 10,649 Class 6+ (average 0-100)

      G Gluten 2,732 Class 2+ (average 0-100)

      IGA to Casein 2+ <1 titer normal

      IGA to Gluten 0 <1 titer normal

      IgG to Dermorphin .95

      IgA to Dermorphin 1.12

The high G Casein score is reflective of antigen antibody pairs binding as his body tries to neutralize what it perceives as antigens in the partly digested casein. The peptides that provoke an antigen response mimic the actions of endogenous opiates such as endorphins. HPCL scores are reflective of level of polypeptiduria. They were low the last two times Chris became psychotic. Both times he was eating both gluten and casein. This suggests that high levels of antibodies are necessary to manage it as reflected, for example in Chris's RAST. Chris's excessively high level of antibodies to casein, 10,649 per given volume of blood, seemed significant to me, especially since immune activation, specifically an increase of IL-2, is implicated in mania and vital brain precursors such as choline and inositol are diminished when the body has to deal with excessive antigens.

According to Dr. Cade, his studies with autism and schizophrenia demonstrated that these peptide levels correlate with the Brief Psychiatric Rating Scale (BPRS). High scores reflect greater psychopathology. In a letter to me he stated that as the total peptide concentration fell during treatment (dialysis and or a gluten/casein free diet) of patients the BPRS scores fell. When the peptides reached normal range the BPRS was normal or close to normal. When total peptides were less than half of normal, the BPRS scores increased with each decrease of the peptides. In a preliminary study with bipolar patients, HPCL scores were high with depression and low with mania.

Dr. Richard Kunin, an orthomolecular psychiatrist, and past President of the International Orthomolecular Society, states the RAST scores indicate enteropathy in the gut, or leaky gut syndrome. Dr. Stricker states that Lyme disease can cause leaky gut. He also says that many people with no psychiatric illnesses have high RAST scores. To me, this suggests that other compensating mechanisms exist in a non psychiatric population that do not exist among those with the syndromes currently labeled as schizophrenia, autism, or bipolar disorder. It does not suggest that the RAST scores are insignificant for Chris or a patient population, particularly in light of Dr. Cade's findings.

Stealth Virus Culture (9/21/01)

"The assay showed a rapid development of a moderate cytopathic effect consisting of vacuolated cells with cytoplasmic inclusions. Although the virus presumably causing the CPE was not further characterized, the positive culture finding could explain signs and symptoms of a multi-system illness, including psychiatric manifestations. They have also been observed in 10% of presumably healthy blood donors."

Dark Field Microscope Anne Bernard (8/15/01)

The photos are said to demonstrate white blood cells that are being "parasitized" by a virus, or the Borrelia burgdorferi. Reportedly the live blood shows the impairment of the white blood cells that are not seen in traditional laboratory assessments. Lyme disease is known to take over white blood cells. Also, Ms Bernard had other photos suggestive of free radical damage, heavy metal damage, and leaky gut syndrome. The debris in his blood suggests that Chris has malabsorption problems, as do a great many "psychiatric" patients. See color photo insert and Appendix 3 for details.

Kalamazoo Psychiatric Hospital (7/12/01)
- Specific gravity 1.031 range (1.001-1.030)
- Amorphous crystals trace

Second Western Blot by IgeneX ordered by Dr. Stricker (1/29/01)
- 30 kDA +, 39 kDA+, 41kDA+, 45kDA+, 58KDA+, and 66KDA+
- CDC criteria require five bands for a positive. Chris got six. On a sample taken July 31, 2002 he got 8, according to IgeneX. On a sample taken August 2, 2002, the findings were "indeterminate," according to the University Medical Center at Stony Brook in New York. These differences demonstrate the ongoing problems with diagnostic accuracy of Lyme disease.

MRI

This was not approved. We were going to pay for it, but by the time it was disapproved Chris had already started treatment, thereby preventing any useful pre-post comparison.

Dr. Stricker's T-Cell Test (1/29/01)
- Monocytes 11.1 (range 2-9)
- WBC 4.83 (Range 4.3-10.8) After three months of forced psychiatric care without supplements it was 3.87.
- Absolute lymphocyte count 1435 (range 1500-4000) After three months of forced psychiatric care it was 1366.
- Specialized ratios were normal. CD57 profile, unlike most Lyme patients, was 100 (range 60-360). Dr. Stricker said the supplements might be improving his immune system.

Great Smokies Diagnostic laboratories (11/10/00)

- Hair Analysis:
  Antimony, .054 (range 0-.03)
  Mercury, 1.07 (range 0-1)
  Iodine, 40 (range .16-1.75 possibility of external contamination)
  Lithium .24 (range .0027-. 032 with possibility of external contamination.) Chris was coming off Lithium at the time.
  Ca/P ratio 1.5 (normal range 2.5-10)
  Na/K ratio 1.1 (normal range 1.5-10)
- Food Antibody Assessment 10/19/00
  IgE 0
  IgG 220.1 (Reference Range 1.3 – 241.3)
  Total IgE 220.1
  Relative antibody levels (Very High 3+)
- Notes from Dr. Ingendaay's conversation with the lab: Urine Amino Acid Profile may be needed as sulphur is low, but this can't be done while taking nutritional supplements which would skew the results. DMSA is recommended for antimony and mercury contamination. We did not do this because we prioritized Lyme disease for treatment. However some of the ingredients in the supplements Chris took such as such as selenium and Vitamin C are known to help detoxify the body.

Associated Pathologists Laboratories (11/29/00)

- Basic chemistry, iron, CPK, lipid profile, thyroxsine, Hemogram, Ferritin, Hemogram and Urinalysis all were normal.
- Differential has two significant findings
  Segmented Neutrophils 81 (range is 42-71%) High
  Lymphocytes 8.6 (range 24-44 %) Low
  Dr. Tang said there was diminished immune function because of Lyme disease or unknown viral infection. For three months Chris had been on Zyprexa, a drug known to cause leukocytopenia, or a shortage of lymphocytes. Chris also had a bad cold or flue during his exam.
- Western Blot (11/29/00):
  The following bands were present: 41,45,58, 66. Band 39 was questionable.
  The following bands were absent: 21,23,28, 30, and 93
- Negative Lyme Immunoblot – IGG (Those I talked with from a local Lyme support group said that the positive 4 ½ bands, and his psychiatric illness was enough for the Lyme diagnosis. One Lyme support group member said the test should have been done at IgeneX and that the test Chris took looked at the wrong bands.)

- Diptheria antitoxoid was .10 IR/ml. This is a significant level of diptheria antibody. Should be .01. Dr. Tang believes immune response to childhood vaccinations may trigger bipolar later in life, I presume through the actions of cytokines on the brain or other immune activity.

IgeneX Inc

- Lyme Urine Antigen Test (11/29/2000) This test came back negative, but I have been told it wasn't done correctly. Chris gave one sample only for this. There was no antibiotic challenge and no follow up for collection for 5 days.

Dark Field Microscope (11/29/2000) This summary is from a verbal description from Dr. Tang.

Cluster fibrin, fibrous needles in serum attributed to undesired chemicals; some clumping of cells which she said could be dehydration or something else; leukocytes that had been neutralized, presumably by Lyme disease or a virus. There were white flecks explained as "waste the liver hasn't removed yet." Some cells had white circles inside the cells. Those were interpreted as the "spleen not doing its job. Some had dark cells which were interpreted as "not being properly cleaned by the liver." Dark field microscopy is an emerging field practiced by respected professionals and charlatans. Results are often inconsistent. There are also cases of unethical practitioners who sell products based on their "findings."

Doctor's Data Inc

- Urine Toxic Elements (15) No elevated findings.
- ELISA/ACT Lymphocyte Response Assay Results
  Strong Reactions to Aldrin, Endrin
  Moderate Reactions to Xylene, Carbon Tetrachloride, Polysorbate 60

These findings demonstrated a chemical sensitivity to the above substances but did not address whether or not these chemicals were in Chris's blood at the time of the test. They do indicate sufficient exposure during his life for him to have developed a sensitivity to them.

Appendix 9 - Books recommended by the author

ADD and ADHD: Complementary Medicine Solutions – Charles Gant, M.D.

This is one of the best books I have read on the physiology of ADD/ADHD and the role of nutrients to dramatically alleviate symptoms.

A Dose of Sanity – Dr. Sydney Walker III, M.D.

In this outstanding book, Dr. Walker, a board certified neuropsychiatrist discusses the reasons why the rate of misdiagnosis in psychiatric illnesses is more than four in ten. He explains how the DSM-IV has resulted in patients being diagnosed as having psychiatric disorders when they actually suffer from hypothyroidism, Lyme disease, and, even poor nutrition.

Breaking the Vicious Cycle – Elaine Gottschall, B.A., M.Sc.

While this book is written for patients with various digestive problems such as Crohn's disease and ulcerative colitis, it is invaluable for the person whose brain has been impaired because of inability to uptake needed nutrients.

Depression Cured at Last! – Sherry A. Rogers, M.D.

This is but one in a number of books by Dr. Rogers that address environmental, nutritional and metabolic factors in depression. It is a comprehensive approach that focus on such neglected issues as foods, chemicals, and molds.

Desperation Medicine – Ritchie Shoemaker, M.D.

In this pioneering book, Dr. Shoemaker describes a new family of environmental diseases and describes innovative and effective ways to treat them.

The Food Mood Body connection - Gary Null, Ph.D.

The book covers a variety of nutritional and environmental approaches to mental health and physical well-being.

His Bright Light - The Story of Nick Traina - Danielle Steel

This moving biography and memoir details the troubled life of the author's son and the impotence of the mental health delivery system to provide hope for him. It is a powerful book that chronicles the author's attempts to try to understand what is wrong with her son and her futile attempts to get him the help he needs. When the system finally gives a label to his malady, childhood bipolar illness, she finds it can do little to reverse his progressive deterioration. He kills himself.

Mad in America - Robert Whitaker

This review of the treatment of the mentally ill is an eye opener. While <u>Too Good To Be True</u> describes one family's experience with the "system," Mr. Whitaker's book provides a big picture view of the system from the past to the present, a portrayal that suggests that if consumers do not bring about change, then the past will continue to be prologue.

Molecules of Emotion: The Science Behind Mind-Body Medicine - Candace Pert, Ph.D.

While this book does not specifically address issues relative to bipolar illness or nutrition, it provides a stunning view on the role of peptides that affect areas of study such as neuroscience, immunology, and endocrinology. I believe these ideas are transforming our understanding of the brain. Had I read this book first, I may well have titled this book <u>Nutrients Quiet the Unquiet Body</u>. However, I chose not to change titles since I wanted the book to be "leading" as opposed to "bleeding" edge.

Nutritional Influences on Mental Illness – Melvyn Werback, M.D.

This is the most complete and exhaustive reference resource on nutrition and mental health on the market that I have found. It is written for professionals and is fairly expensive. Buy it and take it to your doctor.

The Omega-3 Connection – Andrew Stoll, M.D.

This book discusses the macrophage theory of depression and the role of Omega-3 fatty acids in minimizing cytokine production. It is an excellent book, a must-read for the bipolar patient.

Prescription for Nutritional Healing - Phyllis Balch, CNC, James Balch, M.D.

While the subject matter of this book is very broad, there are sections that could be helpful for a person seeking nutritional solutions for bipolar illness or schizophrenia.

Appendix 10 - This Just In

September 21, 2002:

It took three months, but the county finally blinked — right before a jury trial on permanent conservatorship was to begin. Finally Chris was home, or, perhaps I should say, parts of him were home. He was easily confused. He couldn't remember. He was tired. He drooled at night. He slept excessively. Chris now had the opportunity to demonstrate the results of three months of forced hospitalization. He had taken no Synergy supplements and he had been forced to take Clozaril, Haldol, and Depakote for three months. See Appendix 8 for preliminary lab results showing the effects.

He took a new series of tests, including a Western Blot, to see if he qualified for the long term neuro Lyme study by Dr. Brian Fallon at Columbia University. Dr. Stricker ordered a SPECT and this time we obtained it without asking for any preauthorization. We would pay for it if Medi-Cal didn't. The test demonstrated significant hypoperfusion. The radiologist attributed this to "neuro lyme, psychiatric illness, or psychotropic medications." If psychotropic medications could cause such hypoperfusion did that mean that preventing his brain from functioning properly was one of the goals of such a regimen? When I first saw the report I thought of the study involving rats discussed in Chapter 13. Their common response to antipsychotic drugs was proliferation of glial cells and swelling of the prefrontal cortex.

Through MMI members and alternativementalhealth.com I had found a doctor who not only understood what we were trying to do, but who had pioneered nutritional assessment procedures that are now used throughout the United States. Chris had not been willing to see him before his hospitalization. Now he was. His name is Dr. Richard Kunin, an orthomolecular psychiatrist in San Francisco. While Dr. Stricker focused on the germ, Dr. Kunin focused on the soil. Now that the lab work was almost complete, additional evidence of immune dysfunction was becoming apparent, supporting the notion that cytokine mediated processes play a central role in his illness. See color photo insert for details of his SPECT.

Late in September while proofing the final copy of this book, I learned from a post by Dr. Martin to the stealth virus group that the FDA had finally done a study that looked for simian cytomegalovirus (SCMV) in stocks of live polio virus vaccines. Using PCR technology three of eight old polio virus vaccine samples were found to have DNA from SCMV. Looks like the FDA is finding that there are stealth adapted viruses in our vaccines in spite of earlier denials from the CDC.

The other day Chris and I went for a hike in the mountains. He was quiet, and when he spoke his speech was slurred. He wanted to climb a rock wall. I told him I thought that would be dangerous. He wanted to do it anyway. I hoped he wouldn't push the issue. He started to, but then relented. Until all of his frontal cortex is working properly, I will have to serve as his brakes. He didn't say much that day. Although he had cut some of his psychotropic medications in accordance with Dr. Kunin's recommendations, they still caused him to be tired and uncommunicative. It will be another slow process restoring his brain with more nutrients and less drugs.

October 3, 2002:

Got to get this proof in.

More tests. Antinuclear antibodies test (ANA) is 1:80. The score is high and outside the expected range. About 5% of positive ANA tests definitely have lupus, an autoimmune disorder, and — if I hadn't read it I would not have believed it — a potential side effect of Depakote. Is Depakote causing the antibodies to specific brain cells that are listed in the lab work? Chris is tired and still has a rash on his face, two symptoms of lupus. The SPECT of a Lyme patient and a lupus patient are indistinguishable. One more thing to worry about. However, as he has cut back on his medications, the drooling at night has reduced substantially.

Saw the headlines in The Union, our local paper today: "Governor Signs Laura's Law." Laura was Thomas's friend from high school who was murdered at Nevada County Behavioral Health Services shortly after I quit working there. Now the mentally ill can be ordered into outpatient treatment — to take their medicines. I would have a lot more confidence in Laura's Law if I had a lot more confidence in the system of which I have been a part for a good part of my adult life. Now I fear the American Gulag will grow. I hope I am wrong. Who can do the math? Who can calculate all the future Lauras who will be saved? Who can measure all the future Chrises whose spirits will languish, if not expire from the crushing weight of the American Gulag?

After a long silent spell, I heard Chris singing and playing the piano the other day. It made my heart feel good.

Index

Y

Z

Order Form

Too Good To Be True?
Nutrients Quiet the Unquiet Brain
A Four-Generation Bipolar Odyssey

USA

Price per book $21.95

Postage and handling $4.00
Add .50 per additional book)

Canada

Price per book $29.00

Postage and handling per book $4.00
     (Add .50 per additional book)

Please complete the following:

Total number of books   _____
Total price for books   _____
Total for postage and handling _____
Total   _____

Send with check or money order to:
Nu-Tune Press
P.O. Box 691
Penn Valley Ca 95946

Name:_____

Address: _____

City, State or Province: _____

Postal Code_____